PSYCHIATRY AT THE CROSSROADS

Edited by

John Paul Brady, M.D.

The Kenneth E. Appel Professor of Psychiatry
and Chairman of the Department
University of Pennsylvania

H. Keith H. Brodie, M.D.

Professor and Chairman
Department of Psychiatry
Duke University

THE SAUNDERS PRESS

W. B. Saunders Company

Philadelphia · London · Toronto

The Saunders Press
W. B. Saunders Company
West Washington Square
Philadelphia, Pennsylvania 19105

IN THE UNITED STATES DISTRIBUTED TO THE TRADE BY

Holt, Rinehart and Winston
383 Madison Avenue
New York, New York 10017

IN CANADA DISTRIBUTED BY

Holt, Rinehart and Winston of Canada, Limited
55 Horner Avenue
Toronto, Ontario
M8Z 4X6
Canada

Library of Congress Cataloging in Publication Data

Main entry under title:

Psychiatry at the crossroads.

"Taken from a larger collection entitled Controversy in psychiatry."

1. Psychiatry—Philosophy—Addresses, essays, lectures. 2. Psychotherapy—Philosophy—Addresses, essays, lectures. I. Brady, John Paul. II. Brodie, Harlow Keith Hammond, 1939- III. Controversy in psychiatry.

RC437.5.P76 616.89′001 80–50717

ISBN 0–7216–1916–9 (Saunders)

ISBN 0–03–057657–1 (HRW)

First Edition

Last digit is the print number: 9 8 7 6 5 4 3 2 1

Contents

Psychiatry At the Crossroads

JOHN PAUL BRADY
University of Pennsylvania

H. KEITH H. BRODIE
Duke University

Psychiatry is the branch of medicine having to do with the diagnosis and treatment of disorders of behavior and psychological functioning. There is both optimism and pessimism in the field today; psychiatry is at the crossroads.

Some three decades ago psychiatry as a field was seen as the golden key to understanding human problems. It enjoyed wide and enthusiastic acceptance. Effective drugs were being introduced into the field for the first time and the insightful concepts of Freud and his successors were being more fully appreciated. This enthusiasm led us to hope or to believe that in addition to discovering the nature and cure of most forms of mental disorder, psychiatry would provide answers to problems of delinquency, crime, racial prejudice, international tensions, and an assortment of other social and political ills. This premature optimism in the field has waned as solutions to these problems have not evolved. Gradually it has been recognized that most lie outside the understanding of our field and that their solution requires other methods and procedures than those provided by psychiatry as a branch of medicine. There has been, in fact, an overreaction to this disillusionment, and the appropriateness of psychiatric methods for treating psychological illnesses and problems of living has come into question. Some of the most severe and forceful critics of psychiatry in recent years have been psychiatrists themselves. Two of the essayists in the present volume, Dr. E. Fuller Torrey and Dr. Thomas Szasz, have written books in this category: *The Death of Psychiatry* and *The Myth of Mental Illness.*

However, there is renewed enthusiasm and optimism in the field. Over the past decade great strides have been made in our understanding of the genetic, biological, psychological, social, and cultural roots of the major forms of mental illness. Striking progress has been made in methods for treating manic-depressive disease with new compounds such as lithium and the antidepressants. Very recent discoveries concerning the nature and action of neurotransmitters—chemicals used by brain cells (neurons) to transmit messages—hold great promise for increasing our understanding of how the brain works and what goes wrong in persons with schizophrenia and related disorders. The discovery of endorphins makes possible new treatments for schizophrenia, drug addiction, and chronic pain. These discoveries may eventually lead to more effective treatment for mental illness. At the same time there have been major advances in psychological treatment methods, including the development of behavior modification techniques and cognitive therapy techniques which focus on the ways in which patients think about themselves and the world in which they live.

This book focuses on thirteen key issues that confront the field today. Perhaps the most basic issue is whether psychiatry has a future at all. This is addressed by Dr. E. Fuller Torrey, an articulate and outspoken critic of the field as a whole. Particular forms of psychotherapy have also been the subject of study and debate in recent years. Some have argued that psychoanalysis, the form of psychological treatment developed by Sigmund Freud which entails the intensive and prolonged exploration of the patient's unconscious wishes and impulses, is too expensive and specialized a form of treatment for most patients. This question is discussed by Dr. Harley C. Shands, a broadly trained psychiatrist and social scientist. One of the major challenges to psychoanalysis comes from behavior modification therapy, a form of psychological treatment developed largely by non-medical psychologists, which claims to have a more solid basis in scientific method and experimentation than the more traditional forms of psychotherapy. This is another of the crossroads at which psychiatry stands. Will psychiatry move in the direction of behavior therapy or take some middle road which integrates the newer developments in behavioral and cognitive psychology into the main body of psychoanalytically oriented psychotherapy? Dr. Jarl E. Dyrud, a psychoanalyst who is knowledgeable and experienced in the behavior therapy area, provides some provocative thoughts and insights.

Behavior therapy and some of the other newer forms of psychological intervention have been developed largely by psychologists and other nonphysicians. This raises the question of whether psychiatrists need to be medically trained at all. This very controversial question is addressed by Dr. Martin T. Orne, a prominent psychiatrist who is also fully trained and qualified in clinical psychology.

Recent discoveries of the role of genetic and biological factors in schizophrenia, along with the development of drugs that greatly aid in the treatment and management of this disorder, raise the question of whether psychological treatment plays more than a palliative role in the condition. This question is addressed by Dr. Allen Will, Jr., a leading exponent of psychotherapy as a treatment for schizophrenia.

Psychiatry is only one of the several fields and institutions concerned with the behavior of individuals and its effects upon others. The legal profession, civil courts, and the criminal justice system are also involved in these matters and often interact with psychiatry. One of the crossroads at which psychiatry stands concerns the degree to which psychiatry, as a branch of medicine, should address issues of a moral, ethical, and judicial nature. Several of the chapters in this volume concern this borderland. Should homosexuals be allowed to adopt children, should sex change operations be performed, and should psychiatric patients ever be hospitalized involuntarily?

Whether the psychiatrist should have any role in the criminal justice system is currently being debated. It is discussed in this volume by a leading jurist, David L. Bazelon.

Another question which has engaged the interest of psychiatrists is whether marihuana is hazardous to one's health. The psychiatric and other evidence relevant to this issue is discussed in a chapter written collaboratively by a psychiatrist and an attorney, Dr. Lester Grinspoon and Mr. James B. Bakalar. As these authors point out, this is one of those areas in which maintaining one's objectivity in reviewing the data is very difficult.

One trend in psychiatry in recent years has been to look outside the individual and into the family or broader community for the causes of particular forms of psychological disturbance. This has been the case especially with disorders and emotional problems of children. However, some authorities believe that emphasis on the family as the origin of the emotional troubles of children has been overstated. This issue is tackled by a leading child psychiatrist, Dr. E. James Anthony, who looks at the question in historical perspective.

Finally, another crossroad at which psychiatry stands concerns the degree to which psychiatric services should be community-based and have a community orientation. Indeed, some have argued that the psychiatry of the future will be a community undertaking, whereas others have argued that "community psychiatry" is merely a slogan, more political in its connotation and purpose than a substantive way of reorganizing the delivery of mental health care services. This question is addressed by a leading scholar of contemporary American psychiatry, Dr. Daniel X. Freedman.

The decade of the eighties will be one of great promise and great challenge for psychiatry. The biological and behavioral sciences upon which this medical discipline rests are rapidly developing, as are the applications of this new knowledge to the understanding and treatment of psychological illness in man. At the same time the field is being questioned by psychology, the law, and other professions, as well as by the public in general, as to its proper purview and *modus operandi.*

Does Psychiatry Have a Future?

E. FULLER TORREY

National Institute of Mental Health

Psychiatry has the same future as a medical specialty as hand-wind gramophones have as stereo equipment. Both were good ideas at the time they began, yet both have been superseded by technological developments and more advanced design. Psychiatry, like the gramophone, is now obsolete and belongs on the shelves of museums where it can be fondly and nostalgically regarded. This chapter will review the evidence for this thesis.

Before analyzing psychiatry, it is necessary to review briefly the history of ideas and the process by which ideas change. To say that psychiatry has no future as a medical specialty is a rude and jolting experience, for we have grown up believing otherwise. After all, psychiatry is practiced by approximately 25,000 doctors who were trained in medicine; by sheer number alone they must prove it will continue to be a medical specialty. There are now departments of psychiatry in medical schools, psychiatry textbooks by the hundreds, and a specialty society with an annual budget of over five million dollars. Don't these tangible, concrete accouterments prove that psychiatry is viable?

In fact they do not. Rather, they only prove that psychiatry will take longer than it should to pass from the scene. Liquidating tangible assets tends to be a painful job when one is faced with bankruptcy, and for this reason the psychiatric profession is not likely to be graceful in its exit. The more threatened it feels, the more likely it is to cling to the tangible trappings surrounding it, as if by so doing it can put off the inevitable day when its edifice will stand no more. The department offices will be occupied by rival sections of the medical school, the American Psychiatric Association headquarters divided into apartments, and psychiatric textbooks ensconced alongside books on phrenology in second-hand book stores. Such glimpses of the future offend our sensibilities. Stop, we cry, it cannot be because we don't want it to be. The wheels of progress, however, have never been stopped by such cries.

The history of science teaches us that although we grow up thinking that certain things are right, they often turn out to be otherwise. This is true not only of specific facts, but of whole models of knowledge. The idea that the sun moved around the earth was prevalent for thousands of years, and "known" to be "right." As new data was perceived that failed to fit the old model, a period of crisis began which eventually ended with the Copernican model of the earth moving around the sun. Thomas Kuhn, in his brilliant monograph *The Structure of Scientific Revolutions,* analyzes such changes in models of scientific thought as they have been found in all the sciences. It is my contention that we are in the midst of just such a scientific revolution in our thinking about disordered behavior and people whom we currently call "psychiatric patients." Fifty years from now when we look back on them, our current ideas will seem silly, although comprehensible in their historical context.

No Patients

The major reason that psychiatry has no future as a medical specialty is that it will have no patients. Those people now called "psychiatric patients" will be divided into two groups and reassigned. Those who truly have diseases of the brain will eventually be annexed by neurology, and those who do not will be considered under the jurisdiction of education. With nobody left to call a patient, psychiatry will wither and die.

The history of psychiatry in its brief lifetime since "alienists" began gathering those with disordered behavior into asylums is a history of the cause of some disordered behaviors being discovered followed by those people being reassigned in another medical specialty. Pellagra was a common cause of "insanity" until its cause was discovered; then it was turned over to nutritionists and internists. General paresis was also a common psychiatric disease earlier in this century, but when the spirochete was discovered it became the province of internists. Delirium due to infectious diseases was cared for by "alienists" until the underlying infectious diseases were understood, at which time it ceased being a psychiatric responsibility. Patients with epilepsy constituted significant numbers of psychiatric patients in the past; as the different seizure disorders were sorted out, they were turned over to neurology. Brain tumors may cause disordered behavior, but when the presence of the tumor became clear, these patients were assigned to neurosurgery. Mongolism and phenylketonuria both were once considered primarily psychiatric entities, but as their etiology was clarified, they were given to pediatrics.

Where does this leave psychiatry now? It leaves it holding the bag of seriously ill "mental patients" for whom the organic etiology has not yet been clarified. The bag is full of "functional psychoses," a rather nebulous term which is about as illuminating as "idiopathic." The primary division of these "functional psychoses" is into "the schizophrenias" and "the affective psychoses."

It has become increasingly clear in recent years that the "functional psychoses" have primarily organic etiologies, a fact acknowledged by everyone in medicine and psychiatry except those whose early development was arrested at the psychoanalytic stage. The evidence includes indicators of a genetic predisposition, as well as anatomical, neurological, neurophysiological, and biochemical abnormalities in many patients with "functional psychoses." There is also epidemiological evidence that these conditions are primarily organic in origin.

The genetic indicators pointing toward an inherited predisposition to "functional psychoses" consist of twin studies, HLA typing, and biological abnormalities found in first-degree relatives of such patients. Twin studies have shown that the concordance rates for schizophrenia in twins is approximately 50 per cent in monozygotic and 15 to 20 per cent in dizygotic pairs. HLA (human leukocyte antigen) typing done to date suggests that a person with some psychoses may have a genetic predisposition (Cazzullo et al., 1974; Eberhard et al., 1975; Smeraldi et al., 1976; Shapiro et al., 1976). And several examples of the identification of abnormalities in the first-degree relatives of psychotic patients have been reported (Holzman et al., 1974; Meltzer, 1969).

Anatomical abnormalities in psychotic patients have been reported for many years but often such studies have not been able to be replicated (Torrey and Peterson, 1973). Recent work suggests that many psychotic patients have dilated ventricles in the brain (Haug, 1972; Johnstone et al., 1976) and also abnormalities of cerebral blood flow (Ingvar and Franzen, 1974). Abnormal dermatoglyphic patterns and capillary formations have also been described in a disproportionate number of functionally psychotic patients (Torrey and Peterson, 1976). Finally, muscle fiber abnormalities and subterminal motor nerve abnormalities have been reported among schizophrenic patients (Meltzer, 1976).

Neurologically, functionally psychotic patients have been shown to have a broad range of subtle abnormalities ("soft" signs). Tucker et al. (1975), for example, demonstrated in a recent study of 109 consecutive admissions to a psychiatric ward a strong correlation between neurological impairment and thought disorder and between neurological impairment and schizophrenia. This finding is consistent with several other studies in the literature. Neurophysiologically the studies showing abnormalities among such patients are very impressive, including Holzman et al.'s work on eye tracking movements (1974), Meltzer's H-reflex recovery curve (1976), and Landau et al.'s work with average-evoked response to light intensity (1975). Each passing year now turns up new evidence of how functionally psychotic persons are different neurophysiologically from normal control populations.

The list of biochemical abnormalities that have been described among psychotic patients is long indeed. The most prominent among them are dopamine and its metabolites (Meltzer and Stahl, 1976), MAO (Wyatt and Murphy, 1976), creatinine phosphokinase (CPK), aldolase (Meltzer, 1976), and abnormalities in proteins in the serum and spinal fluid of psychotic patients. Which among them are cause and which are effect is not certain at this stage; what is clear, however, is that schizophrenics and affective psychotics are not, biochemically speaking, like a group of mentally normal controls. And finally, there is epidemiological evidence to support a biological etiology. There has now been shown, in studies of more than 150,000 schizophrenics in five countries, to be a seasonality to the birth pattern of these patients (Torrey et al., 1977).

Thus the evidence is rapidly mounting that the "functional psychoses" have primarily organic etiologies. Given the present exponential rate of research knowledge, it is likely that within two decades the organic bases of the majority of "functional psychoses" will be well understood. There will probably be several of them, and they may well involve a genetic predisposition to a specific biochemical, metabolic, nutritional, toxic, and/or infectious agent with the initial insult to the brain occurring as early as the prenatal period.

What is likely to happen to these patients as these etiologies become clarified? They will, of course, follow their predecessors like general paresis, pellagra, and phenylketonuria and be turned over to that medical specialty best equipped to care for them. Biochemical, metabolic, nutritional, and toxic abnormalities of the brain will become the responsibility of neurologists, internists, and all of their subspecialties. If the cerebral insult can be corrected or alleviated by surgical means, then some of them may be given to the neurosurgeons for care, as happened with some epileptics. If the initial insult occurred early in life, pediatrics and neonatology (which by then is likely to be a vastly enlarged specialty) will cooperate to achieve both early detection and prevention.

One may argue that psychiatrists will continue to care for these patients through expanding their training and knowledge. I believe that this is unlikely because there already exist specialists who cover these fields. If, for example, some schizophrenics turn out to have a concentration of a heavy metal in their amygdala, or an inborn error of cerebral metabolism, or a latent viral encephalitis of the limbic area combined with a genetically predisposing HLA type, these patients will need highly specialized care. For a psychiatrist to be retrained to provide this care, he would have to be trained as a subspecialist in internal medicine and/or neurology, but in so doing he would become that specialist. And in fact I suspect that many psychiatrists currently in practice, especially those in the research area, will do exactly this. But the term "psychiatrist" as such for the ongoing care of these patients would lose meaning and cease to have any jurisdiction.

What would psychiatrists be left with? They would be left with all the remaining people whom we currently call "psychiatric patients." Included in this group are people with anxiety, depression, fears, phobias, addiction to alcohol or other drugs, personality disorders, bad marriages, poor interpersonal or sexual relationships, and unfulfilled lives in general. These people can be generically designated as having problems of living. They include people who run a very broad range of discomfort, from the man who is so afraid of relating to others that he chooses to spend his life as a hermit to a highly successful executive who wants to improve his interpersonal relationships so as to increase his chances of becoming corporation president.

Why are these people called "psychiatric patients"? They are called "psychiatric patients" because they have sought, or their relatives have sought for them, care from a psychiatrist, *ergo* they become "psychiatric patients." The simplicity of this labeling process should be kept in mind; if it is forgotten, we tend to deify the label, mistakenly assuming that it was divinely created. The corollary of this is that "psychiatric patients" attain their status by being so designated by a psychiatrist or other member of the medical profession. MacAndrew (1969) summarizes this very nicely for people called alcoholics: "One is an alcoholic by virtue of the fact that a *bona fide* member of the medical profession, acting in his capacity as a member of that profession, has so designated him."

What is actually wrong with these people called "psychiatric patients"? They all are uncomfortable with themselves, or at least their relatives are uncomfortable with them. They have "dis-ease," which is often confused with disease but in fact is quite different. True brain disease implies impairment of neurophysiological or neurochemical function by an organic cause, and when the cause is removed or repaired, the disease ceases to exist. "Dis-ease" implies discomfort, a condition we all experience more or less every day. Some people experience more "dis-ease" more often, and may seek help to learn how to minimize it or at least live with it. Such discomfort is often the consequence of faulty learning earlier in life and may or not be alleviated by relearning.

To date there is no evidence that any of the "patients" in this large group have true diseases of the brain. It is of course possible that a few of them will turn out to, and research should continue to search them out. If and when they do, they will join their brethren and be assigned to the speciality of medicine best able to provide care for their organic disease. It is unlikely that this will happen to more than a handful in the large category of people with problems of living.

Three other arguments are often paraded out to justify the categorization of problems of living ("dis-ease") with true disease. The first is that of genetic predisposition, which states that if a genetic predisposition can be shown for the particular state of "dis-ease" (e.g., "alcoholism" or "neurotic depression"), then that will prove that the condition is really a disease. This is simply not true, for genetic predisposition can be shown for a wide variety of non-disease states (e.g., artistic ability, athletic ability) as well as for disease states (e.g., hypertension, ankylosing spondylitis of the spine). Therefore, if and when there is shown to be a genetic predisposition to "alcoholism," for example, this in itself will not prove that "alcoholism" is a true disease any more than artistic ability is a disease.

Second, it has been argued that since states of "dis-ease" (problems of living) can eventually cause real physical diseases, then the original states of "dis-ease" are also real diseases. For example, since chronic anxiety can produce hypersecretion of acid in the stomach which may precipitate a peptic ulcer, then the chronic anxiety must be a disease. Hives and asthma are other physical diseases in which the person's mental state is commonly cited as being of prime etiological importance. In fact, the more we learn about physical diseases, the more apparent it becomes that people's mental state, including their sense of "dis-ease," has some effect on virtually all physical diseases, including picking up viral upper respiratory infections and some cancers. The mental state may be of relatively greater importance (as in asthma) or of little importance (as appears to be the case for viral upper respiratory infections), but it does assume some role in the etiological chain.

Does this mean that all mental states that may help precipitate real diseases should be considered diseases themselves? This is, in essence, the psychosomatic argument. If so, then *all* unhappiness, anxiety, frustration, ennui, disappointment, etc., will have to be categorized as disease, and that is patently absurd. The concept of true disease loses meaning altogether by coming to include everything that even remotely may be possible precipitating factors in the multifactorial etiological chain.

Finally, it is sometimes argued that problems of living are real diseases because they include neurophysiological or neurochemical processes in the brain—not impairment necessarily, but just processes. Of course, problems of living and states of "dis-ease" include neurophysiological and neurochemical processes, as indeed all brain functions do. Each thought, wish, memory, or impulse consists of a neurophysiological and/or neurochemical change in the brain. The question is whether or not there is *impairment* of the processes, which would be true disease. If we define brain processes as disease, then each thought would qualify and we have arrived at a truly nonsensical state of affairs.

What I have said so far about the large number of "psychiatric patients" with problems of living is simply that their "dis-ease" is logically not true disease. My naïeveté may be great, but I do not believe that logic alone is likely to produce much change in the current state of affairs. All other things being equal, most of this large group of "psychiatric patients" would go on indefinitely seeing their psychiatrists, blissfully unconcerned that logic did not support their activity as being part of true medicine.

But all other things are not equal, and I believe that there are social and economic forces underway which will force us finally to categorize these psychiatric activities as being nonmedical. And when they are finally categorized nonmedically, which I believe is inevitable, then psychiatry will be left bereft of the truly diseased (who will have been given back to the other medical specialities) and bereft of the "dis-eased" (who will no longer be considered as medical patients).

What are the social and economic forces which will force the final demise of psychiatry as a medical specialty? First and foremost is the system of payment. As long as individuals wanted to spend their own money paying private psychiatrists who would sympathetically listen to their problems of living, nobody raised many objections. But as soon as third-party payments began to cover the bill (medical insurance, state programs like Medi-Cal, and Federal programs like Medicaid), then the administrators of the programs rightfully began to ask what was being funded. The answer to date has been a kind of mutually agreed upon hoax, with the psychiatrists labeling their "patients" with medical-psychiatric labels (e.g., chronic anxiety reaction, depressive neurosis, passive-dependent personality) and with their "patients" accepting these labels so that the bills can be paid. If at any point the "patient" asks the psychiatrist, "Am I really sick?" the answer is of course "no." Only a handful of psychiatrists have refused to participate in this pantomime of illness, and the majority of them have been psychoanalysts.

All directions point to increasing, rather than decreasing, third-party payment for medical illness in the United States. As such, questions about who is being "treated," with what diagnosis, and at what cost will inevitably increase. It will not be enough in the future for a solo psychiatrist to say that a person is "sick" and thereby eligible for third-party coverage. The quality and quantity of the "sickness" will become legitimate areas for inquiry and review. The outcome is inevitable; somebody will eventually cry out, "but he doesn't have any clothes on." When this word reaches the higher echelons of decision-making, all the lobbying in the world will not reverse the withdrawal of third-party payments for nonmedical conditions.

Whether or not problems of living are included under National Health Insurance Coverage, if NHI is enacted at all, will influence the outcome only slightly. If they are included initially, there will be a rising cost of the program as people learn of its availability and as the number of providers (psychiatrists and perhaps psychologists and social workers, depending on how the law is written) increases. How many people will not avail themselves of the opportunity to sit down with a sympathetic professional listener and discuss their problems of living, as long as someone else is paying the bill? Current studies purporting to show that psychiatric benefits level off when paid under third-party coverage have serious methodological flaws, including such things as lack of knowledge about services among those covered and limitations of the number of providers (Nelson, 1976). They are reminiscent of projections about how expensive Medicare and Medicaid would be before these programs were enacted, projections which proved to be grossly optimistic and inaccurate. If unlimited psychiatric benefits are included under NHI, then the history of Medicare and Medicaid will repeat itself with spiralling costs, reevaluation, and eventual retrenchment. Sooner or later there will be a general realization that problems of living cannot be covered by medical insurance.

In addition to economic forces, there is also underway in this country an impressive social change which will affect the medical position of people with problems of living. Increasing numbers of people are availing themselves of ways to learn about themselves and gain insight into their lives. Whereas twenty years ago it was only the intellectual and literary elite who could avail themselves of self-knowledge via their psychoanalyst, now the various methods of self-knowledge are as available as the basement of your local church or synagogue. Esalen moved from its bucolic environs into the living room of middle America, and brought with it a veritable outpouring of fads from primal scream to TM to est, and there is no end in sight. A broad spectrum of Americans is realizing that the quality of their lives can be influenced and changed, and that this is essentially an educational activity. With increasing leisure and the movement toward the four-day work week, this trend is likely to continue. The quality of one's life will become of increasing importance in the remaining years of this century, as the quantity of one's life was in the earlier years.

The greater availability of self-educational activities will intersect, at some point, with the economic forces referred to above. The hypothetical person responsible for making the decision on what psychiatric activities should be included under NHI will eventually partake of TM or est or some other set of initials promising self-knowledge. When he/she does, and then realizes that much of what goes on in psychiatric offices is also strivings toward self-knowledge, then only two conclusions will be possible: either all self-educational activities are legitimate medical expenses, or none are. Psychiatrists should not bet on the former for their economic future.

Another force which will push people with problems of living into an educational paradigm is research on "psychotherapy." As I have extensively reviewed elsewhere (Torrey, 1972), there is an increasing amount of evidence that the important ingredient in people's ability to learn about themselves is the personal characteristics of the "psychotherapist" (=teacher). Carl Rogers in particular initiated a series of studies on qualities like genuineness, empathy, and warmth which, when present in the "therapist," produce change in the "patient." When these personal qualities are not present, change is much less likely. It is not that training is of no value; rather it is of secondary importance to the personality characteristics. You can train a cold, hostile person until he is 93 and he will never become a good "therapist." Conversely, you can take a genuine, empathetic, warm person and with only a little training he may be a very successful "therapist."

The most interesting thing about this line of research is that it is proving to be equally true for primary level education. In one study, 120 third-graders were monitored on how fast they learned to read. Their eight teachers were assessed for the qualities of genuineness, empathy, and nonpossessive warmth. It was shown that the children clearly learned to read faster under the teachers who offered higher levels of these three qualities (Aspy, 1965). In another study, first-graders were found to improve on intelligence tests and self-concept as their teachers improved in interpersonal skills (Aspy, 1972a). When teachers listen to their students rather than lecture to them, the students get better grades and learn more. In a comprehensive review of all the evidence available for this, D. N. Aspy concludes that "... a teacher's increased positive regard for students is translated into classroom behavior which elicits higher levels of cognitive functioning from the students (Aspy, 1972b). In other words, what the teacher thinks about the student and how the teacher relates to the student will determine what the student learns. As this research is replicated and becomes more widely known, it will act as a further impetus to the full realization that most psychiatric activities are educational in nature, and have nothing whatever to do with medicine.

The final force tending to push people with problems of living out of medicine is the general unhappiness with the consequences of not doing so. As long as people with problems of living are considered "diseased," they will continue to parade into the courtroom, psychiatrist in tow, and claim they are not responsible for their criminal actions. The ensuing psychiatric burlesque has become standard comic relief in major criminal trials, with the psychiatrists usually exhibiting the finesse of an elephant doing the waltz. The public at large has watched these shows with increasing amusement, and is rapidly (and correctly) concluding that it is not real diseases which are being discussed.

The final chapter, then, would begin. People with brain diseases would be firmly ensconced in medical specialities like internal medicine and neurology. And people with problems of living would be happily becoming educated about themselves. Psychiatry would be left bereft of patients, and without patients it cannot exist. Its future as a medical specialty, then, is nonexistent. To invest in it for the future is to invest in the Erie Canal as an important future transportation system. Psychiatry is not a growth stock. Rather, it will shortly be removed from the big board altogether.

References

Aspy, D. N.: A study of three facilitative conditions and their relationship to the achievement of third grade students. PhD dissertation, Univ. of Kentucky, 1965. For a summary see Truax, C. B., and Carkhuff, R. R.: Toward Effective Counseling and Psychotherapy. Chicago, Aldine Publishing Company, 1967.

Aspy, D. N.: Reaction to Carkhuff's articles. Counsel. Psychol., *3*:35–41, 1972a.

Aspy, D. N.: Toward A Technology For Humanizing Education. Champaign, Ill., Research Press, 1972b.

Cazzullo, C. L., Smeraldi, E., and Penati, G.: The leukocyte antigenic system HL-A as a possible genetic marker of schizophrenia. Br. J. Psychiatry, *125*:25–27, 1974.

Eberhard, G., Franzen, G., and Low, B.: Schizophrenia susceptibility and HL-A Antigen. Neuropsychobiology, *1*:211–217, 1975.

Haug, J. O.: Pneumoencephalographic studies in mental disease. Acta Psychiatr. Scand., *38*:11–104, 1962.

Holzman, P. S., Proctor, L. R., Levy, D. L., Yasillo, N. J., Meltzer, H. Y., and Hurt, S.W.: Eye-tracking dysfunctions in schizophrenic patients and their relatives. *Arch. Gen. Psychiatry, 31*:143–151, 1974.

Ingvar, D. H., and Franzen, G.: Abnormalities of cerebral blood flow distribution in patients with chronic schizophrenia. Acta Psychiatr. Scand., *50*:425–462, 1974.

Johnstone, E. C., Crow, T. J., Frith, C. D., Husband, J., and Kreel, L.: Cerebral ventricular size and cognitive impairment in chronic schizophrenia. Lancet, *1*:924–926, 1976.

Kuhn, T. S.: The Structure of Scientific Revolutions. Chicago, University of Chicago Press, 1962.

Landau, S. G., Buchsbaum, M. S., Carpenter, W., Strauss, J., and Sacks, M.: Schizophrenia and stimulus intensity control. Arch. Gen. Psychiatry, *32*:1239–1245, 1975.

MacAndrew, C.: On the notion that certain persons who are given to frequent drunkenness suffer from a disease called alcoholism. *In* Plog, S. C., and Edgerton, R. B. (eds.): Changing Perspectives in Mental Illness. New York, Holt, Rinehart & Winston, 1969.

Meltzer, H. Y.: Muscle enzyme release in the acute psychoses. Arch. Gen. Psychiatry, *21*:102–112, 1969.

Meltzer, H. Y.: Neuromuscular dysfunction in schizophrenia. Schizophrenia Bull., *2*:106–135, 1976.

Meltzer, H. Y., and Stahl, S. M.: The dopamine hypothesis of schizophrenia: A review. Schizophrenia Bull., *2*:19–76, 1976.

Nelson, S. H.: Current issues in national insurance for mental health services. Am. J. Psychiatry, *133*:761–764, 1976.

Shapiro, R. W., Bock, E., Rafaelson, O. J., Ryder, L. P., and Svejgaard, A.: Histocompatibility antigens and manic-depressive disorders. Arch. Gen. Psychiatry, *33*:823–825, 1976.

Smeraldi, E., Bellodi, L., Scorza-Smeraldi, R., Fabio, G., and Sacchetti, E.: HLA-SD antigens and schizophrenia: Statistical and genetical considerations. Tissue Antigens, *8*:191–196, 1976.

Torrey, E. F.: The Mind Game: Witchdoctors and Psychiatrists. New York, Emerson Hall, 1972.

Torrey, E. F., and Peterson, M. R.: Slow and latent viruses in schizophrenia. Lancet, *2*:22–24, 1973.

Torrey, E. F.: The Death of Psychiatry. Radnor, Penn., Chilton Book Company, 1974.

Torrey, E. F., and Peterson, M. R.: The viral hypothesis of schizophrenia. Schizophrenia Bull., *2*:136–146, 1976.

Torrey, E. F., Torrey, B. B., and Peterson, M. R.: The seasonality of schizophrenic births. Arch. Gen. Psychiatry, *34*:1065–1070, 1977.

Tucker, G. J., Campion, E. W., and Silberfarb, P. M.: Sensorimotor functions and cognitive disturbance in psychiatric patients. Am. J. Psychiatry, *132*:17–21, 1975.

Wyatt, R. J., and Murphy, D. L.: Low platelet monoamine oxidase activity and schizophrenia. Schizophrenia Bull., *2*:77–89, 1976.

Comment

Dr. Torrey's answer to the question is straightforward and unequivocal: psychiatry as a medical specialty is obsolete and will soon go out of existence. His argument is equally straightforward. Any clinical branch of medicine requires patients, and in time there will be no "psychiatric" patients. Patients with so-called "functional psychoses"—mainly schizophrenia, psychotic depression, and mania—will be found to have true diseases of the central nervous system. He supports this by reviewing some of the rapidly accumulating evidence for the organic nature of these afflictions. When this becomes apparent to all, these disorders will go the way of general paresis (syphilis of the central nervous system), pellagra, and other medical conditions and become the province of neurology and internal medicine. What about the other patients the psychiatrist sees—the persons with anxiety, phobias, bad marriages, sexual dysfunctions, etc.? Torrey argues that these individuals do not suffer from medical illnesses but have problems of living. They may have "dis-ease" but do not suffer from a disease. Hence, their problems are educational rather than medical, and in time psychiatry as a medical specialty will no longer be able to lay claim to them. Torrey predicts that a number of societal factors will hasten this change and the demise of psychiatry. The most important of these is the method of paying physicians for these services—the increasing role of insurance in American medicine. These will be forced to recognize that "psychiatric patients," i.e., those with problems of living, are not truly sick and do not have medical (reimbursable) conditions. Torrey believes that these changes are inevitable and desirable.

This is, of course, a minority view among psychiatrists and most other professionals in the mental health field. Many would argue that the medical training of the psychiatrist, and his experience as a physician with the seriously ill or dying patient, gives him a broader and perhaps more human perspective in helping people with psychological problems. The medical background of the psychiatrist also equips him better in diagnosis. In particular, he is more apt to suspect and detect the presence of an underlying physical disorder in a patient who presents himself as a person with purely psychological or social difficulties. He is also better equipped than the nonmedical psychotherapist to adequately treat the person who presents with a combination of physical and psychological disorders. Indeed, an area of increasing interest and activity within psychiatry is the consultation/liaison field. This entails helping the nonpsychiatrist physician, such as the surgeon or internist, understand better and deal more effectively with the psychological and behavioral aspects of his patient's illness.

It is possible that a new medical specialty will evolve which is more clearly medical than contemporary psychiatry and which will address those human problems not easily accessible to the nonmedical psychotherapist. These might include behavioral and psychological management of the medically ill person (liaison and consultation psychiatry), difficult problems in diagnosis in which both physical and psychological disorders coexist, and the application of behavioral and psychological procedures to medical disorders (behavioral medicine). Of course this new specialist may go by another name and resemble the psychiatrist of today no more than the latter resembles the alientists (mental specialists) of the American colonial period who treated mania with blood-letting and depression with emetics.

JOHN PAUL BRADY, M.D.

Does Psychoanalysis Have a Future?

HARLEY C. SHANDS

Columbia University College of Physicians and Surgeons

> The qualification which is the determining factor of fitness for psychoanalytic treatment . . . is whether the patient is educable. . . . By this time you will have received the impression that the field of analytic psychotherapy is a very narrow one, since you have really heard nothing from me except the indications which point against it. . . . It is gratifying that precisely the most valuable and the most highly developed persons are best suited to these curative measures. . . . If you succeed in persuading [the patient] to accept, by virtue of a better understanding, something that up to now, in consequence of this automatic regulation by pain, he has rejected (repressed), you will then have accomplished something towards his education.
>
> Sigmund Freud, 1904

Consideration of the *future* of psychoanalysis presents the question of what psychoanalysis is—the problem of "identity." For a long time it has been routine in the United States to think of psychoanalysis as a "treatment," and until relatively recently (to the distress of Freud, it may be noted) psychoanalysis was officially defined in this country as a medical monopoly. When one examines the data presented below, however, it appears obvious that if psychoanalysis is a treatment, it is a treatment applied by and offered to remarkably small samples of the population. It is "caviar for the general" in a most dramatic sense.

The development of psychoanalysis as a social movement occurred very rapidly in this country. In a kind of explosion after World War II, psychoanalysis spread through the medical schools to the point of "saturating" departments of psychiatry, many of which were brand new; an interesting period of my own career was that spent in such a new department (dedicated to "dynamic psychiatry") at the University of North Carolina. The high point of this development was reached somewhere in the same time period as the high point of American power and influence in the world; since that time the acceleration has been passed to community psychiatry and other forms of psychiatric practice in which psychopharmacologic agents and family therapy have become the focal points of interest. Community psychiatry is obviously a contrapuntal response to the increasing awareness that the official psychoanalytic or psychodynamic orientation has little or nothing to offer the great majority of patients. In an estimate we have recurrently affirmed, the proportion of patients "suitable" for the "talking cure" is somewhere around 2 per cent of the total population, an estimate supported by the data of Scharfstein and Magnas quoted below.

A major influence upon psychoanalysis is now being exerted by the egalitarian sentiment widespread in this country. Traditionally in the United States emphasis has been placed upon equality of *opportunity*, with the disproportion in *achievement* because of various competitive advantages being taken for granted. Now, however, it is apparent that a powerful sentiment in political circles favors the mandating of egalitarianism throughout as much of the society as possible (cf. Jencks et al., 1972). When we consider the "results of psychotherapy" in terms of the loss of symptoms and other indices of medical improvement, it is impossible to demonstrate a positive effect (Malan, 1973). I, for one, believe this lack of demonstrable change to come from the scientific (or quasiscientific) use of "controls" that do not in fact control because all patients and all therapists are lumped together in many studies. Whatever the reason, the lack of demonstrability of results has been widely admitted by psychotherapists.

On the other hand, a conspicuous positive "result of psychotherapy" when such "therapy" has the specific *educational* purpose of training "candidates" (who freely admit to being at least "sick enough" to become psychotherapists) is demonstrated by Henry et al. (1971) to be a remarkable *upward social mobility*. Psychotherapists regularly move from a childhood Class IV level to an adult Class I or II level. Thus, all one has to do to demonstrate the tangible benefits of psychoanalysis and psychotherapy is the simple maneuver of changing the definition from *treatment to training*, therapy to education, and to use *income* criteria.

Psychoanalysis illustrates the ancient axioms that "To him that hath shall be given" and that "Nothing succeeds like success." The demonstrations I propose to set forth below present the extraordinary selectivity psychoanalysts and psychotherapists use in accepting patients for "insight" or interpretative or anxiety-provoking therapy. Peculiarly enough, since the prevailing ethos of psychoanalysis, at least in the United States, is borrowed from a view of medicine that emphasizes not its humanistic but its scientific side, this selectivity has had to be obscured to avoid the obviously appropriate label of "elitist." Psychoanalysis is unquestionably and necessarily elitist—just as the selection of students for advanced degrees in universities is necessarily elitist. It is the most highly trained students that are accepted—and this fact is clearly explained by the consideration that only already well-trained students can "play the game" required.

Psychoanalysis has flourished in, and only in, those countries that can be considered *developed* in the "modern" sense of that term (Inkeles and Smith,

1974). This form of development depends basically upon the presence of a highly educated cadre of persons capable of accepting responsibility for managing very complex industrial and educational institutions. In general, the one supports the other, as industrial concerns (in the present or through the foundations that preserve the results of industrial efficiency) help support the educational institutions through which they recruit and develop their own future officers and managers.

Inkeles and Smith have presented a fascinating description of the process of "becoming modern" in a number of different cultures. Their conclusions are of both positive and negative interest. On the positive side, they document the fact that to become modern it is necessary to have been intensively schooled in a formal setting; on the negative side, they show that becoming modern requires the rejection of the traditional social supports associated with the "embeddedness" of the member in his culture, i.e., (1) the extended family, (2) traditional forms of religion, and (3) the subordinate status of women. In addition, it is possible to see that the abandonment process moves always in the direction of a greater emphasis upon democratic political forms, away from the authoritarianism that is, one must admit, much more peaceful when the population fully submits.

Psychoanalysis offers to the human being undergoing an "identity crisis" a preceptorial relation in which he is educated in the direction of becoming his own primary respondent (or, in the words of a popular book, his own "best friend"). The process uses the "inner speech system" to train the "patient" (student, novice) to take both roles and learn how to "see himself" and to "speak to himself" from points of view other than the "egocentric" one occupied by the naive child. But we immediately find that to do this in the prescribed manner requires that the selected student or novice shall have already developed at least the rudiments of this method. Piaget emphasizes that coordinating points of view and learning to describe behavioral sequences ("operating upon operations") begins to take place only at puberty (in a continuous education) and that if the process is to be completed satisfactorily, the student must be able to continue his education in a formal manner through that period, postpuberty, that in a developed society we call "adolescence."

A Series of Contexts

In the subsequent discussion, I propose to present a series of demonstrations to be understood as more correlative than sequential. It is as though I were scribing a series of Venn diagrams, each of which overlaps part or parts of others; the "game" then is that of interpreting the meaning of the overlapping portions. In this way I shall be presenting some results of insurance funding of psychotherapy, some geographic and social class contexts of psychotherapy and psychoanalysis, a comment upon the urban intellectual of the United States, and, recurrently throughout, aspects of the ethnic composition of psychotherapists. The peculiar correlation that appears and reappears is that of the relation of the Jew and the Protestant (cf. Weber, 1904).

In the modern world, there is an enormous difference between nations, groups, classes, and persons on the basis of "development"; there is a close relation between *personal* development and *national* development, since it is only through the agency of highly trained and cognitively sophisticated persons that a complex civilization can be directed and regulated. The "heart" of the developed system is to be found in its bureaucracy, the "mind" in its intellectuals. Therefore, it seems of considerable usefulness to begin with an attempt to describe and define the relations of *psychiatry* as the broader field in which medical psychotherapy exists and of *psychoanalysis,* the narrow field exclusively concerned with psychotherapy in the "dynamic" mode, to a number of such significant contexts in the developed nations, especially in the United States. Limitation of space prevents a comprehensive review of the various contexts I shall touch upon briefly, but the significant relations appear self-evident.

Insurance Support of Psychotherapy

Scharfstein and Magnas (1975) studied a "high option" coverage for psychiatric treatment as a fringe benefit to federal employees (i.e., bureaucrats). The insurance company paid 80 per cent of the cost, providing a test of the often claimed restriction of the use of psychotherapy-psychoanalysis on purely financial grounds. Three different localities were involved, in significantly different ways. Four per cent of all the members of the group of users were from Ohio and 6 per cent from California, while *21 per cent* were from the District of Columbia (federal district) area. Of those members incurring charges for mental and nervous disorders, 4 per cent were from Ohio, 7 per cent from California, and *37 per cent* from the federal district. Thus it is clear that although there were many more covered persons in the federal district, those persons used the services at a high rate, almost twice as much as would be expected on the basis of the Ohio and California figures. In addition, and perhaps even more remarkably, 65 per cent of all those incurring charges of more than $10,000 were from the federal district, as contrasted with the consistent proportions of 4 per cent from Ohio and 6 per cent from California. The use of psychotherapy in the federal district is thus extremely high in comparison with the two complete states. The authors point out that in Washington, the population (especially federal employees) tends to include very high proportions of *employed, young,* and *educated* persons—all criteria usually associated with mental health.

When we turn our attention then to the frequency of treatment, we find equally astonishing—but significantly different—figures. The authors estimate the frequency of visits from the cost figures on what seems to be a reasonable set of statistical assumptions. Most analysts would insist that three visits a week is the minimum for "analysis." On this basis, treatment frequency wipes out the differences noted above; these figures are consistent in each of the three areas. In all three, 90 per cent of the patients were seen once a week or less, while in all three areas (with very minor differences) only *1 per cent* of all patients were seen three times a week or more.

The significance of this figure is striking: when financial considerations are of no great moment, and when there is a very large number of psychiatrists and psychoanalysts available, as in the federal district (see below), then *only one out of a hundred pairs of therapists and therapees* opts for psychoanalysis. The significance is enhanced when one suspects that some or many of the "patients" being seen more than three times a week were in fact trainees primarily and "patients" secondarily. The emphasis is upon the extraordinarily high *mutual selectivity* of each by the other participant.

Demographic Notes

Let us turn to a closely related problem: where and in what numbers do psychotherapists and psychoanalysts occur? We can approach the question somewhat obliquely by consulting official sources, psychiatrists numbered in recent official publications of the American Psychiatric Association, psychoanalysts by the American Psychoanalytic Association. In the latter case, these are persons officially classified as *orthodox* (and overwhelmingly medical) psychoanalysts of the Freudian persuasion. The prevalence rates were figured on the basis of 1970 census figures.

In a recent paper, Brown (expressing the point of view of the central federal institution having to do with psychiatry and psychotherapy) reviews trends in the prevalence of psychiatrists locally and nationally, then and now. In the latter context, he points to a very high rate of acceleration in the past few decades. The numbers of psychiatrists in the United States (in figures always referring to numbers per 100,000 of the population) run: 1939:2.3, 1950:4.7, 1960:7.7, 1970:11.3, and in a projected figure for 1980:17.8. This amounts to a 7.7-fold increase in 40 years. Despite the well-known liberal trend in the profession (at least in comparison with surgeons), the minority representation remains extremely small: 1.4 per cent black, 1.5 per cent Spanish American, 1.3 per cent from other minorities. Parenthetically, Vidal comments that blacks constitute about 2 per cent of the nation's 350,000 physicians and about the same proportion of the 355,000 lawyers; minorities are "underdeveloped" groups in the professions.

Brown's figures of national distribution are striking: 11 states have less than five psychiatrists per 100,000 population; New York has 25, Maryland 19, and Virginia more than 5 but less than 8. These figures are of special interest in relation to the District of Columbia, contiguous to both Maryland and Virginia, in which are the homes of many of those working in the federal district; the district has 58 psychiatrists per 100,000 population—and Brown emphasizes that this does *not* include the absolute number of 2200 psychiatrists directly employed by the federal government in the district.

The background is that of the bureaucracy in a "company town" in which the exclusive business is that of government. To round out the picture, it is useful to refer to other towns, of which one of the most interesting is Chapel Hill, North Carolina, the seat of the University of North Carolina, in which a four-year medical school was first established in the early 1950's. By personal knowledge, in 1950 there were 0 psychiatrists and 0 psychoanalysts in Chapel Hill; in 1952, one psychologist was providing part-time counselling to students in the university, but he did not continue after the development of the medical school.

Let us begin with the internal relative prevalence in parts of New York City as compared and contrasted with the figures above. The figures give for Manhattan 106 psychiatrists per 100,000 population, for Queens 9, the Bronx 5, Brooklyn 7, Richmond (Staten Island) 10. When we turn the microscope to high power, as it were, and look at psychoanalysts, the numbers are (per 100,000 population) Manhattan 25, Queens 0.5, the Bronx 0.5, Richmond 0.3. The concentration within Manhattan is pronounced, to no one's surprise. By comparison, the number of psychoanalysts in the federal district is 17 (per 100,000 population).

To show startling differences, it is only necessary to move to a small suburb, Great Neck, Long Island, at the edge of New York City, in which there is a universally admired school system supported by very high real estate taxes. This is a suburb from which access to Manhattan is easy. In this town of 40,000 the prevalence of psychoanalysts is notable, 60 per 100,000 population. Following the educational implication and focussing upon Chapel Hill, we find the astonishing figures (in a town of 26,000 "in the boondocks") of 184 psychiatrists (per 100,000 population) and 42 psychoanalysts. By comparison, in Durham (population 95,000), the home of Duke University, 12 miles from Chapel Hill, there are 59 psychiatrists and 11 psychoanalysts per 100,000 population. The local psychoanalytic institute was begun and developed mostly under the auspices of the two universities. In the largest town in North Carolina, Charlotte, with a quarter of a million inhabitants, there were 7 psychiatrists and 0 psychoanalysts (per 100,000 population). To indicate that these figures are significant, it is possible to take a passing glance at the prevalence of psychologists to find a similar distribution: Manhattan 27, the Bronx 0.5; Chapel Hill 89, Charlotte 0.4.

International Implications

The following figures were collected in the early 1960's and indicate the "maldistribution" of psychoanalysts around the world at that time. When the figures ("psychoanalysts" here as members of the International Psychoanalytic Association) are rank-ordered, it is of considerable interest to note that in the 1960 comparison, the United States (with by far the greatest number in absolute terms) comes fourth in a list—Israel 8.8 (per 100,000 population), Switzerland 5.7, The Netherlands 4.5, United States 4.2, Sweden 2.6, United Kingdom 2.0, Austria 2.0. In another interesting figure, Roazen reports that in

1952 64 per cent of the members of the International Psychoanalytic Association were Americans.

It is of special interest in terms of "growth" to note the very low prevalence rates in the Latin countries in 1960—France 0.5, Italy 0.3. To indicate something of the influence of religion, Belgium, in part sharing a language and a border with the Netherlands, but predominantly Catholic, had in 1960 a prevalence rate of 0.9 in comparison with the 4.5 in the largely Protestant Netherlands.

Most countries of the world do not appear on the list at all; one interesting prevalence rate is to be found in India, in which although the absolute number cited is nearly the same as that of Sweden and France, the proportional figure comes out at 0.006 per 100,000 population.

Psychotherapy and Intellectualism

Roazen (1976) quotes Fromm, who describes the early psychoanalysts: "They were urban intellectuals, with a deep yearning to be committed to an ideal, to a leader, to a movement, and yet without having any religious or political or philosophical ideal or convictions."

A further discussion of the relation of intellectual and psychoanalyst can be drawn from Kadushin's books, *Why People Go to Psychiatrists* (1969) and *The American Intellectual Elite* (1974). As indicated above, New York appears as the "capital of psychotherapy." Kadushin estimates that at the time of his writing, there were 3,550 physician-psychiatrists in New York (mostly in Manhattan, as noted above), with 300 members of the American Psychoanalytic Association and in addition 1000 clinical psychologists and 900 social workers employed in psychiatric settings (and mostly having private practices as well). Kadushin cites the well known Midtown study indicating that the overall rate of going to psychiatrists in the midtown, east side neighborhood studies was "over six times the national average."

In the figures noted above, it was apparent that in places where there is a high "production" and "consumption" of psychotherapeutic services there also tends to be a similar trend in educational services. In this context, it is interesting to turn to Kadushin's conclusions on the distribution of intellectuals, by definition very high producers and consumers of educational services. The author comments that

> 70 per cent of the editorial offices of the top 25 intellectual journals are within 10 miles of the Empire State Building. Over 50 per cent of the American intellectual elite themselves are still located within 50 miles of the Empire State Building. . . . Reflecting American tradition, New England (especially Boston-Cambridge) still has a large concentration of intellectuals, though its 14 per cent does not put it in the same class with New York. The rest is a scatter, except for Washington, D.C., which while it cannot rival European capitals, still can boast a surprising 11 per cent of the total.

Kadushin goes on to emphasize the proportion of Jews in the intellectual elite, noting that "Jews are indeed much more strongly represented among leading intellectuals than in the population at large. They compose about half of the American intellectual elite; Catholics are vastly underrepresented, but Protestants, who are one third of the group, are also relatively underrepresented." If one takes the proportion of Jews in the population of the United States as about 2.5 per cent, then the fact that 50 per cent of the intellectuals are Jews means that one fortieth of the population produces half the intellectuals. Sowell points out that more than a quarter of all Nobel prize winners in the United States have been Jews.

The astonishingly high proportion of psychoanalysts in Great Neck goes, in this context, precisely along with its designation as a "Golden Ghetto," i.e., a geographical locus in which a very large proportion (perhaps a majority) of well-to-do Jews live. In turn, again, these distributions reflect the traditional interest in education of Jews, the "people of the book." The predominance of the educational over the ethnic is demonstrated in the Chapel Hill instance.

What appears in this series of parallelisms is the significance of educational-intellectual development in Jews; it has long been evident that psychoanalysis is mainly of professional interest to Jews. Henry et al. (1971) note that 51.5 per cent of all psychotherapists are of Jewish "cultural affinity"; psychoanalysts as a special group show the same trait at the level of 62.1 per cent. A further demonstration of the astonishing statistical consistency of the group is shown by these authors' figure that 78.1 per cent of Jewish psychoanalysts were second-generation Americans, while only 7.1 per cent of the much less frequent protestant psychoanalysts were second generation. Still another feature is of major note, in that 66.0 per cent of the fathers of Jewish psychoanalysts were of Eastern European origin—a fact especially notable with reference to "modernity" (Inkeles and Smith). This figure becomes more notable when contrasted with the figures of 2.5 per cent from Western Europe and 10.6 per cent from Germany and Austria. In contrast, the relatively small number of Protestant psychoanalysts tend to come from old American families.

A recent comment by the critic George Steiner emphasizes the extremely small sample used by Freud in reaching his theoretical conclusions:

> (T)he important point to be made concerns the specificity, the linguistic-social historicity and even localization of the material. Freud is a Viennese Jew. . . . His circle is that of other Viennese Jews or of the emancipated Jews and half-Jews coming to Vienna from the very particular language spaces of Budapest-German and Prague-German. . . . (T)he speech acts which Freud listens to and analyzes are those of the more or less leisured middle class, of a Viennese middle class and of women. Each of these parameters—the social, the ethnic, and the sexual—is language-specific in profound and manifold ways.

Steiner concludes, in a reference to this extraordinarily restricted sample, "The consequences of this historical specificity have never, I believe, been fully grasped, nor, I think, has psychoanalysis quite faced the paradox inherent in the foundation of a universal, normative model of meaning and behavior on so particular a semantic base."

Roazen emphasizes that the premier usefulness of Jung to the early psychoanalytic movement was associated with his gentile origin. Freud is quoted in a letter to Abraham in explaining why Jung had been "formally adopted . . . as an eldest son" and anointed as his "successor and Crown Prince":

> Please be tolerant and do not forget that it is really easier for you than it is for Jung to follow my ideas for in the first place you are completely independent, and then you are closer to my intellectual constitution because of racial kinship, while he as a Christian and a pastor's son finds his way to me only against great inner resistances. His association with us is the more valuable for that. I nearly said that it was only by his appearance on the scene that psychoanalysis escaped the danger of becoming a Jewish national affair.

In another comment to the same end, the Jewish scholar, Bakan, has analyzed the Freudian theoretical system to demonstrate the number of ways in which it derives from Hassidic theology.

Epistemological Considerations: Relative Maturity

Piaget and psychoanalysts alike concentrate their efforts on highly selected subjects (patients, students). Such subjects are well-educated members of a developed society: "normal" standards so established are highly artificial ones, grossly influenced by the selection process.

We have been deeply interested for many years in the selection process by means of which in psychoanalysis-psychotherapy the vast majority of the population is eliminated by subtle procedures of which the eliminator is himself usually quite unaware (Shands, 1958). The conclusion has been progressively supported that testing *cognitive* sophistication gives a measure that is highly useful in predicting, *not* outcome, but the probability that a psychotherapist will be interested in establishing a long-range relationship with the subject in question (Meltzer, 1972).

We (Shands and Meltzer, 1975) have found that persons displaying the characteristic features of a somatization reaction (as a variant of a conversion reaction) in the disability state following an industrial accident show a profound limitation in the ability to find simple similarities on which to establish categorical classification, the initial step in any intellectual analysis. Asked as to how a banana is similar to an apple, such persons invariably say, "Nothing is similar; the one is long and yellow, the other round and red." The taxonomist has to begin with the similarity between two somewhat different "objects"; but these persons say that there is no similarity between a dog and a lion, for instance. An interesting "concrete" answer was that the lion is fierce and has a long tail, while dogs are "nice"; the interviewee then added, egocentrically, "I am a dog lover myself." Such a person is unable to construct the simple category "fruit" or "animal." In spite of this severe limitation, persons of this sort often give a satisfactory work history of many years and have proven themselves to be parents and family members of prior stability. They are not, however, "good candidates for psychotherapy." In Piaget's classification, the inability to form classes (and failure in serial subtraction of 7 from 100) categorizes these working class persons as pre-operational, that is, functioning in this special cognitive test at below the age of 7!

In contrast, the techniques of "free association," the capacity to "develop a transference," and the mutual usefulness of interpretation requires that the "patient" have developed the kind of intellectual techniques Piaget refers to as formal operations (Shands, 1977). Formal operations usher in the stage of "reflective thinking," and the beginning of this stage is correlated with the specifically testable ability to conserve volume, i.e., to understand that a change in shape of a liquid does not change its amount. The astonishing demonstration given in published material is the small number of persons who reach this level of sophistication in the general public.

Elkind established experimentally the proportion of American youths who had reached the level of conservation of volume. Testing 11- and 12-year-olds, he found that only 27 per cent succeeded in conserving volume. In a second study with somewhat older (12 to 18) subjects, he found that while 87 per cent demonstrated conservation of mass (normal 8 years) and weight (normal 10 years), only 47 per cent conserved volume. In still a third study, this time using college students, he found that only 58 per cent could conserve volume several years after the supposed critical time. In a study of black and white adults in a night class, Graves (1972) found a remarkable restriction of cognitive ability (even in voluntary students). Only 78 per cent had achieved conservation of mass, 67 per cent that of weight, and 24 per cent conservation of volume.

To emphasize the appraisal of these figures, it has been estimated that some 20 per cent of the people in the United States have had some college work. Generalizing Elkind's last figure for a very approximate guess, 58 per cent of 20 per cent is about 12 per cent of the whole population that has reached Piaget's "normal" stage of intellectual sophistication at the beginning of adolescence. In this particular context, less than 12 per cent of the people of the United States are estimated to be at the level of Piaget's well-educated 12-year-old. At most, then, this is the group from which analysands are drawn.

Education or Therapy?

As suggested above, the data presented from a number of overlapping studies suggest that the interpretation Freud gave in 1904 remains current. Psychoanalysis is a "very narrow" field in which the analysand comes from a "highly developed" group characterized primarily as "educable."

The ethnic theme appears and reappears. Weber emphasized the close relation of capitalism and the protestant ethic, and he called particular attention to the derivation of protestant thought from the Old Testament, noting that influential English protestant sects were called "English Hebraists."

"Development" in the modern sense is associated not only with protestantism and capitalism but also with democratic theory, scientific research, industrial-technological progress, and with greater and greater emphasis in recent years on egalitarianism and civil rights. All these are associated with a central ideological emphasis upon *individualism.*

What has been ignored for the most part in this ideological context is the fact that to develop the concept of an "individual" and especially to develop a self-concept—myself as individual—is a major problem in *cognitive* context. One reason, again, is that in the oligarchy most responsible for generating and promulgating ideas of individualism, cognitive development at a high level can be taken for granted; ethnocentricity then tends to obscure "objective" recognition of the group's own consistently high educational superiority. The idea that perhaps only 12 per cent of adult Americans are capable of formal operational thinking is stunning, almost as much so as our estimate that only some 2 per cent of the population are intellectually capable of playing the psychoanalytic game (although it is probable that a not much greater percentage of the population is capable of playing a really competent game of chess).

Piaget's *conservation* is a variant of what has often been called "context-independence." In various different ways, the child learns that *quantity* can be quite independent of the *qualitative* context of "shape." In a very similar way, the scientific emphasis upon measurement focuses on quantity independent of context, in traditional statement "reality" instead of "appearance."

Bruner has emphasized the importance in individualistic self-differentiation of the significance of studying written records and descriptions in school, commenting upon the implicit training in knowing what clearly is *not* present (except in record and imagination.) Cross-referencing again, Piaget comments that the (educated Swiss) adolescent "delights in considerations of what is not," that is, in fantasies; and fantasies are to a very considerable extent the "raw material" of psychoanalysis (cf. Marty and de M'Uzan, 1963).

For the development of an "individual," Bruner (1973) comments that "implicit in this notion is the distinctness of onself and one's own point of view. Thus, the individual must conceptually separate himself from the group; he must become self-conscious." It is of some considerable significance here to note that "becoming self-conscious" in one sense is equivalent to objectifying the self; on the other hand, the central characteristic of the state of *anxiety* that is the main concept in psychoanalysis is that of a paralyzing self-consciousness.

Interminable Education

A point that brings together these diverse strains is that psychoanalysis represents perhaps the most extraordinarily extended group-educational training known in human history. The discipline and its institutional forms select human beings not only tolerant of, but in a sense "addicted to," education. According to Henry et al., the postresidency training of the psychoanalyst requires *less than 4* years in only 16 per cent of cases, 4 to 7 years in 58 per cent and *more than* 7 years in 26 per cent. These figures are to be added to 24 years of medical training.

As a part of a larger (and still somewhat informal) study of the experience of psychiatrists particularly interested in psychotherapy, I sampled the personal experience of psychoanalysis in a small group of close associates, all of whom carry significant responsibility in the psychiatry, psychology, nursing, and social work services in a general hospital. The number of years in psychoanalysis or psychoanalytic-type therapy in this group runs: 10, 10, 9, 8, 7, 6, 3, 3, and several of those asked are still in "treatment" without immediate prospect of "cure."

Since, by the criteria outlined by Vaillant in relation to "mental health," *all* in this group would be characterized as outstandingly "healthy" in the sense of social and personal success and reasonably stable human relations, the extraordinary commitment to "treatment" precisely bears out Freud's comment, "the optimum conditions for . . . [psychoanalysis] exist where it is not needed—i.e., among the healthy." A good deal more significance can be introduced by noting the reversibility of Freud's statement that psychoanalysis has to do with *re-educational* techniques to "overcome" internal resistances: the opposite side of the picture is that education (to hyperliteracy) is specifically concerned with inculcating and reinforcing those same "internal resistances" through the systematic educational "repression" of "doing what comes naturally."

Conclusion

The material quoted above shows, conclusively in my opinion (the data can be indefinitely extended, to the same end) that psychoanalysis, far from being a general psychology, is an extraordinarily narrow theoretical system, drawing its reciprocal role-occupants from the most highly educated levels of the population. What is further noteworthy is the remarkably differential success of psychoanalysis in the United States, in a version of the theory that has been vehemently criticized by Lacan as "philistine," particularly because of the American habit of integrating psychoanalytic theory with sociological and behavioristic notions.

This local flourishing-with-modification seems to be a peculiarly American characteristic; the United States is a country that greatly supports innovation, although to a very great extent the original impetus in many such contexts comes from abroad. The United States appears to be extraordinarily fertile "transplant medium," perhaps in a fashion that reflects the traditional acceptance of aliens and immigrants. This country is a composite of immigrants, of whom the "old Americans" go back no more than three hundred years at most. The short history of a country that has, if it has, only just ceased to incorporate new states, together with the diverse kinds of persons constituting its population, has required a very different kind of "national personality" than those Western European nations from whom it originally borrowed inspiration for its radically novel institutional forms.

A most interesting combination of factors has to do with the differential success of persons identifiable as "WASPS" and Jews. Both groups have demonstrated differentially high rates of success best seen in the context of advanced intellectual work. In Roe's (1965) sample of 64 highly successful scientists (biological, physical, and social), the origins of 5 are given as Jewish, 1 as from a "free thinking" family, and 58 (90 per cent) from Protestant family origins, including many from ministerial families. On the other hand, the data quoted above indicate that intellectuals and psychoanalysts come differentially from Jewish families. Both the intellectuals and the scientists demonstrate an extensive loss of religious faith. Inkeles and Smith comment that becoming modern seems easiest for Nigerian Ibos, East Indian Parsees, Eastern European Jews, and Swiss Protestants.

Servan-Schreiber (1967) commented upon the trend for American multinational firms to invade European industry; he cites the powerful influence of the emphasis on education in the United States, with three times as many university students per 1000 population as in Europe. At that time Servan-Schreiber emphasized as well the extraordinarily different interest in education and research by the federal government as a major support to the developmental impetus of American industry.

Any system dedicated to "freedom" has what statisticians call many more "degrees of freedom." This means that the level of uncertainty, i.e., anxiety (cf. Shands, 1957), is high, and that a vastly greater amount of data-processing is required to make a decision. By contrast, members of preliterate cultures display an extensive unconscious submissiveness to tradition and an avoidance of innovation or freedom. Carothers notes that in the African native, "Behavior is minutely governed from childhood on in a host of particular, concrete situations by meticulous rules and taboos, and not on the basis of a few broad principles which require personal decisions for their application." There is no notion of an "individual": "(A) man comes to regard himself as a rather insignificant part of a much larger organism—the family and clan—and not as an independent, self-reliant unit; personal initiative and ambition are permitted little outlet; and a meaningful integration of a man's experience on individual, personal lines is not achieved." Carothers also notes that in contrast to this lack of intellectual freedom, the native is expected to express "emotions" freely in an "extroverted" fashion.

The goal of psychotherapy (more and more so in its modern variants) is that of achieving a greater degree of spontaneity and personal "liberation." The process moves toward the free expression of emotions, i.e., toward the norm in uneducated persons. Thus we find the paradox that the extended education of the psychoanalyst has the purpose of reproducing the "expressiveness" of the uneducated. At the same time, however, it is apparent that an intensive education in a highly dependent relation to a preceptor is significantly associated with the production of society-institute groupings that display remarkably authoritarian and restrictive "codes," with an insistence on following the "party line." The analogy between the libertarian ideals of both psychoanalysis and Marxism, with the regimentation visible in the social forms of both, appears to represent a "repetition compulsion." The demonstration is that of the "deep structure" of human group formation, always "irrational" even when dependent upon ostensibly rational theoretical systems. In a personal communication, Roazen recently commented upon the complaint made by a "bright analyst" who felt that the extended "adolescence" had interfered with his ability to develop his own professional identity. "Forty is too late to *begin* to think for oneself."

Of perhaps even greater interest has been the recent development of a consensus as to the apparently specific inability of patients with certain kinds of "psychosomatic" diseases to describe feelings (Shands, 1958, 1975, 1977a, 1977b; Sifneos, 1967; Sifneos and Nemiah, 1970) or to use fantasies (Marty and de M'Uzan, 1963) in working in interpretative psychotherapy. This inability ("inarticulateness," in the description of a rheumatologist) has been observed and described in the United States, France, Germany, and several Scandinavian countries so that it would appear to be a "fact." The most interesting feature of this inability is the demonstration of a major deficit in introspective capacity, without development of the kind of "private world" that "suitable" patients and psychotherapists take for granted. An attempt to summarize all these tendencies into a single construct emphasizes that psychoanalysis must be understood as existing in a particular and peculiar sociocultural niche, in a specific epoch that has now lasted so short a time that all we can say about its future is that "change will continue."

The Dominant Minority

Finally, it may be of interest to note that the problem of the dominant minority in an egalitarian culture is not unique to the psychological universe of discourse. The comment quoted below has to do with the accelerated development of the computer in developed societies, with the implicit generation of an elite familiar with the technology of that fantastic data-processing machine. After first commenting upon the manner in which nineteenth century scientific ideas have now reached "common sense" levels (at least in the highly educated group of the population), Weizenbaum emphasizes that the metaphors implicit in materialistic scientific theories have "been influential in shaping our entire civilization's imaginative reconstruction of the world." It is of some interest to note here in passing that this is a restatement of the so-called "Sapir-Whorf hypothesis" that relates the universe known to the means whereby it is known.

Continuing, the author writes,

> The computing metaphor is as yet available to only an extremely small set of people. Its acquisition and internalization, hopefully as only one of many ways to see the world, seems to require experience in program composition, a kind of computing

literacy. Perhaps such literacy will become very widespread in the advanced societal sectors of the advanced countries. But, should it become a dominant mode of thinking and be restricted to certain social classes, it will prove not only repressive in the ordinary sense, but an enormously divisive societal force. For then classes which do and do not have access to the metaphor will, in an important sense, lose their ability to communicate with each other. We know already how difficult it is for the poor and the oppressed to communicate with the rest of the society in which they are embedded. . . . (T)he communication difficulties, which have grave consequences, are very largely due to the fact that the respective communities have unsharable experiences out of which unsharable metaphors have grown.

This problem seems to me to be that one to which the future of psychoanalysis, with its incredibly small metaphor-sharing community is most significantly related. What is clearest is the proliferation of psychotherapies; Hildebrand, writing on the future of psychoanalysis, cites Harper's estimate of 36 separable psychotherapies derivative from the basic psychoanalytic system, mostly in the United States. A trend still evident in psychoanalytic institutions is that of progressive sectarian splitting. All of these trends very much suggest that it is the politicoreligious implications of psychoanalysis that progressively work themselves out in the evolution of what must be seen primarily as a *social movement* always significantly related to its context, and again we find the paradox that methods of education emphasizing context-independence require the kind of ideological climate that constitutes a major form of context-dependence.

References

Bakan, D.: Sigmund Freud and the Jewish Mystical Tradition. Princeton, N.J., Van Nostrand, 1958.

Bernstein, B.: Social class, speech systems and psychotherapy. Br. J. Sociol., *15*:54–64, 1964.

Brown, B.: The life of psychiatry. Am. J. Psychiatry, *133*:489, 1976.

Bruner, J. S.: Culture and cognitive growth. *In* The Relevance of Education. New York, W. W. Norton and Co., Inc., 1973.

Carothers, J. D.: Culture, psychiatry, and the written word. Psychiatry, *22*:307–320, 1959.

Elkind, D.: Children's discovery of the conservation of mass, weight and volume. J. Genet. Psychol., *98*:219–227, 1961.

Elkind, D.: Quantity conceptions in junior and senior high school students. Child Dev., *32*:551–560, 1961.

Elkind, D.: Quantity conceptions in college students. J. Soc. Psychol., *57*:459–465, 1962.

Freud, S.: On psychotherapy. *In* The Standard Edition of the Complete Psychological Works of Sigmund Freud, vol. VII. London, The Hogarth Press Ltd., 1953.

Graves, A. J.: Attainment of mass, weight and volume in minimally educated adults. Dev. Psychol., *7*:223, 1972.

Henry, W. E., Sims, J. H., and Spray, S. L.: The Fifth Profession. San Francisco, Jossey-Bass Inc., Publishers, 1971.

Inkeles, A., and Smith, D. H.: Becoming Modern. Cambridge, Mass., Harvard University Press, 1974.

Jencks, C., Smith, M., Acland, H., Bane, M. J., Cohen, D., Gintis, H., Heyns, B., and Michelson, S.: Inequality: A Reassessment of the Effect of Family and Schooling in America. New York, Basic Books, Inc., Publishers, 1972.

Kadushin, C.: The American Intellectual Elite. Boston, Little, Brown and Co., 1974.

Lacan, J.: The Language of the Self: The Function of Language in Psychoanalysis. Trans. Anthony Wilden. Baltimore, The Johns Hopkins Press, 1968.

Malan, D. H.: The outcome problem in psychotherapy research. Arch. Gen Psych., *29*:719–729, 1973.
Marty, P., and de M'Uzan, M.: La Pensée Operatoire. Rev. Fr. Psychoanal., *27*:345–356, 1963.
Meltzer, J. D.: The Suitable Patient: Talking, Thinking, and Therapy. Ph. D. Dissertation, New York University, 1972.
Piaget, J.: Intellectual evolution from adolescence to adulthood. Human Dev., *15*:1–12, 1972.
Roazen, P.: Freud and His Followers. New York, American Library, 1976.
Scharfstein, S. S., and Magnas, H. L.: Insuring intensive psychotherapy. Am. J. Psychiatry, *132*:1252, 1975.
Servan-Schreiber: The American Challenge. New York, Atheneum Publishers, 1968.
Shands, H. C.: An approach to the measurement of suitability for psychotherapy. Psych. Q., *32*:500, 1958.
Shands, H. C.: Some social and biological aspects of anxiety. J. Nerv. Ment. Dis., *125*:459–468, 1957.
Shands, H. C.: How are "psychosomatic" patients different from "psychoneurotic" patients? Psychother. Psychosom., *26*:270–285, 1975.
Shands, H. C.: Suitability for psychotherapy I: Transference and formal operations. In press, 1977a.
Shands, H. C.: Suitability for psychotherapy II: Unsuitability and psychosomatic disease. In press, 1977b.
Shands, H. C., and Meltzer, J. D.: Disproportionate disability: The Freud-Charcot syndrome rediscovered. J. Psychiatry Law, *3*:25–37, 1975.
Sifneos, P. E.: Clinical observations on some patients suffering from a variety of psychosomatic diseases. Acta Med. Psychosomat., 3–10, 1967.
Sowell, T.: New York Times Magazine, August 8, 1976, p. 14.

Comment

Dr. Shands focuses on psychoanalysis as a form of treatment, looking at both its practitioners and their analysands. Shands regards psychoanalysis as an elitist treatment, since it is available to a very small and highly selected portion of the population. He documents this by looking at the demographic, economic, intellectual, and cultural characteristics of persons who undergo psychoanalysis, pointing out that it is more a form of education than of treatment. Paraphrasing Freud, he notes that it is the most highly developed (cultured and educated) members of society who are best suited to the experience. Shands points out that psychoanalysts are also highly select individuals who mirror their patients intellectually and culturally. Shands notes whimsically that although it is difficult to demonstrate loss of symptoms or other indices of medical improvement, a conspicuous positive result of psychoanalysis is the upward social mobility of its training candidates.

The future of psychoanalysis will be determined in no small part by the economic conditions of our time. Currently, economists in Washington are developing blueprints for a national health insurance program which most likely will not contain reimbursement for psychoanalysis. The movement of psychoanalysis away from the mainstream of medicine through the increased training of nonphysicians as clinical practitioners will serve to undermine the medical credibility of the discipline. In short, the future may be grim from an economic standpoint; however, as a theory of personality and a research tool, psychoanalysis will continue to play a vital role in the training of mental health professionals.

JOHN PAUL BRADY, M.D.
H. KEITH H. BRODIE, M.D.

Is Behavior Therapy a Fad or a New Direction for Psychiatry?

JARL E. DYRUD

The University of Chicago

> In contrast with natural objects—even with the higher animals—man is unique in that he is dissatisfied with himself; he is the discontented animal, the romantic, argumentative, aspiring animal. Consequently, his behavior can only in part be described by scientific principles or laws.
>
> Frank Knight

It can hardly be disputed that behavior therapy is a current fad in psychiatry. This is our perennial fashion of reacting to new views that hold some promise for the field, undoubtedly related in part to the fact that our treatment methods are numerous and neither as reliable nor as effective as we would like. In addition, psychiatry is particularly vulnerable to fads because our patients, varying from the worried well to the profoundly psychotic, present us with problems that hold to no neat classification scheme. They can be characterized but not contained. Apparently durable traits keep turning up state-dependent. That is one reason we are already finding fault with the Diagnostic and Statistical Manual III before it is even in print.

I suppose I have been asked to discuss whether behavior therapy, bubbling over to us from our mother science, is just another of the eccentric, aberrant forms proliferating there in a decadent period when the great forms have been disappearing, or is different and better. I use the term "decadent" in the ecological sense of deteriorating, drying up. Some psychologists may be busy and happy exploring primal screams and encounter groups, but scientific psychology has been having a hard time. The great family trees of verbal report research appear to have reached a disappointing limit of growth (Fiske, 1974). A desert has been forming where James had expected the science of consciousness to flourish (James, 1890). My reason for referring to behavior therapy as a form of psychotherapy, that is, a form of psychological treatment rather than a new class of intervention closer to the biological, is that I see it as a beginning reversal of the trend. As rough grass planted in a desert, it may well give us new access to a science of consciousness—not by extending an animal model of behavior manipulation to man, but by developing a powerful pragmatic technology for studying man's self-referent symbolic behavior and his use of it in controlling his own and others' behavior (Hunt, 1975).

I know of no good explanation for why fish "school," but I have a pretty good idea why people do. In the first place, it is so much easier to copy than to think. In the second place, it is one thing to be a solitary investigator coming up with new and challenging ideas, but a practitioner needs a like-minded community to help him define "usual and customary good practice." A case could be made for the necessity of fads in the practice of psychiatry so that responsibility for innovative practice be shared by a larger number, but I favor the first explanation. It is not clinicians only who are carried away by fads. My colleague Herbert Meltzer, M.D., told me that at the neurosciences meeting just concluded, the pack of basic scientists is now off and running after endogenous opiates, having seemingly lost the scent for classical neurotransmitters.

During a fad excesses occur owing to misunderstanding and misapplication as well as to the inevitable disappointments that come with testing a paradigm to its limits. My own view is that we rarely come close to testing a paradigm to its limits in psychiatry, but we do get a lot of mileage out of the placebo effect of the initial enthusiasm for any new procedure. There is always the hazard that good advances will be neutralized by the excesses of true believers. Excessive faith in any theory or system amounts to superstition and often acts against the evidence of our senses. This presents us with a paradox. We know that there are many nonspecific, or rather unspecified, factors at work in any form of psychotherapy. As Martin Orne has pointed out (1975), unless you have *some* belief in your specific factor, which you may call your particular brand of treatment, your nonspecific factors won't work. Therefore, the good psychiatrist must always split two roles in himself, the therapist-believer following his conscious model, and the researcher-critic seeing how this process relates to everything else going on.

It is my hope that behavior therapy, or as I prefer to call it, behavior analysis, will persist, not as a new direction for psychiatry, but as a valuable "course correction."

Behavior techniques have to do with keeping track of observable behavior in a context, looking for what may be making it happen, keeping it happening, or terminating it. This is more intricate than it sounds. A pigeon pecking at a disc attached to a cumulative recorder gives us a record of events over time in which we can have a lot of confidence. But what is a unit of human behavior? How do we arbitrarily cut the stream of on-going behavior into discrete episodes? Much of what makes behavior therapy seem strained and rigid to other therapists lies in efforts to cope with this problem.

During the period of excessive preoccupation with psychoanalytic concepts in our field, we had drifted far from the course of looking at and accounting for observable data. We had become so preoccupied with listening to words and inferring what was not being said that the art of clinical observation had suffered neglect. I have been told that one of the techniques of examination of a University of Pennsylvania veterinary student is to have him look out from an upstairs window to watch a horse being led across the inner courtyard, at which point he is asked to make a diagnosis. Veterinarians must be extremely good observers. We have the advantage of being able to talk with our patients, but many psychiatrists in training seem to have a hard time looking at their patients and reporting the nuances of what they see. Accurate observation is the equivalent of accurate thinking if you have a language in which to think. Clinical theory needs to be closely tied by its terminology to such careful observation.

I am not proposing that we view behavior solely from its surface manifestations. Such observations may be easy to categorize, but not to comprehend. At the Second International Schizophrenia Conference in Rochester in May, 1976, I heard John Romano quote Yogi Berra's comment, "You can observe a lot by just watching." I am confident that when he made the statement, Berra was looking for the functional relationship between the movement of the pitcher's arm and the ball traveling through the strike zone rather than looking at the topography of resemblances of one pitcher's movement to that of another. I want to emphasize this concept of the functional relationship because it is at the heart of the operant paradigm. It presents us with the possibility that our sequences of maladaptive behavior are not on a magnetic tape that can only be erased with great difficulty, but that to a surprising extent behavior floats free of the conditions that instated it. In most instances it is supported by current environmental contingencies that can be changed. This is the source of the optimism and specificity of behavioral diagnosis and intervention. Today when there is a clear-cut behavioral deficit, or an undesirable behavior of high habit strength, the principle of parsimony would suggest that a behavior analysis should be tried first to scout the territory for adjustable environmental contingencies.

To illustrate the point of optimism while at the same time working in a simple, direct, and pragmatic fashion, I think of a young lady named Monica in the three-year-old group of a normal nursery school where Cathryn Levison and I were observing. In this group of 15, Monica was distinguished by sitting in a corner and sucking her thumb during more than 80 per cent of the half-day session. None of the other children in her room knew her name. As one observed her, one could see that this was a sober, sad child who had, after six weeks, failed to adapt to the conditions of the nursery school as her peer group had. If one put on one's inferring hat, one might think something dreadful has been going on at home. She is an unhappy child—perhaps there is a new baby at home. There may be tension in the family that we have no notion of. If one put on one's prognostic hat, one might say that this is a child who will be school phobic by the time she is six or seven. Certainly whatever is wrong with her is serious and requires intervention.

Our first intervention was to arrange for her to spend 15 minutes at the beginning of each session alone in a playroom with another child from the group who had demonstrated in our baseline study the highest level of spontaneous engagement of other children in play and conversation. This led to a marked increase in her responsiveness and even initiation of play in the 15 minute session, but had no impact on her behavior in the larger group over a period of two weeks. We thought she was by then "primed" for the larger group, so in that time slot we set up a 15 minute group game in which the children competed and Monica wore the apron that had in its pocket the prize for the winner of the game. She would award the prize. Within 10 days to two weeks, every child knew her name, she had stopped sitting in the corner sucking her thumb, and her spontaneous play in the group had reached the mean of the group. Six months later, toward the end of the nursery school year, she was observed to be continuing to function at an appropriate level for the three-and-a-half-year-old nursery group. This is a homely story lacking in elegance, but it was a success. For a comparison, we might consider Professor Wayne Booth's story illustrating "symbolic exchange" as cited by Joseph Schwab in his essay "Education and the State" (1976):

> A child, Monique, had for six weeks in a classroom said no word to anyone, had not participated in a single game, her only activity some private playing with blocks and puzzles. On one occasion, the class, on an outing, had proceeded more than a block before Monique's absence was noted. The teacher, going back, found her by the fountain where they had stopped for a drink. Monique had simply stood there, saying nothing.
>
> "Then," said Booth, "a therapist is called in, one who believes that what children like that need may very well be some kind of genuine personal intrusion, some kind of genuine symbolic exchange in which two persons really meet. She begins to play with the girl with no guide but her own sense of this child here in this hour."
>
> The therapist began by playful touching of the girl's ankle, hand, ribs. Then a question about what she would like to play with. Monique gave no response. The therapist then pointed to one and another game or toy. Finally, Monique nodded "yes" to a pointing toward a puzzle involving matching of shapes and colors.
>
> Monique and the therapist played with the puzzle until it was clear that Monique understood the game and could do it well. The therapist then pretended that the rectangle of the puzzle was a circle. Monique cried out with a playful annoyance, "No-o-o." In moments, Monique and the therapist were involved in a game of error by the therapist and correction by Monique.
>
> "In thirty-five minutes," remarked Booth, "a miracle had occurred but the miracle is the everyday reality we tend to forget: persons by nature can respond to symbolic offerings and it is fun for them when they do."
>
> The case described by Booth was therapeutic, but symbolic exchange is therapeutic because it is an invitation to a human person to join in humanity. It involves all that symbols and exchange of symbols can be to people.

I like his story better, not only because of its elegance, but because it took only 35 minutes. We have no follow-up of that case vignette, but let us assume that Monique went on as well and happy as Monica. To paraphrase Wallace Stevens, then it would truly be a romantic story in the sense of being more wonderful than probable. Psychotherapists of my acquaintance would have a hard time accepting that moment of successful encounter as sufficient in and of itself. Most of them would consider it an auspicious beginning of a longer therapeutic relationship. In any event, the moral of the story would seem to be that constructive entry into the assumptive world of the child may be made either at a symbolic level or at a behavioral level.

We must bear in mind that the organism is unitary, and behavioral interventions can change meaning as reliably as symbolic interventions can change behavior—not with perfect reliability, in that thought and action fortunately are rarely directly linked, but the relationship is reciprocal. It may well be that both interventions simply interrupted an automatic and maladaptive sequence of socially learned behavior and, in a favorable climate, brought other options to the child's attention.

Behavior therapy is no panacea. As the first flush of enthusiasm has worn off and follow-up studies begin to improve in number and in length, claims for lasting results inevitably become more modest. Obtaining durable therapeutic gains from the treatment situation that carry over to life lived without the therapist is a problem in all forms of psychotherapy. For this reason, I sincerely hope our period of psychoanalytic preoccupation will not be compensated too heavily by a period of behavioral preoccupation. It seems to me that as American psychiatry has swung from one polar illusion of certainty to its opposite, we have on each turn tended to throw out the good with the bad. As psychiatrists, I think we have a particular obligation not to do that. One may have a particular interest and expertise in biochemistry, behavioral analysis, or psychoanalysis, but as a psychiatrist he must act as a critical evaluator and consumer of other people's science, always looking for the application of new findings and new insights to his care of patients.

I mentioned biochemistry because this question of the place of behavior therapy in psychiatry comes at a particular time when the whole idea of psychological intervention in psychiatry is being questioned in some quarters. It comes at a time when medical students are being bombarded by the information explosion in cell biology and residents' heads are being filled with exciting new advances in neurobiology in general and brain chemistry in particular. Curriculum committees question time spent on talking with patients, to say nothing of one's particular style of talking with patients. In Miami (May, 1976) Abraham Wikler, M.D., from Lexington spoke for many psychiatrists when he proposed that all of psychotherapy be turned over to non-M.D.'s, leaving the psychiatrist free to become an expert on organic brain disease—not in the sense of irreversible tissue damage, but in the newer understanding of perhaps reversible disordered brain chemistry and physiology. This, he said, is the psychiatry of the future.

Granted that we now have some interesting biological leads that Kraepelin didn't have (although he spoke at the turn of the century in much the same fashion as Wikler), how wise is it to narrow the field of training at this time? Isn't that what was wrong with academic psychiatry before World War II? Wasn't that narrowness overcorrected by the generation of psychoanalytic domination of training programs following the war?

We must hold firmly in mind what psychiatry is, and what it is not. Psychiatry is not a science. It is a branch of medicine that cares for that subset of human misery that cannot be alleviated by the knife or a pill. As physicians we are consumers and deliverers of the product of science, although, in addition, many physicians are in fact scientists. We trade in many sciences, but our vocation requires us to remain open to all of human nature. At the very time neurochemistry promises us such exciting prospects, we must remember that the social sciences remain as important to us as ever.

Ours is a perpetually open system in which closure is always a temptation, always a risk. It is only human to be more often threatened than challenged by ambiguity. It is so much more comfortable to take a polar position, for instance, on stimulant medication for hyperactive children. We probably do prescribe too much, yet there are some who really need it. It is very difficult to tell which is which. One of our main concerns should be to avoid the wholehearted adoption of any marginally effective treatment, whether it be pharmacological, behavior analytic, or psychodynamic, because so often this blanket endorsement leads to the indefinite postponement of the basic studies necessary if the true worth and appropriate application of the treatment is to become known. In many areas of medicine it is now almost impossible to run a control group on a treatment for "humane or ethical considerations," even though the treatment itself may have little more than a 50–50 chance of helping rather than harming.

Much of what we do is based on opinion. Opinions at best are the culminating use of facts. Yet we know that in the practice of medicine, strong opinions are held and taught in the absence of adequate data. If you feel uneasy about our differences, listen to the debates on the use of anticoagulants in the management of patients with myocardial infarction, antibiotic prophylaxis in emphysema, or even plain old ulcer diets.

It would be tedious in the extreme to attempt to evenhandedly address all of the possible applications of behavioral theory in all areas of psychiatry. My strategy will to be make some generally orienting statements about behavior therapy as I view it and then to develop the discussion further under the headings of in-patient and out-patient practice.

The term "behavior therapy" has come upon us by common usage, partly, I think, to avoid the negative connotation of manipulation and control given by the term behavior modification. My personal preference is the designation "behavior analysis" coined by John B. Watson, because it gives a more precise description of what the behaviorist does in his shrewdly watching for clues to what is going on between the organism and its environments.

Behavior therapy was defined by Joseph Wolpe (1969) as "the use of experimentally established principles of learning for the purpose of changing maladaptive behavior"; this is, of course, an exaggeration. It is true that experimental psychologists have applied a variety of theories of learning to the data of their experiments with animals in the laboratory. But when it comes to the clinical situation it is apparent to me that behavior therapy as well as other kinds of psychotherapy are still art forms. Howard Hunt, my collaborator of many years, has expressed this position in a most economical and eloquent fashion in a paper read at the 1975 Kittay Conference entitled "Recurrent Dilemmas in Behavioral Therapy":

Does the behavioral approach help because it is "scientific"?

In my own clinical experience, I have not found behavioral approaches to psychotherapy to be as simple, straightforward, "scientific," and unambiguous as behavioristic protagonists sometimes have implied.

The logical problems in clinical application differ somewhat from those of the laboratory. In the laboratory, we work from theories or hypotheses that suggest how behavior, as a dependent variable, should be affected by manipulations of independent variables—causative or antecedent variables—that we can control. If things do not work out, we can go back to the drawing board, develop new hypotheses, and rerun the whole enterprise with new, "naive" subjects substantially equivalent to the ones already studied. Here, the context of justification or confirmation flows naturally out of the context of discovery or invention (Reichenbach, 1938). Our theories tell us what should happen, and we can find out if it does, exploring the problem repeatedly under supposedly comparable conditions until the data satisfy the conventions of scientific proof.

In contrast, in the clinical situation we are confronted with behavior (the dependent variable) and must guess as to what could have produced it—guess as to what independent variables it is a function of. Then, in the light of that guess, and with the aid of hypotheses as to how changes in contemporary or intercurrent factors in patients' lives may alter their behavior, we start to work and hope for the best. Because no two patients and no two situations are alike, we have fewer opportunities for reruns, for corrections of mistaken guesses. Further, with human subjects in clinical settings some socialization experiences and learning may be irreversible; impressions are formed, patients develop theories, skills are acquired in changes that are so enduring that the patient cannot be returned to a condition of naivete that permits a replicated experiment with that patient in an own-control design. Thus, practical applications remain largely in the context of discovery, with firm scientific data in the context of justification most difficult to come by (Reichenbach, 1938).

In addition, we can control only a fraction of the important independent variables in patients' lives. Patients already have histories. Patients work and live in social contexts that have their own dynamics and necessities. Further, the human capacity and propensity for symbolic behavior and internalized representations permits a decoupling of important behavior from controllable external conditions, and over the broadest range. Such behavior includes expectations, interpretations, theories about the self and the world and the future, and fantasies. These are related in complex and poorly understood ways to external conditions and to other, more overt behavior. Indeed, the current excitement over problems of cognition, thinking, and language in psychology testifies to the importance of these covert aspects of human behavior and to our uncertainties about them.

With all these qualifications, a cynic might say we have simply discovered that we have been speaking prose. Many of the techniques of behavior therapy have in fact been in prior use, such as assertiveness training with its behavioral rehearsal, modeling, and even aversive conditioning (remember the ducking stool), but now we not only have terms but a considerably more orderly way of keeping track. Aristotle spoke of education by blows and kindness, but I think we at least now have a more precise way of making connections among the behaviors, the blows, and the kindnesses.

One of the major upsets in the field came when Stampfl and Levis (1967) found that systematic desensitization worked just as well when you turned the hierarchy upside down, called it flooding or implosion, and went right on curing phobic symptoms. For this very reason there is something essentially scientific about the approach. Hypotheses can be tested as they did. This is very different from the all-too-common practice of changing one's diagnosis rather than one's hypothesis when the patient fails to respond.

Even though the bogeyman of symptom substitution has been laid to rest with regard to the behavioral removal of symptoms, professionals in the field know that the gains have been modest. Even stutterers who under laboratory conditions achieve fluency at 100 per cent rates show a high degree of recidivism. Among his parting remarks to his successful stuttering patients Goldiamond says: "We have given you a new suit of clothes (fluency). We are not taking away your old one that is full of holes. After treatment you may wear whichever one you want. If you wish to wear the old one and embarrass your friends, you will." The words, "will," "want," and "wish," relics of the old psychology, nestle comfortably here in the midst of the practical summing up of a behavior intervention. We know that some of the new prosocial behaviors are simply inadequately reinforced in the patient's environment. This is not a reason to despair, but to do studies that may help all forms of psychotherapy learn more about the specific circumstances in which improvement is maintained, and those in which it is lost.

It is the model of single organism study over time taken from the observations in a Skinner box to the study of the vicissitudes of an individual life that gives the behavior paradigm its power. There is more to the operant behavior paradigm than linear causality. Personality theory may be reopened as a lively topic with the study of adjunctive behavior. Much of the texture of individual style can be approached by mapping concurrent interacting behaviors.

In a conversation recently, David Shakow told me of Kluckhohn and Murray's classification of data substantively in this fashion:

> There are three levels of data about people. The first level is what can be said of all people. For instance, that we are a symbol using species. The second level is what can be said of some people; typologies, diagnostic categories, etc. The third level is what can be said about the individual.
>
> I doubt if our particular field can be advanced very directly by studies at the first level. On the second level, Kraepelin was able to sort out everything a vast number of patients had in common. What he seemed unaware of was that in the process he lost the individual. I doubt if this seemed important to him because he was dedicated to finding the biological laws of psychiatry. Biology does not easily tolerate the individual; the purely biological method, seeking to discover the laws governing natural phenomena, cannot apprehend these laws unless individual variations are fully discounted so that it becomes possible to make a proper generalization.

I do not fault Kraepelin in this. One life is about the same as another; the variance in length can be handled by an actuary. It is simply the meaning we attach to it that has any significance at all. We have a problem, both as behavior analysts and as psychoanalysts, in wanting very much to be scientific while working with third level data.

I would like to quote from H. D. Lewis's essay "On Poetic Truth" (1946), in which he would appear to be speaking very directly to our situation:

> Science can tell us much but it cannot tell us the particularities of the here and now....

> Plato saw reality exemplified best by mathematics. The aim of life should be to draw ourselves away as much as possible from the insubstantial fluctuating world of facts and reach for what is comprehended by thought and not sense. Plato was a realist in the sense that it is by way of breaking away from the world of facts that we make contact with reality. . . .
>
> On the other hand, only the individual and the particular can give us a solid reality that does not wholly dissolve itself into the conceptions of our own minds.

In our field, we do not progress except by particulars. In that sense, Freud and Skinner had really very much in common. Each was a meticulous observer of individual data: Freud, the subjective data of consciousness; Skinner, the objective data of observable behavior. They were both seeking to apply and extend the search for deterministic natural scientific laws to the psychology of the individual. The economist Frank Knight (1947), in his essay "Fact and Value in Social Science," viewed this as a questionable strategy. He said:

> The fundamental revolution in outlook which represents the real beginning of the modern natural science was the discovery that the inert objects of nature are not like men, i.e., subject to persuasion, exhortation, coercion, deception, etc., but are "inexorable." The position which we have to combat seems to rest upon an inference, characteristically drawn by the "best minds" of our race, that since natural objects are not like men, men must be like natural objects. . . .

Perhaps we could compromise with Knight and say, as we did in the cases of Monica and Monique, that studying the more automatic sequences of human thought and behavior may not give us natural laws but they do give us conventions that permit us to proceed in a stochastic fashion toward increasingly relevant responses.

At their best, neither Freud nor Skinner extended his theory beyond the data his system was designed to observe. Unfortunately, disciples almost invariably do treat theories as if they encompassed more phenomena than they do. William James pointed this out to the Spencerians by reminding them that Darwin recognized spontaneous variation as the other unexplored half of evolution but chose to concentrate his attention on natural selection (James, 1905). No one can have a scientific theory of what he does not admit into his range of observation. In his Nobel Prize acceptance speech, E. P. Wigner (1964) said:

> Physics does not endeavor to explain nature. In fact, the great success of physics is due to a restriction of its objectives: it only endeavors to explain the regularities in the behavior of objects. This renunciation of the broader aim, and the specification of the domain for which an explanation can be sought, now appear to us an obvious necessity. In fact, the specification of the explainable may have been the greatest discovery of physics so far.

Radical behaviorism, to use B. F. Skinner's term, began similarly with the renunciation of the broader aim to explain all of human nature and confined itself to the specification of the explainable. This modesty and limitation of goals has been hard for his followers and even for B. F. Skinner to maintain. We now have his version of behavioral man as we have Freud's model of psychoanalytic man or the economist's models of economic man. While granting them poetic license, it is well to bear in mind Wittgenstein's notation in the diary he dictated to George E. Moore on their walking trip through Norway (Wittgenstein, 1969). He said, "All our theories are grids cast across the face of the unknown and our logic is only the logic of the relationship between two points on our grid."

The unbridled optimism I mentioned earlier has led to exaggerated claims of effectiveness and power over people's lives that has given the behavioral enterprise a very poor public image. In the September, 1976, issue of *Resident and Staff Physician,* Charles A. Ragan, Jr., M.D., wrote an editorial entitled "Behavior Control in Medicine: A Frightening Possibility." He made the observation that obesity, tobacco, alcohol and drug abuse, and noncompliance with therapeutic programs all seem unresponsive to usual health education efforts. He noted that some attempts at behavior modification have been suggested. In his closing paragraph he stated:

> Behavior control and behavior modification are now considered more and more, not only in closed population centers such as psychiatric and penal institutions, but in the general population as well. This application is frightening to me and it is difficult to determine when health education becomes behavior control. Behavior control in its totality has few advocates—only some true fanatics—but great vigilance will be needed to call a halt before education becomes behavior control.

Dr. Ragan's response may be extreme but it is not atypical. At the moment, there is at least a 50-50 chance that bungling amateurs, particularly those who run brutal prison programs in the name of behavior modification, will get the behavioral enterprise stopped or at least severely compromised and restricted before the professionals get behavior techniques comfortably established so that they can supply us with those modest but useful tools we need.

In-patient treatment

It would seem apparent that prospects for behavior therapy are best in the laboratory or in the pyschiatric ward where the behavior therapist has the most control. On the psychiatric ward he has, at least in theory, a 24-hour-a-day opportunity for observation and intervention. When one reflects on it, we realize that in-patient units are behavioral of necessity. In the vast majority of our acute cases it was a behavioral complaint that brought the patient in. Behavior management is the first thing the staff has to attempt. Behavior modification is a goal devoutly sought after. Some form of analysis of that behavior is inevitably done.

Acute patients do generally well and tend to improve on the usual and customary in-patient unit. Many of the people in this category have a self-limited disturbance, others simply needed a time-out from a stressful environment. Still others find a friendly, supportive environment adequate to help them deal with their demoralization and to begin again to hope and plan.

There are at least two parallel diagnostic systems in operation on any psychiatric ward whether one acknowledges it or not. The usually informal behavioral assessment provides current data for planning psychosocial interventions and can be up-dated on a day-to-day or even shift-to-shift basis. Formal, conventional diagnosis based on inferences from observation of manifest behavior ties in more directly with medication prescription than with psychosocial intervention on most units. This seems to be because it is based on looking at a person badly out of his social context. He has been uprooted from one context and has not yet found his way into another when the diagnosis is made. Medication falls into three major categories. With the acute patient we rarely need hypnotics any more. The sedative effect of antipsychotic medication tends to diminish behavioral output enough, but at the same time hopefully the drug improves cognitive functioning. Antidepressant medication as it takes hold over a longer time tends to reduce response latency and thus "ups" behavioral output.

What I am saying is that 70 per cent or even more of one's acute patients on a well-staffed and well-motivated general hospital ward tend to have a worthwhile experience. For this reason, I am inclined to say that the usual good ward needs behavioral principles to be taught to its staff rather than techniques. It is important to teach our staffs that usual social control in a hospital environment includes under it a variety of negative, behavior-reducing responses. The very fact of confinement, the necessity of seclusion, restraints, prohibition, and disapproval are all conventional acts that occur on a psychiatric ward where psychopathology is the focus of attention, and is to be discouraged. The opposite also occurs with less frequency when patients are encouraged to "get out" the bad behavior. This attitude is less apt to be seen on the short-term ward of a general hospital, but it still persists in longer-term treatment settings where it is referred to as "going through regression."

By teaching behavior principles to our staff, I mean very much the same sort of thing I meant earlier when speaking of teaching psychiatrists to look at their patients. Our staff needs to see what Howard Hunt told me he saw when he looked at patients' behavior on the most disturbed unit at Columbia's Psychiatric Institute. He saw that even there more than 75 per cent of a patient's daily behavior fell within normal limits. Yet if you read the shift notes, you would have seen that only the most strikingly aberrant behavior was recorded. This is because natively we tend to characterize or epitomize rather than to report observations.

We need to teach what a truly responsive environment is. Years ago, Dr. Will Menninger of the Menninger Clinic devised his never-published "Guide to the Order Sheet," which included a series of diagnosis-related attitude prescriptions for staff, such as "kind firmness" and "love unsolicited." This was a groping beginning, but what our staff has to see in a responsive environment is precisely what behavior on the part of the patient their responsiveness *is* rewarding. Israel Goldiamond's paper, "A Constructional Approach to Treatment," gives us a basis for identifying what needs to be done and a language to communicate concretely with our staff about how to reinforce prosocial behavior (Goldiamond, 1975).

I can imagine a purist saying "But why don't you want a total behavioral unit? Why don't you use a token economy? Why are you suggesting that we use behavior principles only to provide a rational rather than an intuitive or common sense basis for staff behavior?" The answers lie in my earlier remarks about behavior therapy being best characterized as single subject research. Most in-patient units have very heterogeneous populations and the application of a total and standard behavioral program to a heterogeneous population would at best be a Procrustean bed. People with little choice in the matter might submit to such a system, and under such conditions I can guarantee you would get good ABA reversals because the moment the contingencies were lifted they would revert again to being a heterogeneous population. I am confident that this is why token economies and rigorously behavioral wards have shown their greatest successes to be with homogeneous populations, either the severely retarded, as in Travis Thompson's Faribault, Minnesota study (Thompson, 1972), or in chronic schizophrenics, as in Ayllon and Azrin's study at Anna State Hospital (Ayllon and Azrin, 1968). Robert Schuster reminded me that, to be effective, token economies must be tailored to the individual. Nevertheless, my observation has been that in any group setting the individual may initially be captured by the system by attention to his particular necessities, but the system is unitary, monopolized by the goals of a strong central authority as surely as were the Greek city-states of 2500 years ago when coinage was introduced. All control over other people is ideally immoral. When we take it, as we must, over the lives of patients who, for the time being, are incapable of rational consent, it must be with the intent to return control and full human status to the patient as rapidly as possible.

Evidence that we do not routinely need that degree of total control was given in Arnold Lazarus' report at the London Ciba symposium on the role of learning in psychotherapy (1968), in which he told about setting up some behavioral interventions on an in-patient service and his attempt to set up a placebo therapy control ward. He devised something he called graded structure to be the placebo therapy. This began with an initial lowering of expectations of the patient's behavior, and then a stepwise increase in expectations over time. It turned out that graded structure was as therapeutic as or more than the experimental techniques. This should come as no surprise to psychiatrists with any interest in the history of in-patient treatment of the mentally ill. Graded structure has been with us for a long time, whether it be in the practices of the York retreat, Japanese Morita therapy, or the dynamic psychotherapist initially lowering expectations so as to establish trust and then gradually increasing expectations in small achievable steps as therapy proceeds.

"Moral" therapy of the nineteenth century involved graded structure. One problem with it was that when the numbers began to grow larger in the twentieth century, people stopped moving through the structure and the system was paralyzed. Instead of starting the patient out on the right step of a ladder, the hospitals provided a graded set of behavioral units into which they could place patients at any level of regression and maintain them at that level. Particularly in large state hospitals the idea of movement up and out was lost. There were wards not only for paranoids and hebephrenics, but for soilers. This was an example of second level data collecting in which patients could be categorized and placed without individual characteristics or prospects being taken into account. Older psychiatrists who lived through even a small part of that period have a proper distaste for diagnosis stemming from the nontherapeutic uses that were made of symptom classification at that time. Since World War II we have found ways to get people moving through the system again. Designing active treatment environments in smaller units, located usually in general hospitals closer to the patient's home, gave psychiatrists the opportunity to reinvent graded structure. More acute patients, family involvement, and the new psychotropic drugs all converged to improve the patient's prospect. It can be seen, then, that from the standpoint of programing, what the good general hospital ward today needs is a competent behavioral consultant. When usual and customary good practice fails and medication seems to be of little or no effect or, as is more often the case, when the medication is of some effect but it is not enough, then a fine-grained analysis of staff-patient interaction can often lead to a series of planned interventions that dramatically increase the probability of improvement for this group of patients.

Out-patient therapy

At first viewing, it appears that behavior therapy has an infinitely poorer prospect of success in out-patient work because the therapist has infinitely less control over contingencies than he does on the best but still imperfectly controlled in-patient unit. Except for the hour or two a week the patient spends with his therapist, he is at the mercy of the usual social contingencies which have served him so badly that he has come for treatment. Yet a powerful therapeutic factor is working on behalf of the treatment. The patient has come seeking help. This is different from many of the involuntary admissions to an in-patient unit. The out-patient is a much more likely candidate to be enlisted as a collaborator in observing his own behavior and exploring new ways of thinking about self-control.

We all know that the style of history-taking by the therapist is a very crucial variable. A patient interviewed by Joseph Wolpe has a high probability of finding phobic areas in his life that would seem worth working on. The same patient being interviewed by a psychoanalyst would be more apt to find unhappiness and ennui. In either case, I think it is important to find something reasonably small to start working on that has some prospect of success, because the experience of a small success is the first major step in dealing with the patient's demoralization and helplessness. It may be as small as being able to talk about one's self to someone who listens.

It is more important to decide what you are going to work on together than to arrive at a Diagnostic and Statistical Manual diagnosis when one is using Type III (individual) data to be of therapeutic help. A person may appear quite schizophrenic to one interviewer and quite rational to another.

It is not so much that one is right and the other wrong as it is that we have a very poor prospect of good assessment when we are making it on the basis of observation of behavior without taking into account the context, particularly the interviewer's contribution. Even a structured interview gives us no guarantee of escape from this problem. Some years ago, an elderly man was admitted late at night to a state hospital. The resident on call gave him a mental status exam which included the question "Do you hear voices?" The old man said "yes." The next question was "Male or female?" The man replied, "Don't you know what you are, son?" The next morning I was surprised to read that the elderly man was reported as suffering from hallucinations and was rather negative, so that the examiner concluded he was a paranoid schizophrenic. It did not occur to him that the man thought he was being asked about his hearing. This is a somewhat extreme example of the problems inferring can get one into or, to put it another way, the problem of having to use a descriptive language of things unseen in making a diagnosis.

In out-patient treatment, the bulk of our patients do not require chemotherapy, and even the most meticulous history taking often fails to come up with clear-cut behavioral deficits. This point was illustrated by Arnold Lazarus' paper in *Psychological Reports* entitled "Where Do Behavioral Therapists Take Their Troubles?" (Lazarus, 1971). He was trying to arrange a meeting and found that the majority of the group of leading behaviorists he was trying to convene had difficulty planning a time because they were in psychoanalytic treatment. He accounted for this on the basis of their having no clear-cut behavioral deficits, but problems of meaning.

Like it or not, we must acknowledge that today a large segment of our psychobiologically malfunctioning patient population is not seeking relief from phobias, pain, or discomfort, or even relief from anxiety, but is seeking relief from boredom and meaninglessness. Lazarus' paper strikes me as an excellent demonstration that really good behaviorists are flexible, pragmatic, and not crippled by theoretical bias. They may well be developing conceptual tools rather than a school of thought. Another illustration of the absurdity of making one theoretical system a total system was given many years ago by J.B. Watson (1924). In a brilliant polemic he damned psychoanalysts as having no more scientific basis than phrenologists and confidently predicted the early and rapid disappearance of this fad. He then went on to say that he hoped none of his psychoanalytic friends would hold this against him at a time when he might need help.

One of the more prominent out-patient behavioral specializations in recent years has been in the area of sex or marital therapy. Generally speaking, this involves speaking directly about sexual performances and practices. As an educational device, it eliminates some misunderstandings but, I think more significantly, it does seem to work to strip away an excessive crippling overburden of meanings. In that sense, sexual failure is also treated as a form of phobia. As a further illustration of the unitary nature of the meaning-behavior system, Taylor Segraves, M.D., Director of our Marital Therapy Clinic, reports to me that no matter how strictly behavioral the therapist is in his approach, the patient is often determined to report dreams and fantasies as a part of his overall experience of treatment for his performance problem if the therapist will only listen.

Even in psychoanalytic therapy, much of what goes into making a good patient may be viewed in behavioral terms. My teacher, Lewis Hill, used to say, "I can analyse anyone in a month but sometimes it takes me two or three years to get them in shape for it." We have not paid sufficient attention to specifying what goes on in that shaping process.

Conclusion

In an essay of opinion, conclusions are apt to appear in every paragraph, or at least they have in this one. Obviously, I appreciate what behavior therapy has to offer us. I enjoy its optimism, pragmatic flexibility, and lack of an overarching theory. One may use a tape recorder, a kitchen timer, or a cumulative recorder to capture not only units of behavior but mental events as evanescent as images and elusive as affects. It gives us Marianne Moore's "imaginary gardens with real toads in them." This cannot be a rigorous science. Perhaps the most scientific remark one can make about behavior therapy as it is practiced in all its diversity would be to borrow from signal detection theory and observe that "talented" behavior therapists do have a higher hit rate than mediocre behavior therapists. This may well have more to do with their having had a variety of fortunate life experiences that extended their range of sensibilities than with rigorous adherence to a particular technique.

There are a limited number of ways in which humans are capable of interacting. Thus, it seems reasonable to me that the fact of one person's benignly influencing another person's behavior for the better, which we currently call psychotherapy, has been going on within those limits for a long, long time. I'm not really questioning progress or discovery. I think Freud's discovery of the dynamic unconscious was the culminating event of the nineteenth century's emerging preoccupation with the individual. In a similar vein, I see B. F. Skinner's explication of the operant paradigm as the great psychological discovery of our era.

When we look beyond the discoveries to the question of why tremendous schools of thought and devoted adherents have built up around each of these men, we must look at issues of contemporary style in Western civilization. It is curious to note that the overelaboration of meaning without new discovery that occurred in some of the psychoanalytic psychologizing between the wars had a surrealism about it very similar to the surrealism of that period in art. Freud's discovery of the "color perspective" of unconscious affects was at risk of being diminished by the striving after novel effects of those who sought to improve upon it.

In this pragmatic and technological phase of our culture, psychoanalysis has been moving rapidly toward a more operational, clinical, event-oriented theory in the hands of George Klein (1976) and now Roy Schafer (1976), yet it appears that behavior therapy is truly modern in the sense that abstract art is modern. It seeks to tease out the operative principle that underlies the meanings. It is the isosceles triangle that peaks at the Virgin's left eye, done as an isosceles triangle rather than as Leonardo's "Madonna of the Rocks."

We need not ask ourselves, is it the triangle that works or is it the color perspective? In the art of psychotherapy, as in art criticism, there is no final truth. Our models and views are all incomplete and serve limited purposes. The only serious question is, does the particular model of treatment proposed conform enough to the realities of the particular patient so that rather than being a sterile exercise within a model, it provides him with a vehicle (perspective, strategy and tactics) for solving his problems?

References

Ayllon, T., and Azrin, N. H.: The Token Economy. New York, Appleton-Century-Crofts, 1968.
Fiske, D. W.: The limits for the conventional science of personality. J. Pers., *42*:1–11, 1974.
Goldiamond, I.: Personal communication, 1976.
Goldiamond, I.: Toward a constructional approach to social problems: Ethical and constitutional issues raised by applied behavior analysis. Behaviorism, 2:1–83, 1974.
Hill, L.: Personal communication, 1947.
Hunt, H.: Recurrent dilemmas in behavior therapy. New York Kittay Conference, April 8, 1975.
James, W.: The Principles of Psychology. New York, H. Holt & Co., 1890, p. 136.
James, W.: The Will to Believe. New York, Longmans, Green & Co., 1905, pp. 188–189.
Klein, G. S.: Psychoanalytic Theory: An Exploration of Essentials. New York, International Universities Press, 1976.
Knight, F. H.: Fact and value in social science. *In* Freedom and Reform. New York, Harper and Brothers, 1947, pp. 226, 237.
Lazarus, A. A.: Where do behavior therapists take their troubles? Psychol. Rep., *28*:349–350, 1971.
Lazarus, A. A.: Behavior therapy and graded structure. *In* Porter, R.: The Role of Learning in Psychotherapy. Boston, Little, Brown & Company, 1968, pp. 134–143.
Lewis, H. D.: On poetic truth. Philosophy, *21*:154–155, 1946.
Orne, M.: Psychotherapy in contemporary America. *In* Freedman, D. X., and Dyrud, J. E. (eds.): American Handbook of Psychiatry, vol. 5. New York, Basic Books, Inc., Publishers, 1975, p. 5.
Ragan, C. A., Jr.: Behavior control in medicine. A frightening possibility. Res. Staff Phys., p. 49, Sept. 1976.
Schafer, R.: A New Language for Psychoanalysis. New Haven, Yale University Press, 1976.
Schwab, J.: Education and the state: Learning community. *In* The Great Ideas Today, 1976. Encyclopedia Brittanica, Inc., 1976, pp. 262–263.
Shakow, D.: Personal communication, 1976.
Skinner, B. F.: Cumulative Record. New York, Appleton-Century-Crofts, 1961.
Stampfl, T. G., and Levis, D. J.: Essentials of implosive therapy: A learning theory-based psychodynamic behavioral therapy. J. Abnorm. Psychol., 72:496–503, 1967.
Thompson, T., and Grabowski, J. (eds): Behavior Modification of the Mentally Retarded. New York, Oxford University Press, 1972.
Watson, J. B.: Behaviorism. New York, W. W. Norton & Co., Inc., 1924, p. 246.
Wigner, E. P.: Events, laws of nature and invariance principles. Science, *145*:995, 1964.
Wittgenstein, L.: Notebooks 1914–1916. London, B. H. Blackwell, Ltd., 1969, pp. 35e and 43e.
Wolpe, J.: The Practice of Behavior Therapy. New York, Pergamon Press, Inc., 1969.

Comment

Behavior modification therapy as a distinctive and systematic approach to psychiatric and psychological problems is less than three decades old. During this brief period, numerous scientific and professional societies, journals, and training centers have developed. Some professionals regard it as an entirely new direction for the field which in time will largely supplant the older, less "scientific" ways of conducting psychotherapy. Others regard behavior therapy as a fad which will have only a small, lasting influence on the field. **Dr. Dyrud's** position is somewhere between these two extremes. Taking an historical and philosophical perspective, and making some comparisons with the development of psychoanalysis, he is concerned that the behavior therapy movement has some fadlike characteristics. He is concerned specifically that some of the benefits of this approach to the field may be neutralized by the excesses of its true believers. A chief benefit of the behavioral movement, according to Dyrud, is its influence in restoring the place of clinical observation in psychiatry, and more particularly, of "keeping track of behavior in a context." Thus Dyrud sees behavior therapy not as a new direction, but as a much needed course correction in the field. He hopes that one impact of behavior therapy will be to train the psychiatrist to observe his patient more closely, especially in his immediate social environment, so as to identify some of the factors that may be maintaining current maladaptive behaviors. In in-patient settings, he hopes that staff will come to appreciate what constitutes a responsive environment and to identify better what specific behaviors are being reinforced. In out-patient settings, Dyrud notes that there is often opportunity to get the patient to collaborate with the therapist in observing his own behavior and developing new and better ways of managing it. Clearly Dyrud views behavior therapy as a model, a strategy, or a perspective which is useful in the treatment of some patients, some of the time.

Is behavior therapy a truly new direction that will change our ways of assessing clinical problems and conducting rational psychotherapy or is it a course correction in the field? The data are not in but are rapidly accumulating.

JOHN PAUL BRADY, M.D.

Does Psychotherapy Change the Outcome in Schizophrenia?

OTTO ALLEN WILL, JR.
Richmond, California

On Controversy

In view of the fact that what follows is written for inclusion in a book entitled "Controversy in Psychiatry," a few remarks on the significance of the title to me should not be out of place. In the dictionary, *controversy* is defined as dispute, quarrel, strife, or a discussion marked by the expression of opposing views.

Disputes, quarrels, and strife may lead more frequently, in my view, to the clouding of issues than to their illumination. Sometimes we become engaged in such behaviors in response to our own feelings of insecurity and our needs for prestige. Here I speak for myself—not necessarily for others. I have spent many years of my professional life as the psychotherapist of people diagnosed as schizophrenic; I should not have engaged in this work had I not considered it to be significantly beneficial to some of the patients. As in most human endeavors, of course, the desired goals were not always achieved, and treatment was not, in my terms, successful. In taking a look at my experiences I should not like to think that they constitute a form of personal illusion, whereby what I call therapy is no more than a kind of nonsense of no tangible value to the persons with whom I am concerned. To entertain such a view persistently would certainly increase my sense of insecurity and threaten whatever self-esteem I might possess. Finding myself "embattled," I could then take part in quarrels and strife, defending "my position" and attacking those of others, with, perhaps, more regard for my own "reputation" than for the matters with which I should be more properly concerned—the phenomena of schizophrenia and psychotherapy and their relationship to each other.

For the moment, at least, I am not inclined to attack or defend, but I should be able (painful as it often is for me) to attend to opposing views and to engage in a discussion of them. This seeming disavowal of convictions should not be taken too seriously, however; there are certain rudimentary persuasions to which I hold. These may as well be stated once again; their repeated expression is not likely to affect events in our field, but will, at least, produce no harm.

I find that with the passage of time I am not so certain, as once I thought I was (or hoped to be), of a number of matters. Among these are:

a. the "nature" of man and his purposes;
b. the certainty and simplicity of cause and effect relationships;
c. the objectivity of the "reductionistic" concept;
d. "mind" as purely an expression of brain; and
e. a "final explanation" of human behavior through any theory, known or to be known.

In short, I have had to come to some restless tolerance of ambiguity, uncertainty, unpredictability, and the ill-defined. I am greatly impressed—particularly in my work as a therapist—by the ever-present and unavoidable influence of the observer on the field in which he acts, even as he attempts to see and comprehend. I seek with a patient to clarify his sense of identity, but in so doing I must realize that I have no certainty about where I came from, who I am, or what shall become of that which I now think of as "myself." With the increase of knowledge, the mystery of our lives is increased rather than diminished.

Having given recognition to ignorance and unending uncertainty, we then can turn to the more immediate task of finding what can be done to reduce, if not cure or eliminate, some of the extravagances of human suffering and disorder. We attempt to discover and define a degree of predictability in the midst of the largely unknown; the fact that we cannot know "all," or control all events, does not deter us from seeking to understand and manage circumstances in the service of improving the welfare of man—and, of necessity, his environs. The words *control* and *manage* suggest the use of power, hopefully arising from, and tempered by, knowledge. Here it is that both knowledge and power must be subject to wisdom, which includes the recognition of ignorance and fallibility. We have some knowledge about human behavior, and, in some instances, a great deal of power in exercising control over it. We know something about forms of living that we label mental disease, and we can change some of those forms, for better or worse, through the use of a variety of procedures. With this power to affect the life of another person comes the obligation of responsibility. We must define what we consider to be illness and health, and recognize the possible disadvantages and costs, as well as advantages and gains, that are associated with the substitution of the one for the other. The work of the psychotherapist cannot be separated from ethical and moral issues, any more than can the disorders of his patients be separated from them. Schizophrenia, from the point of view expressed here, is not "simply" a disease; it is seen to be largely an expression of the vicissitudes of a person's development, a reflection of his society and culture, and a caricature of the problems of existence with which all of us must come to terms, one way or another, in our growing up. The psychotherapeutic approach is designed to modify forms of behavior that seriously interfere with development and productivity, are destructive to the welfare and self-sufficiency of the person, and are usually painful to him, as well as to his society. But the psychotherapeutic process is not some bland "nothing" that can be tossed into the hopper—or blender—of treatments, with the falsely comforting notion that "if it does no good it can do no harm." The process is not neutral; from it can come hurt as well as help. The therapist, then, assumes the heavy burden of responsibility in a field which is, in many respects, not well defined; in an indeterminate existence he must work with determination.

Now—finally—to make a simple and concise statement. Psychotherapy—the use of the human relationship as a therapeutic instrument—*does* alter the course of some people who are schizophrenic, or are on the way to becoming so. I say "some" because many people have very little available to them in any form of treatment, and others are so locked away in the confines of their despair and diminishing, or lost, opportunities, that they turn away from what we can offer as being more hurtful than helpful. To me, the question which is the title of this section is a strange one. The human relationship is a primary factor in the growing up of each of us—in our happiness, our sorrow, our sickness, our health, and the acquiring of our beliefs. We are to a large extent created by these relationships, and the course of our lives is not only altered by them, but dependent upon them. Psychotherapy is a form of that relationship. A person, by virtue of being schizophrenic, has not somehow become immune to the personal influence of other human beings. To the contrary, he is unusually dependent on his fellows extraordinarily sensitive to what they do, and in great need of intimacy with them at the same time that he fears closeness with them.

Personal Comments (with Limitations) on the Writer's Identity

If one is to express his views on a subject, particularly on one that is controversial, he should, to some extent, identify himself. By his so doing the reader may gain a better understanding of the genesis and the significance of the ideas that are being expressed. The need for such identification is particularly evident when we talk about psychotherapy, in which the detachment and objectivity of the reporter are greatly limited by his involvement in what he does. How does a person become interested in medicine, in psychiatry, in schizophrenia, and finally in psychotherapy? The social-psychological mode of therapeutic intervention in schizophrenia is not an enterprise that is likely to attract large numbers of people who wish to earn big incomes, find peacefulness and predictability in their lives, and be rewarded regularly by the affection and gratitude of their patients and the appreciation and respect of professional colleagues. As for myself, I don't think that I "went" into this field as much as I "fell" into it.

When I was young, my father was ill with pulmonary tuberculosis, and much of his time was spent in and out of sanatoria or bed-ridden at home. Physicians came to be important in our lives. They were people who healed (or dared to make the attempt), were not afraid of sickness and death, were understanding, supportive, and protective; I admired them and wanted to be like them, but hesitated to attempt to enter a profession that appeared to be so difficult, demanding, taxing, and somehow "above" me.

I left college after a few months of the first year; lonely, angry, and frightened, I was the nonconformist, rebelling against my version of the establishment. At this time a psychiatrist came to our town, and because of my obvious disgruntlement with my life (and my troublesomeness to my elders), I was led, or pushed, to his office. I met with him some twenty times or so, and he listened to what little I had to say, seeming to have more respect for my remarks than I did myself—and making some apparent sense out of them, also. The crippling anxiety was lessened, and eventually I returned to school. Later, this psychiatrist spent time with my mother and supported her during her periods of depression and withdrawal. Her times of upset had been frightening and incomprehensible to me; I thought that I should do something for her, but I could do nothing useful, being near-paralyzed by my ineffectiveness in the face of such great need and by a sense of horrible guilt and responsibility that was then inexplicable to me. She talked with the psychiatrist and sometimes told me something of what was said. All did not go well with her, but she found life to be more tolerable then, as it also became for my father and for me. Of greatest importance to me was the concept that her troubles were life-size; they had something to do with her own background, with my father and his illness, with me, with her frustrations and disappointments, and her rage at the increasing constrictions of a life that could not be escaped or changed. The behavior could no longer be dismissed or "explained" as madness derived from some source unknown. It was more terrible than that; it was a very part of our living—of all of us concerned with her, now and in the past, and extending into the future; it was a strange, yet not entirely foreign, expression of ourselves—our loves, fears, hates, doubts, puzzlements, hopes, illusions, and disillusionments. What little I saw and understood was not pleasant, but my distress was lessened, to some extent, by the recognition of the fact that meaning could exist in the nightmare. Knowledge, however awful, was found to be more acceptable than the emptiness of ignorance, which could be filled so readily with the phantasmagoria of misconceptions. So it was that, should I become a physician, I should also be a psychiatrist.

In medical school I worked hard at learning how to be a "good doctor"—to be objective, scientific in attitude, and detached enough from the suffering of others that I should not be overcome by it, flee from it, deny it, or take it all upon myself. Where I studied in those days, it seemed to me that psychiatry as a subject of study was not given much attention; it was rather low on the totem pole of professional prestige, the surgical specialties occupying the highest position. I had heard about dementia praecox while in college, and had even attended demonstrations of its various wonders as revealed to students of "abnormal psychology" at a local state hospital for the insane. At those times I was more often embarrassed than professionally enlightened. I couldn't make much sense of the various explanations of psychotic (or other) behavior, and I felt painfully awkward and uncomfortable when faced by a patient. There was much learning available, but I failed to profit greatly from it.

With the advent of insulin coma therapy for schizophrenia I felt more at ease. The procedure involved risks, was accompanied by a theory (however faulty), required laboratory tests with which I was familiar, and was apparently beneficial to some patients. In the application of this treatment my still fragile identity as a physician found some transient support. This did not last long. Insulin programs, being expensive, time consuming, and not always helpful were replaced by Metrazol, which was terrifying to patients unpleasant at best for those who administered it, and often accompanied by the complications of fractures. The use of nitrogen was soon replaced by electically induced convulsions; I had a great deal of experience with that form of therapy, and saw it used to produce states of regression and to control obstreperous and undesirable behavior.

I gave some thought to what I knew of Dementia Praecox (Schizophrenia) [we often wrote the diagnosis thus, giving acknowledgment to both Kraepelin and Bleuler] and the methods of its treatment that I had witnessed, applied myself, or the results of which I had seen. There was the period in which "foci of infection" were sought and removed – teeth, tonsils, sections of the bowel, and so on. There were the uses of intrathecal horse serum, transfusions of "normal" blood, gold therapy, artificially induced fever, prolonged sleep, dietary modifications, and more. Later came the prefrontal lobotomies, transorbitals, topectomies, and their variants. And now we are in the chemical age – with the benefits and the disadvantages that accompany any misuse of powerful medications. Each treatment has a cost that must be recognized and paid.

The therapies of schizophrenia, as I had seen something of them, did not hold my interest. I was somewhat intrigued by the possibility of discovering some biochemical or neurophysiologic disorder that might throw light on this problem, but I lacked the skills, knowledge, and interest that would enable me to enter such fields of investigation. I had some slight acquaintance with the writings of psychoanalysts, but I continued to feel ill at ease if I seemed to be straying far from the medical model within which I desired to work. Schizophrenia was, for me, a "disease of unknown origin," and for a time I found more satisfaction in pediatrics and internal medicine.

A series of events, which need not be described here, enabled me to spend a great deal of time with a deeply psychotic young man, diagnosed as schizophrenic and previously treated with subcoma insulin, electroshock, barbiturate-induced prolonged sleep, and hydrotherapy. At first he would have nothing to do with me and lay in restraints or wet sheet packs as I sat in his hospital room. I didn't say anything very useful, as I recall those days, except, perhaps, to admit that I was puzzled by all of this outlandish behavior and wouldn't object to learning something of what it was all about. At least, I stayed around. With time the more violent upsets ceased, the long period of muteness came to an end, and we could talk together. We were, for a while, not afraid of each other. In the long run this attempt at therapy didn't work out as well as we could have wished. I became too pleased with what I considered to be progress, and I did not realize that the goals that I had set up as a psychiatrist were not ones that the man had set for himself, or wished to attain. He left the hospital, but would no longer meet with me, saying that he would not tolerate my attempts to impose my values upon him. I felt hurt and offended; I had worked hard and I did not think that I was trying to force my views on anyone. On further consideration, however, I realized that I had been pushing him to live some semblance of my conception of the way in which the "average American middle class" male should live. I acted as if I thought that what I favored (but did not always practice) as a way of life was suitable for anyone, and was, somehow, to be equated with good mental health. The patient found my lack of awareness of—and respect for—his own needs to be intolerable.

From this experience there were derived some ideas that were long known in the field of psychiatry, but had not been to that time clearly recognized by me. Among these ideas were the following:

1. The young man who had at first appeared to me as a "case of schizophrenia" was seen to be someone struggling, however inadequately, with the common problems of growing up, separating from his family in an effort to find his own life, developing relationships of intimacy, and gaining a dependable concept of himself and of others. Something—I did not know what—was making it extraordinarily difficult for this man to deal with these commonplace (but not necessarily simple or painless) problems of living, and particularly of adolescence.

2. The attempt of the therapist, unwitting or not, to impose his ways on the patient constitutes a form of assault and may destroy any likelihood of useful outcome from the procedure designed to be therapeutic.

3. It is more important for the therapist to be able to learn from the patient than to "know everything" about the disorder which he is attempting to "treat." Knowledge is necessary and useful in this task (an understatement, indeed) but it should never be used as a substitute for careful observation, or become so honored that it defies change and interferes with further learning.

4. Patience is needed in this therapeutic procedure—on the part of all participants (nurses, psychiatrists, administrators, relatives, and others). Many years are required to learn how to be successfully schizophrenic. Time, often a great deal of it, will be consumed in the effort to modify long-established patterns of crippling behavior in a fashion that will enable further personality growth to take place.

5. The therapist cannot turn to the schizophrenic patient for comfort,

congratulation, and approval. He will often feel anxious and lonely and will find it useful to consult with experienced colleagues about what he does.

6. As the motivations of the patient are obscure (at least in part) to himself and others, so may be those of the therapist. Personal analysis will not lead to everything being clear, but it can help a therapist to find out more about what he is doing—and it may help to keep him a bit on the humble side.

I gave these ideas some of my attention and was so greatly impressed by how little I knew about psychiatric patients (and other people, including myself) that I turned my time to the strange learning process of becoming a psychotherapist. It seemed to me then that I had seen a lot of "pathology" without recognizing it as a manifestation of human living, and possibly as a form of coping with disorder (developmental, interpersonal, social) rather than being simply a disorder in itself. In the years that followed I spent much of my time with patients who were so troubled that hospital care was required, in some instances for long periods. Some of these people did well and went on to live what is conventionally called the "productive life." In many instances I did not know just what the troublesome behavior meant, what its origins were, or what I (and others) did that proved helpful or otherwise. One elemental concept did come to have great importance for me: the human relationship is a requirement for the survival of the human infant and is a major factor in facilitating human growth or in hindering or destroying it. The schizophrenic process is, to a large extent, the reflection of years of a person's efforts designed to maintain some form of life-sustaining relationships without his becoming unbearably anxious and frightened in them. This is a very difficult task for someone who has grown from infancy (despite seemingly contradictory outward appearances) to be shy, distrustful, anxious, and afraid. It is not remarkable that ways of acting developed to deal with this intricate and enigmatic requirement are often in themselves complicated, obscure, devious, and seemingly mad. It seemed that psychotherapy—a special form of the human experience—should be of help in understanding and favorably modifying some of the extravagant and destructive behaviors created in response to other human experiences. That thesis was—and is—reasonable to me.

As the years have gone by, the disorder and the psychotherapeutic approach have made more "sense" to me and I have come to feel more at ease with what I do. Theory and practice are inadequate, but their essential feature—the importance of the human relationship as a major influential agent in change—is, for me, well established and dependable.

Developments in Psychiatry that Contribute to the Making of "Sense"

During the last fifty years there has been an increase in clarity and precision in the formulation and interrelating of concepts that further our understanding of the schizophrenic experience. These observations and studies have contributed significantly to the making of sense—the bringing of meaning—in my work as a psychotherapist. The developments that are of particular concern to me are the following:

1. Systematic studies of the hospital social system—the "psychiatric milieu" (Caudill, 1958; Edelson, 1970; Moos, 1976; Stanton and Schwartz, 1954).

2. Investigations of family structure (Lidz, 1963; Lidz et al., 1965).

3. Social-cultural studies enriched through interdisciplinary collaboration (Hall, 1976).

4. Direct observations of human infant development (Bowlby, 1969, 1973; Mahler et al., 1975; Murphy and Moriarty, 1976; Spitz, 1957, 1965).

5. The concept of the social field and general systems theory (Von Bertalanffy, 1968).

6. Existentialism, with its concern with the human condition and the acceptance of grief, despair, loneliness, and death as essential aspects of our lives rather than being simply pathological aberrations—ideas that admit the schizophrenic person to a more human status (Boss, 1963; Havens, 1973; May et al., 1958).

7. The extension of psychoanalytic theories and practices to include a wider range of people—the young, the aged, the psychotic, and others of the marginal groups (Marmor, 1968; Witenberg, 1973).

8. Chemical agents for the modification of behavior (Grinspoon et al., 1972; May, 1968).

9. Studies of primate lives other than human (DeVore, 1965; Scott, 1958).

10. Reports of psychotherapy (Arieti, 1974; Blatt and Wild, 1976; Freeman et al., 1958; Hill, 1955; Jackson, 1960; Lidz, 1973; Schulz and Kilgalen, 1969; Searles, 1965; Sullivan, 1962).

The references listed are selections from a large amount of available literature and will serve to present the interested reader with a useful introduction to the field. Comments on genetics and the biochemical theories of schizophrenia are given in the volume edited by Jackson (1963), although there are, obviously, many later studies.

A View of Psychotherapy

The term psychotherapy as used these days covers a wide range of activities, and it should be useful to comment on its meaning in this report. In a general sense the word refers to the treatment of mental or emotional disorders by psychological means. To put the matter simply, I suggest that the therapist seeks to develop a relationship with a troubled, frightened, doubting person who has experienced so much emotional stress in his growing up that he shies away from the human contacts that he needs for his further growth and more effective functioning. In such a therapeutic relationship it is expected that anxiety will lessen, and self-confidence and trust increase, to such an extent that the patient will be able to observe more accurately and dispassionately what he thinks and how he behaves with other people, finally coming to a better understanding of these observations in terms of his own past history and the society in which he lives. Such a statement, of course, is not very enlightening about psychotherapy as it exists in practice. For our purposes here something more needs to be said.

There are many therapies in psychiatry, such as group, milieu, encounter, drug, shock, and so on; each of these involves, to some extent, a form of the human relationship. The emphasis here, however, is on the work done by the designated therapist and the patient, with recognition of the fact that other people play more or less direct parts in these events.

Common to all definitions of psychotherapy is the concept of change. The procedure is designed to modify behavior labeled by someone—preferably the patient himself, but sometimes only others—as personally or socially painful, troublesome, and undesirable. It is well to keep in mind the fact that there may be no precise agreement about the nature of some complex of behavior—whether it is "good" or "bad," sick or well, useful or not, desirable or otherwise, and so on. Thus it is that we set what limits we can to "obviously" destructive acts, attempt to find out the meanings of them to the patient and others, and search for the learning and use of more satisfying and effective ways of living.

The psychotherapeutic process is a special instance of the interpersonal relationship; from this point of view it is well suited for intervention in disorders thought of as arising themselves from involvements of human beings with each other. This relationship is not an impersonal, artificial contrivance: it becomes a replica, often obscure, of the early binding of mother to infant, of the parallel play of childhood, of juvenile and preadolescent attachments, of adolescent strivings for intimacy and adult love, and of the separation and loss that accompany, inevitably, all of our intense ties to one another. The procedure is one of learning in interpersonal and social situations. It is designed to correct, in part (never completely), misadventures of earlier years from which arose mistrust and self-doubt, grave misapprehensions of human living and the self, and dangerous oversimplifications or complexities of behavior.

The therapeutic approach being talked about here includes the following concepts: (a) that past experience is a major factor in determining how a person acts in the present; (b) that variants and distortions of what has gone before may be continued into the present, despite their seeming (or actual) lack of relevance or value in terms of current events; (c) that what one does is influenced by his expectations of the future, as well as by what has occurred in his past and what goes on in his present; (d) that previous experience affects the ways in which one views the present, and that the therapist, for example, will often be the target of motivations developed in the patient's past, which may go unrecognized; (e) that behavior is goal-motivated, however obscure and poorly understood that motivation may be, and should not be ignored as somehow unpsychological or "senseless"; and (f) that relearning can occur at any age, although in some instances the damage derived from past experiences may be so profound (or current opportunities for growth so poor) that the work required to produce change cannot be provided, or (to put the matter brutally) is not worth the effort in terms of the many human needs that require attention (a dangerous choice, or decision, is here involved).

The therapist's task is, as I view it, not to "cure" some sickness or to discover the actual or possible causes of the troublesome ways of living with the idea that in so doing they can be dispelled. In psychotherapy there is no cure in the sense that the patient returns intact to a previously enjoyed state of good health. The disorder is, to a large extent, a culmination of past interpersonal and social misadventures, expressed as an inability to deal adequately with the necessities of the current situation. If treatment goes well, the patient will, through his exchanges with the therapist (and others), come to see more clearly how he behaves and may be able to adopt ways of behaving that are less expensive to him (and others). In all of this the patient is not a passive recipient of treatment applied to him by the therapist; the patient is an active participant in the process and has something to say about his wish and ability to accept the discomfort and pain that accompany "getting well," just as he had something to do with accepting or choosing the road to "sickness."

On this subject wrote John Whitehorn: ". . . (T)he actual therapeutic potential is to be found and elicited in the patient, not applied by the psychotherapist. . . . (I)n the psychotherapeutic process or in the process of assisted recovery, as I prefer to call it, the patient regains some capacity to learn, to hear what is said, and to participate in interpersonal transactions with the openness of mind that makes possible further learning and growth. Insofar as the learning process, in this sense, brings greater human understanding of one's self as well as of others, it appears appropriate to call the result insight. . . . (I)nsight in general appears, when it does occur, to be a *product* of assisted recovery rather than the crucial *instrument* of recovery" (Whitehorn, 1956).

Comments on the Schizophrenic Process

By this time it may seem to the reader that the topic of this paper has been forgotten, avoided, or ignored. What is schizophrenia? It seems to me that "it" is a grouping of behaviors that help keep a person alive and in some human contact, but eventually become so devious, obscure, or stereotyped that communication is greatly disturbed and needed relationships are further attenuated or lost. It is a state of great loneliness and despair, extending in its most extreme forms to social, if not biological, death. That isn't a very precise statement, of course.

I turn here to Grinker and Holzman: "Pending the outcome of a number of focused laboratory studies, we believe that the following qualities distinguish the young schizophrenic patients from those who are not so diagnosed: (1) the presence of a disorder of thinking, even though it is subtly present; (2) a striking quality of diminished capacity to experience pleasure, particularly in interpersonal relationships; (3) a strong characterologic dependence on people; (4) a noteworthy impairment in competence; and (5) an exquisitely vulnerable sense of self-regard.

"We would suppose that these five qualities reflect a more basic, hypothetical dysfunction in maintaining the kind of organization necessary for appropriate, adaptive orientation to one's surroundings and to oneself. This basic disorder, we would further hypothesize, need not lead inevitably to psychosis. The loose adherence to stable organizations may sometimes lead to reorganizations of reality that may even have social, artistic, or scientific value. We would suggest, however, that a significant degree of competence among other factors would be necessary for such an outcome" (Grinker and Holzman, 1973).

This "basic disorder" may reflect, in part, stress in the early infant-mother relationship, resulting in persisting problems in so-called object relationships, body image distortions, basic distrust, and easily roused anxiety—all related to the five characteristics listed by the authors. It should be noted that these five traits in their extreme may be readily identified as evidence of florid psychosis; in their more subtle degree they are by no means foreign to many people who may be shy and cautious, but are never identified as psychiatric patients. That is, in our patients we find not strangers but ourselves.

The schizophrenic people with whom I have become acquainted are shy, mistrustful, and hesitant (at best) to expose themselves to anyone, fearing attack, rebuff, or abandonment. They are lonely; the human intimacy that they need is feared, and they tend to retreat from, or push away, tenders of friendship or love. Thus they may appear "cold," "self-centered," arrogant, bitter, hostile, and detached from the concerns or exigencies of their fellows. The anxiety engendered in human contact interferes with accuracy of perception (of self and others), with the necessary control of what is "in the mind," and, as a result, with the ability to concentrate on a subject and to think clearly.

The following brief excerpts from the writings of a few workers in this field are of interest in terms of the above.

David Shakow: "(T)here is good reason to believe that the schizophrenic difficulty begins to develop early, among the first relationships with the mother. . . . We must . . . always keep in mind that we are dealing with profoundly anxious and frightened persons whose security can only be established at a slow rate, sometimes maddeningly so, through the gradual development of the feelings of safety that come when understanding and love are provided by persons . . . whom they consider sufficiently strong to provide them" (Shakow, 1971).

Theodore Lidz: "Schizophrenic reactions are a type of withdrawal from social interaction, and the thought disorder is a specifically schizophrenic means of withdrawal. Everyone is delimited by the meanings and logic of his culture. . . . The schizophrenic patient escapes from irreconcilable conflict and unbearable hopelessness by breaking through these confines to find some living space by using his own idiosyncratic meanings and reasoning, but in so doing impairs his ego functioning and ability to collaborate with others" (Lidz, 1971).

Harry Guntrip: "The schizoid feels faced with utter loss, and the destruction of both ego and object, whether in a relationship or out of it. In a relationship, identification involves loss of the ego, and incorporation involves a hungry devouring and losing of the object" (Guntrip, 1968).

Harry Stack Sullivan: "The etiology of a schizophrenic illness is to be sought in events that involve the individual . . . events relating the individual with other individuals more or less highly significant to him. Interrelation with significant people constitutes the most difficult sort of action required of us. People are decidedly the hardest thing we have to deal with" (Sullivan, 1962).

Ronald Laing: ". . . (I)t seems to us that *without exception* the experience and behavior that gets labeled schizophrenic is a *special strategy that a person invents in order to live in an unlivable situation.* In his life situation the person has come to feel he is in an untenable situation. . . . He is, as it were, in a position of checkmate" (Laing, 1967).

The main themes of these comments are those of anxiety, fear, insecurity, and the dread of losing contact not only with vital human relationships but with one's sense of self and personality organization. The origins of these grim apprehensions are likely to be found in the experiences of infancy. The later withdrawal, shyness, suspicion, distortions of speech, and so on, may be looked upon as methods of making it possible for the troubled person to maintain some semblance of affiliation with other human beings without becoming overwhelmed by a feeling of disintegration of his self and his world.

The Beginnings of Schizophrenia—One View

The view of disorder, expressed very briefly here, is derived from the accounts of patients, from their ways of behaving with the therapist and others in their current lives, and from reports of direct observation of infant-child development.

The human being is unique in the animal world for his long period of dependency on those who care for him during his maturation, for his ability to construct and use symbols and speech, and for the culture that he creates as part of his heredity. The infant is exposed to the anxieties, beliefs, values, idiosyncrasies, prejudices, "truths," and so on, of his family; it is in that medium that his view of himself and his world is formed. When the relationship of infant and mothering person is marked by anxiety, inconsistency, lack of clarity, ambivalence, persistent maternal depression and withdrawal, and a lack of confidence in the personal worth of the participants, the emerging child will have serious doubts about the motivations of himself and others, and will have no abiding, reliable concepts of his body, the nature of his perceptions, and the separation of himself from other people. He will continue to be unusually troubled in relationships with his fellows, being haunted by ever-present anxiety, which becomes extreme when he feels himself to be "too close" to someone, or when he fears that he will lose all human contact. The extremes of infantile deprivation and hurt may be seen in states of marasmus and death, autism, and childhood schizophrenia. Less severe situations may eventuate in the child who is shy, timid, cautious, doubting of the good in himself and others, both clinging and fearful in his social contacts, introverted, and relying more on his "private world" for security than on the "real world." Not all of such children become clinically schizophrenic; the troubles of early life may be alleviated by later fortunate experience with people, and the person is thus saved from becoming a psychiatric case.

My own experience has been primarily with those people who have passed through the changes of puberty without developing major psychiatric disorders that have greatly disrupted their lives. They have not been able, however, to meet satisfactorily the requirements of adolescence. Among these are the reliable patterning of sexual behavior, ideological if not physical separation from home and parents (in our culture, at least), the finding of a career, a reevaluation of personal standards and values, the reduction of autistic thinking, and the development of intimacy with another human being. Adolescence is a time of accelerated changes—interpersonal, biological, and social; it is one of the "critical" periods in life.

The demand for intimacy brings with it the need for self-exposure. Old self-doubts, anxieties, misperceptions, family mythologies, and suspicions, hitherto held in abeyance and at least partially concealed through the contrivance of a fragile structure of activities ("defenses") that are socially tolerable, if not acceptable, come again into awareness, often seeming foreign, strange, frightening, and not part of the personality as known. The person in such a situation feels that he is becoming involved in a nightmare; he must do something in order to escape, but he does not know the nature of the problem—only that it is one of terror and urgency. The behavior displayed in these instances is likely to appear desperate, odd, irrational, incomprehensible, and mad. Speech itself, used then more for protection than communication and associated with events of early life that cannot be expressed in language, becomes peculiar and less informative; its ability to convey meaning is reduced.

The person, now becoming a patient, feels caught in an intolerable predicament. He is irrevocably attached to other human beings, but his need for intimacy with them (or some sense of acceptance by them) frightens him, with the result that he withdraws from them or pushes them away. Resolutions of this state include suicide, the withdrawal characteristic of catatonia, the rejection of people by the paranoid response, the collapse of personality shown in the hebephrenic reaction, and the development of poorly defined conditions of schizophrenic chronicity marked by increasing isolation and despair—a social deterioration. Some of these people improve "spontaneously," probably, I think, through the forming of fortunate, and often unobserved, relationships with other people, in which are made possible an awakening of hope, confidence, and self-respect, and a reduction of loneliness. Others may be helped through formal psychiatric care. Our interest here is with psychotherapy.

A Person Identified As Patient

In an effort to avoid being lost in what may seem to be nothing but abstractions with little relevance to life, I shall describe, very briefly, a young person who became schizophrenic, and then a patient.

Jane's birth, development, and early life were said by her parents to be uneventful. She was highly intelligent, loved, happy, and fairly sociable, had friends, did well in school, and was considered to be a success. At the age of seventeen she appeared to be "moody," kept more to herself, did poorly in school, was often strangely irritable, lost weight, and found her sleep disturbed by troublesome dreams and nightmares. She graduated from high school and was then depressed and seclusive. She went to college, but there she was restless, preoccupied, friendless, and unable to study. She wandered about the town—alone, at night. For several weeks she secretly cut and burned her skin; then she attempted suicide with drugs. She was hospitalized, medicated, discharged, briefly met with several psychiatrists in succession, found each somehow to be distasteful to her, left them, and again tried to deal with an awful, unrecognized, and urgent problem through suicide. Hospital once more.

Jane met with me five times each week for two years of hospitalization; for about one more year she was an outpatient. For a long time she said that she did not like me, trust me, or want to see me. She derided my work, was on a few occasions assaultive, and so accurately perceived and attacked the peculiarities and shortcomings of my personality that I frequently felt that I must get away from her and the discomfort occasioned by her behavior. I did recognize, however, that her approaches, withdrawals, and "negativism" were occasioned by her great need to place trust in someone, and her equally great fear of betrayal and hurt.

Jane and I kept at our meetings with the collaboration of colleagues knowledgeable in these enterprises—nurses, social workers, psychologists, psychiatrists, and others. There was the help of her parents, with whom Jane later made her peace. This is not the place to describe the vicissitudes of a treatment procedure, except to say that it reflected the planned, coordinated use of human relationships in bringing about useful change; there was no use made of electroshock, but medication was occasionally used at times of the patient's extreme anxiety. She did improve, her anxiety subsided, she seemed to comprehend her behavior better, and she went on to college. There was no "miracle," no magic; there was some hard work, and a need for confidence, compassion, understanding, and persistence on the part of all of us.

It seemed to me, the therapist, that despite her earlier apparent successes in living, Jane was a lonely, insecure, frightened person. I came to know her parents fairly well and they gave me their confidence. Jane's early life, and the family in which she grew up, were more troubled than they seemed to be on first accounts. In late adolescence she could no longer maintain a facade of normalcy; she could not emerge as an adult, and retreated to a state of increasing isolation in efforts to avoid human associations that roused the fragments of past painful and nightmarish experience. Out of her fears she had fled from necessary human relatedness. We—my associates and I—invited her to dare that relatedness and intimacy once again. She did dare, and entered upon a course marked by recurrent exacerbations of anxiety, by regression, and by the exposure and a sort of reliving of painful (as well as pleasurable) aspects of her past. We did not "cure" her, but we did help her to gain a degree of understanding of what had happened to her, and opened with her the doors to further learning and growth.

Social-Therapeutic Responses to Schizophrenic Behavior

The schizophrenic person may go unnoticed in our society, causing no great public disturbance, effecting at least a marginal adjustment, and quietly disappearing from the earth. The loss of his potential productivity is probably large, but difficult to measure. Other schizophrenic people cause some sort of disturbance that may constitute a public nuisance; then they become patients and objects of therapeutic—or other—concern. The schizophrenic behavior is distressing not only because of its economic-interpersonal-social costs, but because it is a revealing, mocking caricature of our own lives. It seems to deride certain of our most cherished beliefs and values—the goodness of the home, the worth of love, the rewards of success, and the prospects of the future becoming an improvement over the past. It highlights the ambivalences that many of us (all of us?) feel about the importance of our existence and that we ignore as best we can. These revelations are among the reasons that working with such people is not an extraordinarily popular occupation—or pastime.

The common approach to the schizophrenia problem has been, and is, to control it, ignore it, eliminate or conceal its manifestations, or eradicate it. Thus the shutting away of patients in hospitals (or, nowadays, often substandard foster homes and "halfway houses"). In some societies the too obstreperous deviants are killed, by one means or another; that simple fact cannot be ignored, nor should we ignore the death wishes often directed toward these people who seem to insist on becoming our wards, making us feel "responsible" while they reject what we offer and fail to respond to our efforts to understand and be of help. The distress and pain of the patient are not only his burden; they are ours and we should alleviate them as best we can. But we should also attempt to learn from it and not simply destroy it.

If schizophrenia is a disease in the older, and honored, medical sense, we might find its cause(s), treat it, and finally prevent it. But diseases have a way of recurring, subtly and in protean forms. As we seek to control them, they must, in turn, act to control us. Perhaps, it has been said for many years, we shall some day discover a genetic fault, a constitutional weakness or vulnerability, a neurophysiological-chemical deficit or malfunction with which we can deal more precisely and adequately than can be done at this time. Such may be the case, and when that day comes there comes with it a further increase in our responsibility as to the powers we may exert in controlling and modifying the behaviors of ourselves.

The "Problem" of Schizophrenia

Schizophrenia is the most common of the grossly crippling psychiatric troubles. Each year, 100,000 to 200,000 people in the United States are diagnosed, for the first time, as schizophrenic. Approximately 62 per cent of these would require care in hospitals, or other facilities, were the programs available. "(T)he cost of schizophrenia has been estimated at $11.6 to $19.5 billion annually. About two thirds of this cost is due to lack of productivity by schizophrenic patients and about one fifth to treatment costs. . . . The cost in human suffering to those with schizophrenia is inestimable. It is our expectation that, however costly they are, those interventions which must alleviate human suffering and preserve human dignity will, in the long run, be most efficacious in promoting useful and productive lives for our patients" (Gunderson and Mosher, 1975).

The problem, personal and social, is immense, and grows with the increases in population and the complexities of our societies. There is no purpose in attempting to review here the well-publicized attempts being made to provide care for the many, and the financial stringencies that become ever more evident as the demands for help are enlarged. The outlook for the schizophrenic person—or for any of us—is not necessarily bright, in terms of current ecologic, economic, and social changes.

Psychotherapy and Schizophrenia

In this article I have not addressed myself directly to the title. I have attempted to present a view of schizophrenia as a form of human living—one of its many extremes. I suspect that this disorder is the result of a complex of "causative" factors—biologic, interpersonal, social, cultural. It does appear that the way a person grows up has a great deal to do with what becomes of him, i.e., who he is. From this point of view it is practical to emphasize and pursue studies of human development; intensive psychotherapy is a form of treatment and is also a method of study and investigation.

In my experience—as a therapist and by observing the work of others—the psychotherapeutic approach is useful to many schizophrenic people who have not benefited adequately from other methods of treatment. The acutely ill, "first-break" people often do not enter such a program; efforts are made to end quickly their disturbances through a change in the environment, brief hospitalization, the use of medication, and so on. The relapse rate is high. (In 1972, 72 per cent of the admissions of schizophrenic people to hospitals were readmissions [Gunderson and Mosher, 1975].)

These "first-break" people usually are a bit hesitant about the psychotherapeutic approach because of the fear that a nightmare experience will be opened up again; they don't want that to happen. The outlook for the profoundly paranoid person, or the one seemingly resigned to a hebephrenic dilapidation, is not ordinarily promising, as the patient has found some relief from the miseries of his life, although that relief is a costly one. A great deal can be done for the patient who is still engaged in a struggle and has not yet settled into one of the death-like pseudo-"solutions" to living. I should not dismiss a patient as hopeless in any case, and I am no optimist. There are patients who find great help through attendance in "daycare" and "aftercare" programs in which emphasis is placed on understanding, personal concern, and the setting of needed limits.

I know that "intensive psychoanalytically oriented psychotherapy" (what a term!) cannot be available for everyone, and that there is no evidence that in its most elaborate form it would be helpful to "everyone." Its principles, however, as suggested in my earlier remarks, are applicable, in my view, to a wider range of therapeutic procedures—in and out of institutions.

This presentation will certainly not persuade anyone to become enthusiastic about psychotherapy. That is not my intention. This is a field better suited to continued hard work than to enthusiasms which are likely to be ephemeral. I frequently hear that a few schizophrenic patients can be helped through the "dedicated" efforts of a very few "gifted, empathic, compassionate" therapists. Such statements can be a way of dismissing the problem, as they imply some sort of magic rather than the availability of knowledge, theory, and techniques associated with these—tempered, of course, by wisdom and a sense of humor. Psychotherapy is work, not wizardry. Harry Stack Sullivan said something like the following to me: "I don't see that you are the possessor of any great perceptiveness or gifts for understanding other people. But perhaps you are curious about some of these events. In that case some patients may overlook your not being so clever, and your being at other times obtuse, and will try to teach you something. In the course of educating you they will very likely find their own lives to be improved."

At first I was discouraged by that remark, but with the passage of time it has encouraged and sustained me in this work.

The future of the human race—even the relatively near future—is at best uncertain, and foreboding of further conflict for survival (Heilbroner, 1974). In order to cope with—and to perhaps form—what may come, we are well advised to learn what we can about who we are and why we do what we do. In schizophrenic behavior is exposed a skewed account of human development; we see in it, sharply outlined, the human predicament—how to live with ourselves, our fellows, and our environment without recklessly destroying all through our ignorance, our mythologies, and our clinging to the symbolic structures that we have created and, in some instances, dangerously enshrined. We must learn, as our patients must learn, that we are not simply expressions and victims of our biological-social-cultural heritage; we are also, to some extent, creators of our futures.

References

Arieti, S.: Interpretation of Schizophrenia. New York, Basic Books, Inc., Publishers, 1974.

Blatt, S. J., and Wild, C. M.: Schizophrenia. A Developmental Analysis. New York, Academic Press, Inc., 1976.

Boss, M.: Psychoanalysis and Daseinanalysis. New York, Basic Books, Inc., Publishers, 1963.

Bowlby, J.: Attachment and Loss. Volume 1. Attachment, 1969; Volume 2. Separation-Anxiety and Anger, 1973. New York, Basic Books, Inc., Publishers.

Caudill, W.: The Psychiatric Hospital as a Small Society. Cambridge, Mass., Harvard University Press, 1958.

DeVore, I. (ed.): Primate Behavior. New York, Holt, Rinehart and Winston, Inc., 1965.

Edelson, M.: The Practice of Sociotherapy. New Haven, Yale University Press, 1970.

Freeman, T., Cameron, J. L., and McGhie, A.: Chronic Schizophrenia. New York, International Universities Press, 1958.

Grinker, R. R., and Holzman, P. S.: Schizophrenic pathology in young adults, a clinical study. Arch. Gen. Psychiatry, *28*:168–175, 1973.

Grinspoon, L., Ewalt, J. R., and Shader, R. I.: Schizophrenia: Pharmacotherapy and Psychotherapy. Baltimore, The Williams & Wilkins Company, 1972.

Gunderson, J. G., and Mosher, L. R.: The Cost of Schizophrenia. Am. J. Psychiatry, *132*:901–906, 1975.

Guntrip, H.: Schizoid Phenomena, Object Relations and the Self. New York, International Universities Press, 1968, p. 48.

Hall, E. T.: Beyond Culture. New York, Doubleday & Company, Inc., 1976.

Havens, L. L.: Approaches to the Mind. Boston, Little, Brown and Company, 1973.

Heilbroner, R. L.: An Inquiry Into The Human Prospect. New York, W. W. Norton and Company, Inc., 1974.

Hill, L. B.: Psychotherapeutic Intervention in Schizophrenia. Chicago, The University of Chicago Press, 1955.

Jackson, D. D. (ed.): The Etiology of Schizophrenia. New York, Basic Books, Inc., Publishers, 1960.

Laing, R. D.: The Politics of Experience. New York, Pantheon Books, Inc., 1967, pp. 78–79.

Lidz, T.: The Family and Human Adaptation. New York, International Universities Press, 1963.

Lidz, T.: Egocentric Cognitive Regression and a Theory of Schizophrenia, presented at the 5th World Congress of Psychiatry, Mexico City, December 3, 1971, unpublished. (The theme of this paper is developed further in Lidz, 1973.)

Lidz, T.: The Origin and Treatment of Schizophrenic Disorders. New York, Basic Books, Inc., Publishers, 1973.

Lidz, T., Fleck, S., and Cornelison, A. R.: Schizophrenia and the Family. New York, International Universities Press, 1965.

Mahler, M. S., Pine, F., and Bergman, A.: The Psychological Birth of the Human Infant. New York, Basic Books, Inc., 1975.

Marmor, J.: Modern Psychoanalysis: New Directions and Perspectives. New York, Basic Books, Inc., Publishers, 1968.

May, P. R. A.: Treatment of Schizophrenia: A Comparative Study of Five Treatment Methods. New York, Science House, 1968.

May, R., Angel, E., and Ellenberger, H. F. (eds.): Existence, A New Dimension in Psychiatry and Psychology. New York, Basic Books, Inc., Publishers, 1958.

Moos, R.: The Human Context: Environmental Determinants of Behavior. New York, John Wiley & Sons, Inc., 1976.

Murphy, L. B., and Moriarty, A. E.: Vulnerability, Coping, and Growth, from Infancy to Adolescence. New Haven, Yale University Press, 1976.
Schulz, C. G., and Kilgalen, R. K.: Case Studies in Schizophrenia. New York, Basic Books, Inc., Publishers, 1969.
Scott, J. P.: Animal Behavior. Chicago, The University of Chicago Press, 1958.
Searles, H. F.: Collected Papers on Schizophrenia and Related Subjects. New York, International Universities Press, 1965.
Shakow, D.: Some Observations on the Psychology (and Some Fewer on the Biology) of Schizophrenia. J. Nerv. Ment. Dis., *153*:300–316, 1971.
Spitz, R. A.: No and Yes: On the Genesis of Human Communication. New York, International Universities Press, 1957.
Spitz, R. A.: The First Year of Life. New York, International Universities Press, 1965.
Stanton, A. H., and Schwartz, M. S.: The Mental Hospital. New York, Basic Books, Inc., Publishers, 1954.
Sullivan, H. S.: Environmental factors in etiology and course under treatment of schizophrenia. *In* Schizophrenia as a Human Process. New York, W. W. Norton and Company, Inc., 1962, pp. 246–255.
Sullivan, H. S.: Schizophrenia as a Human Process. New York, W. W. Norton and Company, Inc., 1962.
Von Bertalanffy, L.: General Systems Theory. New York, George Braziller, 1968.
Whitehorn, J. C.: Understanding psychotherapy. *In* Fromm-Reichmann, F., and Moreno, J. L. (eds.): Progress in Psychotherapy—1956. New York, Grune and Stratton, Inc., 1956, pp. 62–69.
Witenberg, E. G.: Interpersonal Explorations in Psychoanalysis: New Directions in Theory and Practice. New York, Basic Books, Inc., Publishers, 1973.

Comment

Schizophrenia remains the single greatest challenge in psychiatry. It afflicts almost 1 per cent of the population during their life and accounts for more hospital beds in the United States than any other medical condition. The course of schizophrenia is highly variable and unpredictable. Some patients have a single episode lasting a few months and appear to recover completely and permanently. Others have multiple relapses and remissions. This variable course of schizophrenia makes evaluating therapies difficult. There is now enough evidence, based on well-controlled research studies, to say that certain drugs (neuroleptics) can favorably influence the course of the illness. They are not a panacea, however, because not all schizophrenia patients respond adequately to them and they sometimes induce serious and persistent side effects. It has been much more difficult to demonstrate that psychotherapy has a significant effect on the outcome of the disorder. There is little doubt that psychological treatment can be helpful in the management of a particular episode and in maximizing the personal, social, and vocational adjustment of persons with this often chronic disease. The scientific evidence for its effectiveness in altering the long-term outcome of the disorder is more equivocal.

The ideas and opinions expressed by **Dr. Will** in his essay do not contradict the limits of our scientific knowledge on the efficacy of psychotherapy in the treatment of schizophrenia. In contrast to a hypothetical-deductive frame of reference, Will's approach is experiential and humanistic. He would answer the question in part by calling attention to the continuity of the schizophrenic experience with the state of being human. He regards schizophrenia as one extreme form of being human. As he states, "In our patients we find, not strangers, but ourselves." Dr. Will regards psychotherapy as the use of a human relationship as a therapeutic instrument. Inasmuch as schizophrenic persons, much like other persons, are sensitive and responsive to human relationships, they are sensitive and responsive to psychotherapy. Put another way, we are all largely a product of our interpersonal relationships. It can reasonably be expected that the course of our lives will be altered by such encounters, including those intensive ones called psychotherapy. Is it not reasonable to assume that those persons regarded as schizophrenic may also have the course of their lives altered by such relationships? For direct evidence that this is the case, Will draws upon his own personal experience of working intensively with schizophrenics for many years, as well as the experience of other clinicians who have worked in this difficult field. His arguments are eminently reasonable in the terms in which he discusses them. Although not so stated, it seems that the question is to be answered by the naturalistic observations of the therapist while he interacts with his patients rather than by quantitative behavioral and psychological data collected in the framework of clinical research.

JOHN PAUL BRADY, M.D.

Is Marihuana Hazardous to Your Health?

LESTER GRINSPOON AND JAMES B. BAKALAR
Harvard Medical School

Use of marihuana continues to increase, and arrests for possession and sale or intent to sell remain at a high level (reaching a high of 445,000 in 1974 and declining slightly to 416,000 in 1975, according to the FBI), while doubt becomes more insistent about whether its effects on mental and physical health justify the criminal laws regulating it. The position of advocates of continued prohibition has become defensive rather than offensive. Many old claims about marihuana's deleterious effects have proven unwarranted and are being quietly abandoned; the new ones are often advanced tentatively and based not on clinical observation but on experiments or laboratory analyses that are difficult even for specialists to interpret. At the same time, the increase in recreational use of marihuana has helped to revive interest in its medical uses, many of them recognized for millennia by folk medicine and commonly known in the nineteenth century but ignored in recent years. Although the possible dangers of marihuana when taken for pleasure and its possible usefulness as a medicine are two different issues, they are historically and practically interrelated: historically, because the arguments used to justify public and official disapproval of recreational use have had unwarranted influence on opinions of its medical potential; and practically, because the more evidence accumulates that marihuana is relatively benign even when used chronically in large quantities, the more clear it becomes that the first requirement for a medicine—that it be safe—is satisfied.

In this article we will review the common contentions about health hazards of marihuana use, dealing briefly with those that are obsolescent and more fully with the more up-to-date ones. We will also consider the medical potential of the drug as revealed by its history and by recent clinical studies. The enormously increased amount of research on cannabis since 1970 has affected public understanding of these issues. People are beginning to recognize that prohibition is not desirable and does not work anyway; interest in the medical uses of cannabis and cannabis derivatives is at its highest point in years. We hope to contribute to that recognition and intensify that interest.

The following statement, based on numerous studies, including elaborate and thorough investigations like the Indian Hemp Drugs Commission Report of 1894 and the LaGuardia Committee Report of 1939 to 1944, was written in 1971:

> While there can be no question that the use of psychoactive drugs may be harmful to the social fabric, the harm resulting from the use of marihuana is of a far lower order of magnitude than the harm caused by abuse of narcotics, alcohol, and other drugs. Marihuana itself is not criminogenic; it does not lead to sexual debauchery; it is not addicting; there is no evidence that it leads to the use of narcotics. It does not, under ordinary circumstances, lead to psychoses, and there is no convincing evidence that it causes personality deterioration. Even with respect to automobile driving, although use of any psychoactive drug must perforce be detrimental to this skill, there exists evidence that marihuana is less so than alcohol. Marihuana use, even over a considerable period of time, does not lead to malnutrition or to any known organic illness. There is no evidence that mortality rates are any higher among users than nonusers; in fact, relative to other psychoactive drugs, it is remarkably safe (Grinspoon, 1971, p. 347).

On balance, work done since then has substantiated these conclusions and confirmed that cannabis derivatives are "remarkably safe" compared to many other substances, both drugs and nondrugs, that are not subject to criminal penalties. Most impressive are the controlled investigations of heavy cannabis users in Jamaica, Costa Rica, and Greece that have already begun to dispel old prejudices and influence public policy in the United States and elsewhere. During these same years, experiments and tests have been reported that suggest new potential deleterious effects of cannabis—on the tissues of the brain, on the immune system, on sexuality and testosterone levels, or on chromosomes; but these reports are at worst completely unconvincing and at best too inconclusive to serve as a basis for public policy.

The dangers to be considered fall into the categories of acute and chronic psychological and behavioral, and physiological effects.

Acute Psychological and Behavioral Effects

Effects on cognition and motor coordination

Many studies show mild, dose-related impairment of short-term memory, reaction time, attention, time estimation, motor coordination, and number facility (Klonoff and Low, 1974, pp. 122–124). Cannabis reduces driving skill (Klonoff, 1974), but possibly not as much as alcohol at intoxicating doses; and unlike alcohol, it does not increase aggressiveness (Dott, 1974). Nevertheless, similar precautions should be taken about driving under the influence. Experienced users of marihuana often contend that they can control the degree and quality of the intoxication by "coming down" when it is necessary to perform some task, and there is evidence that they are right (Babor, 1974; Cappell and Pliner, 1974; Cohen and Rickles, 1974).

Acute anxiety reaction and psychosis

The most common adverse reaction to marihuana is a state of acute anxiety, sometimes accompanied by paranoid thoughts, which may rarely reach the proportions of panic. The sufferer interprets the perceptual and emotional effects of cannabis as signs that he is ill, dying, or losing his sanity. He may also begin to think that others present are critical, hostile, subtly ridiculing him, or planning to inform on him to the police. These paranoid ideas are usually tenuous and easily dispelled by simple reassurance—the best treatment for the acute anxiety reaction in any case. Someone who is taking the drug for the first time or in an unpleasant or unfamiliar setting is much more likely to react this way than an experienced user who is comfortable with his surroundings and companions; it is very rare where marihuana is a casually accepted part of the social scene. The likelihood of the reaction varies directly with dose and inversely with the user's experience; thus the most vulnerable person is the inexperienced user who inadvertently (often precisely because he lacks familiarity with the drug) takes a large dose, which produces perceptual and somatic changes he is unprepared for. Anxiety and paranoia are heightened and to some extent justified in this country by a quite rational fear of arrest; these symptoms are less prominent in areas where penalties for the use of hemp are nonexistent or less severe. The acute anxiety reaction is in no sense a psychosis: there are no "true" hallucinations, and the ability to test reality—necessary if the "treatment" by reassurance is to succeed—remains intact.

The anxiety and paranoid thoughts which characterize this adverse reaction resemble an attenuated version of the frightening parts of an LSD or other psychedelic experience—the so-called "bad trip." Some proponents of the use of LSD in psychotherapy have asserted that the induced altered state of consciousness involves a lifting of repression. Although the occurrence of a global undermining of repression is questionable, many effects of LSD do suggest important alterations in ego defenses. These alterations presumably make new percepts and insights available to the ego; some of these percepts and insights, particularly those most directly derived from primary process, may be quite threatening, especially if there is no comfortable and supportive setting to facilitate the integration of the new awareness into the ego organization. So psychedelic experiences may be accompanied by a great deal of anxiety, particularly when the drugs are taken under poor conditions of set and setting; to a much lesser extent, the same can be said of cannabis. Frightening LSD experiences are sometimes followed by flashbacks, and these have also been reported, albeit rarely, in connection with cannabis. It is thought that cannabis users who have used LSD or other psychedelics are more likely to experience flashbacks. It is possible that flashbacks are attempts to deal with primary process derivatives and other unconscious material which have breached the ego defenses during the psychedelic or, less commonly, the cannabis experience.

Two kinds of psychosis, not always carefully distinguished, are reported in the cannabis literature: a toxic delirium from the ingestion of a very large dose and a syndrome described variously as hemp insanity, cannabis insanity, and cannabis psychosis. There is enough evidence in the Eastern literature to make it plausible that cannabis, especially in the form of large doses of hashish that are eaten rather than smoked, is like many other drugs in its capacity to produce an acute toxic psychosis of short duration, resembling the delirium of high fever, with restlessness, confusion, disorientation, apprehension, illusions, and hallucinations. Emotionally unstable people are most susceptible to this reaction. It is not likely to occur when cannabis is smoked, probably because smokers find it easy to regulate their intake.

Hemp insanity or cannabis psychosis is generally described as a more prolonged derangement with symptoms peculiar to hemp drugs, caused mainly by chronic heavy use rather than by the ingestion of a single toxic dose. As such, it would presumably be a very serious matter. But this syndrome has proved to be peculiarly elusive as a clinical entity. It has never been reported in the West, and diagnostic and record-keeping practices in the Indian and Near Eastern hospitals of the late nineteenth and early twentieth centuries, where it used to be a common diagnosis, were extremely inadequate. In some cases one would assume from the record that half or more of the patients in a hospital were cannabis psychotics. Further investigation reveals that the diagnosis was often copied directly from reports of police, who were required to state a reason for admission and routinely put down "hemp insanity" as the simplest. There was also a practice of assigning cannabis as the cause of a psychosis if any evidence could be discovered that the patient had used it; in this way a large proportion of the schizophrenics and manic patients in these hospitals were misdiagnosed. No clearly defined symptoms differentiate "cannabis psychosis" from acute schizophrenia or the manic phase of manic-depressive illness (Grinspoon, 1971, pp. 251–262). Procedures of this kind may give some idea of the number of psychotics who use hashish, but they say nothing about how many hashish users become psychotic. What reliable evidence there is—for example, a study of cannabis smokers and drinkers by the Indian authors I. C. and R. N. Chopra—suggests that the rate of psychosis in this group is no higher than in an average European or North American population (Grinspoon, 1971, p. 259).

Research over the last 30 years in the United States and elsewhere has failed to confirm the existence of a cannabis psychosis. Occasional findings to the contrary, when closely examined, can be attributed to pre-existing psychiatric disturbances or the use of other drugs. To mention just one piece of evidence, Dr. David E. Smith of the Haight-Ashbury Medical Clinic wrote in 1968 that in 30,000 patient visits to the clinic "no case of primary marihuana psychosis was seen" among its client population of heavy cannabis users (Grinspoon, 1971, p. 270). A survey of 36,000 American soldiers also concluded that cannabis alone almost never produces a psychosis (Tennant and Groesbeck, 1972); recent studies of chronic heavy users in Jamaica, Greece, and Costa Rica are in agreement. In particular, a study of *ganja*, the powerful cannabis preparation smoked in Jamaica, found no evidence that it was a cause of admission to mental hospitals. People who persistently suffer acute anxiety reactions are regarded as "not having the head for *ganja*" and simply avoid it; there is no recognized *ganja* psychosis (Rubin and Comitas, 1975, p. 155). A recent review of the literature on cannabis and psychosis concludes that results are "limited and often contradictory" (Halikas, 1974, p. 292). Undoubtedly cannabis can precipitate psychosis in a few people whose egos are so vulnerable that any severe stress or alteration in consciousness, like those produced by a serious automobile accident or an alcoholic debauch, would have the same effect. But now that there are 13,000,000 people in the United States who smoke marihuana regularly, as well as many heavy chronic cannabis consumers abroad, if the drug precipitated a psychosis with any regularity we would have some unequivocal evidence of the fact.

For some people all this accumulated evidence was less significant than a paper published by Drs. Harold Kolansky and William Moore (1971). The reception of this study is a part of social history rather than a part of medical and scientific history; although long since discredited as scientific work, it is still occasionally cited by opponents of marihuana use. Kolansky and Moore reported on 38 patients seen in their psychiatric practice; all had used marihuana and later suffered from some form of psychopathology; eight had become psychotic. The study was not prospective and therefore could not establish a causal connection with any certainty; however, even the inferior retrospective form of experiment can provide controls to eliminate extraneous variables, but Kolansky and Moore failed to do this. There is also a place for anecdotal studies in clinical research as a way to provide clues for further testing; but the symptoms Kolansky and Moore describe are too varied and ill-defined and too insecurely related to cannabis use even to supply hints for further research. For example, when a boy is seduced homosexually by an older man who also introduces him to marihuana and the boy later develops a psychosis, most psychiatrists would consider the seduction to be of primary importance; but Kolansky and Moore see only marihuana. They further imply that when the boy is hospitalized and recovers, it is withdrawal of marihuana rather than the treatment or the natural course of the illness that restores him to health. The fact that the patients themselves and their parents often attributed their symptoms to marihuana is irrelevant; the parents may have been displacing their own feelings of guilt, and the patients may have been unconsciously providing Kolansky and Moore with the data they needed in order to fulfill a desire to please the therapist that is one consequence of the transference phenomenon. The *Journal of the American Medical Association* would not have accepted this paper for publication if it had had only reasonable medical considerations in mind. It is safe to say—there has actually been some progress since 1971—that it would not accept a paper of similar quality on this topic today.

An article by V. R. Thacore and S. R. P. Shukla (1976) compares 25 cases of what the authors call a paranoid psychosis precipitated by cannabis with an equal number of paranoid schizophrenics. The cannabis psychotics are described as patients in whom there has been a clear temporal relationship between prolonged abuse of cannabis and the development of a psychosis on more than two occasions. All had used cannabis heavily for at least three years, mainly in the form of *bhang*, the weakest of the three preparations common in India; it is usually drunk as a tea or eaten in doughy pellets. In comparison with the schizophrenics, the cannabis psychotics are described as more panicky, elated, boisterous, and communicative; their behavior is said to be more often violent and bizarre, and their mental processes characterized by rapidity of thought and flight of ideas without schizophrenic thought disorder. The prognosis is said to be good; the symptoms are easily relieved by phenothiazines, and recurrence is prevented by a decision not to use cannabis again. The syndrome is distinguished from an acute toxic reaction by the absence of clouded sensorium, confusion, and disorientation.

Thacore and Shukla do not provide enough information to justify either the identification of their 25 patients' conditions as a single clinical syndrome or the asserted relationship to cannabis use. They have little to say about the amount of cannabis used, except that the patients' relatives regarded it as abnormally large; they do not discuss the question of why the psychosis is associated with *bhang* rather than the stronger cannabis preparations *ganja* and *charas*. The meaning of "prolonged abuse on more than two occasions" in the case of men who are constant heavy cannabis users is not clarified, and the temporal relationship between this and psychosis is not specified. Moreover, the cannabis-taking habits of the control group of schizophrenics are not discussed—a serious omission where use of *bhang* is so common. The patients described as cannabis psychotics are probably a heterogeneous mixture of acute schizophrenic breaks, acute manic episodes, severe borderline conditions, and a few symptoms actually related to acute cannabis intoxication: mainly anxiety-panic reactions and a few psychoses of the kind that can be precipitated in unstable people by many different experiences of stress or consciousness change. Thacore and Shukla end their paper by writing: "The history of drug abuse among the patients was invariably known to the observers, and this situation could have influenced their observations. Therefore, this study may suffer from limitations that more sophisticated methods could overcome." The modesty of this conclusion is justified and welcome.

Crime and violence

The contention that marihuana use causes crime has been familiar since the days of Harry Anslinger's notorious campaign against the drug; it has now been thoroughly discredited, presumably beyond the hope of revival. On the matter of aggression, Jared R. Tinklenberg concludes: "There is no convincing evidence that the pharmacological properties of marihuana incite or enhance human aggression," defined as intentional acts leading to physical injury (Tinklenberg, 1974, p. 354). All efforts to show that either the acute effect of large doses or some character change caused by prolonged use inclines people to criminal acts of any kind have failed (Grinspoon, 1971, pp. 302–311).

Acute Physiological Effects

These are recognized to be slight. Marihuana causes a dose-related increase in heart rate, reduces systolic blood pressure slightly, reddens the conjunctiva, lowers body temperature, and dilates the bronchi. It affects breathing very little. It has one of the highest known ratios of lethal dose to effective dose: in the range of 20,000 to 40,000 to 1. There is *no* well-authenticated case of death from cannabis ingestion in a human being (Grinspoon, 1971, pp. 227–228). In one recent incident, a small girl swallowed the enormous dose of 1.5 grams of cannabis resin (about 225 mg. of delta-1-tetrahydrocannabinol, the main active principle, an amount equivalent to 25 or 50 ordinary marihuana cigarettes and rarely obtainable in such concentrated form): her condition was normal after a day (Bro et al., 1975).

Chronic Psychological and Behavioral Effects

Once this was the target on which most accusations were concentrated, and the issues were often confused by law-enforcement zeal and hysterical misrepresentation. Today the results of older work like that of the LaGuardia Committee and newer controlled research in Jamaica and elsewhere have become familiar, and it is much harder to persuade people by means of appeals to diffuse fear or social and racial prejudice that prolonged use of marihuana has deleterious effects. When these fears and prejudices are dispelled, there is very little argument for any of the charges; and in fact many of them are being quietly abandoned by advocates of marihuana prohibition.

Addiction and tolerance

Cannabis is not physically addictive. Something resembling mild withdrawal symptoms has been reported in laboratory animals given enormous doses of THC (delta-l-tetrahydrocannabinol) for a long time and even in human beings in a laboratory situation (Benowitz and Jones, 1975); but as a clinical phenomenon in ordinary recreational use a cannabis abstinence syndrome simply does not exist, even among Jamaicans who use up to 420 mg. of THC a day (Rubin and Comitas, 1975, p. 130). There is equally little evidence of pharmacological tolerance in human beings at recreational doses; in fact, it appears that experienced users are more sensitive to the desired effects at lower doses. "Behavioral tolerance," probably a matter of learning to compensate for or direct the effects of high-dose intoxication when necessary, has been reported in laboratory animals and undoubtedly arises in human beings as well; presumably it enables Jamaicans to do hard physical labor while taking large doses. Some experiments on human beings also reveal dose-related tolerance to various psychological and physiological effects (Benowitz and Jones, 1975). Whatever the nature or degree of the tolerance or reverse tolerance that arises in various circumstances during marihuana use, it does not present a problem to the user or to society. There are no reports of a need to increase the dose to recapture the original euphoria or to prevent a relapse into misery.

Although it is accepted that cannabis is not physically addictive and does not give rise to significant tolerance, it is often said to create a psychological dependency. But this term does not tell us much; almost any habit that satisfies a need or desire, whether related to drugs or not, can be described as a psychological dependency. Some dependencies are trivial, some benign; the significant question is whether the habit does any harm to the individual or to society. One test of this (not, of course, the only one) is whether the person who has the habit wishes he could give it up but feels unable to do so. Marihuana users rarely feel that way; they usually state that they can take the drug or leave it and they do not feel tormented craving in its absence. Undoubtedly there are exceptions; some people, especially those suffering from anxiety, depression, feelings of inadequacy, or certain character disorders, may be susceptible to a psychological dependency on cannabis as to other kinds of psychological dependency. But the inadequacy is more important than the use of cannabis to compensate for it. Certainly the medical evidence suggests that dependence on cannabis is preferable to dependence on, say, alcohol or tobacco.

Stepping-stone hypothesis

In the propaganda campaign directed by the Federal Bureau of Narcotics from the 1930's through the 1950's, the notion that smoking marihuana somehow leads to the use of opiates and other dangerous drugs succeeded the contention that it causes crimes of violence. Since few people take this idea seriously now, it might almost seem superfluous to discuss it. Nevertheless, for the record: There is no good evidence that any property of marihuana produces a peculiar susceptibility to heroin addiction or that marihuana users tend to "graduate" to heroin. It is true that most heroin users have smoked marihuana first, but an even greater proportion of them have used alcohol, and almost all have drunk milk and Coca-Cola; retrospective associations of this sort provide no evidence of a causal connection. (It is interesting to note that one prominent early propagandist of the stepping-stone hypothesis was convinced that the descent to hell began with tobacco smoking, which caused the marihuana use that led to heroin (Grinspoon, 1971, p. 239). The evidence for this three-step version was undoubtedly as good as that favoring the more popular two-step version; but the Federal Bureau of Narcotics, when it belatedly took up the stepping-stone idea around 1950 in its quest for new reasons to continue the war against marihuana, showed no interest in this plausible extension of the theory.)

It should hardly be surprising to find, and it usually is found, that anyone who uses any given drug is more likely to use others and that in particular, by a process of cultural selection rather than anything inherent in the drugs, anyone who uses a given *illegal* drug is more likely to use other illegal drugs. When allowances are made for this, the relationship between marihuana use and heroin use proves to be remarkably slight, more obviously so as marihuana becomes more popular and readily available. For example, from 1960 to 1968 opiate arrests in California declined while marihuana arrests increased 400 per cent (Mandel, 1968, p. 215). If any progression from marihuana to other drugs does occur (and this is doubtful), it is likely to be toward psychedelics like LSD rather than toward heroin, which offers a different kind of euphoria and is generally condemned by the intellectual and cultural leaders who favor use of marihuana.

The stepping-stone hypothesis, which used to have "a life of its own apart from the published data" (Mandel, 1968, p. 216)—a life largely pumped into it by law-enforcement officials—is now dead or at least playing possum. But it is useful to keep in mind this theory and its fate when considering other charges against marihuana that may be inspired by a need to find justifications for a fixed conviction that prohibition is necessary.*

Other prolonged adverse reactions

One of the most common contentions made by opponents of marihuana use, and one of the most difficult to prove or disprove, is that in the long run it causes mental, moral, or emotional deterioration of some kind—either cognitive and psychomotor impairment or a personality change like the vaguely defined impairment of mind, emotions, and will known as the "amotivational syndrome." The problems that arise in connection with the stepping-stone theory exist here too: intervening variables and cultural bias. Does smoking marihuana cause personality change or, in our culture, is it the other way around? If there is a personality change, from whose point of view and by what implicit standards is it assumed to be a deterioration? Objective measures of this phenomenon are in short supply, and so are prospective studies that might extricate a causal role for marihuana from the complex web of associations tying social and psychological conditions to drug use.

Given all the ambiguities, it is impossible to make a definitive pronouncement. But it is safe to say that the conclusion of the seven-volume report published by the Indian Hemp Drugs Commission in 1894, the product of one of the most extensive surveys of cannabis use ever conducted, has been repeatedly confirmed: "There is no evidence of any weight regarding mental and moral injuries from the moderate use of these drugs" (Grinspoon, 1971, p. 277). Later studies confirming this include the report of Mayor La Guardia's Committee on *The Marihuana Problem in the City of New York* (1944), a study by H. L. Freedman and M. J. Rockmore of 310 marihuana users published in 1946, and a study by W. Bromberg

*See Grinspoon, 1971, pp. 237–252 for the story of how the stepping-stone hypothesis was developed and promulgated and a discussion of the evidence refuting it; see also Carlin and Post, 1971.

comparing 67 marihuana-using criminals with a similar non–marihuana-using group (Bromberg, 1939). In more recent work, a survey of a random sample of UCLA students made in 1972 (Hochman and Brill, 1973) showed no difference between users and nonusers in grade-point average. Homer B. C. Reed, Jr., found no difference on tests of general intelligence and specific cognitive and motor capacities between casual and heavy users of marihuana (Reed, 1974). The report of the National Commission on Marihuana and Drug Abuse (1973) and the Canadian Government's Le Dain Commission (1974) have also denied the existence of an amotivational syndrome. On psychological tests and neurological examination, 47 Greek subjects who had used cannabis heavily for an average of 23 years showed no deficit when compared with controls (Stefanis et al., 1976). In a rare controlled prospective study of American college students, C. M. Culver and F. W. King found no deterioration even with frequent cannabis use in scores on a set of psychological tests, including the Wechsler Adult Intelligence Scale and tests of spatial perception; this result is subject to the qualification that the period between tests was only a year (Culver and King, 1974). A recent controlled study of chronic heavy cannabis users in Costa Rica (Satz et al., 1977) found no deficit on neuropsychological, intelligence, or personality tests. The results of a prospective study of subjects who smoked large amounts of marihuana daily in a research ward at UCLA for 94 days were similar: no significant effect on learning, performance, or motivation (Lessin and Thomas, 1976).

Possibly the most substantial evidence on this subject so far is contained in a study that has already influenced legislation in the country where it was undertaken and may be on its way to becoming a classic: *Ganja in Jamaica*, by Vera Rubin and Lambros Comitas. Rubin and Comitas compared 30 heavy chronic cannabis users with 30 controls matched for age, residence, and socioeconomic status; all were admitted to a hospital for six days of medical examinations, psychological questionnaires and tests, and psychiatric interviews; their life histories were taken, and their work habits were observed in the field. There was no evidence that continual heavy use of cannabis (up to 420 mg. of THC a day, far more than most heavy users take in the United States) caused violence, psychosis, poverty, mental deterioration, or apathy and indolence. *Ganja* does not produce an "amotivational" condition but on the contrary is used to provide the will and energy to work. *Ganja* users showed no significant differences from controls on indices of mental status, social deprivation, extraversion, and neuroticism (Rubin and Comitas, 1975, pp. 104–106). There were no signs of brain function impairment of any kind and no differences between the two groups on fifteen intellectual and verbal and fifteen neuropsychological tests—including many that are sensitive to the acute effects of cannabis (Rubin and Comitas, 1975, p. 118). *Ganja* users expend slightly more energy than nonusers in performing some tasks, because the cannabis makes their movements less efficient; but Rubin and Comitas regard this as much less important than the fact that they often take the drug *in order to* work (Rubin and Comitas, 1975, p. 68). It is worth noting, in view of the conclusion of the Indian Hemp Drugs Commission that "moderate" use of cannabis is harmless, that the daily consumption by these Jamaicans is probably the highest in the world (Rubin and Comitas, 1975, p. 192) and yet on the evidence does not constitute immoderate use. The results of this study should make us regard with some skepticism the anecdotal reports from the Old World, and especially from Egypt, suggesting what would otherwise be plausible: that cannabis, like alcohol and opium, destroys the mental and physical health of a few who take it to excess. There seems to be no condition among *ganja* users corresponding to that of the alcoholic or the heroin addict.

The question now arises of how to evaluate numerous studies showing personality differences between marihuana smokers and nonsmokers, especially those made in the United States in the late 1960's and early 1970's. For example, a survey of a random sample of blacks by L. N. Robins found more psychopathology among those who used marihuana (Halikas, 1974). Brill and Christie found that college students who had used marihuana for seven years or more were more likely than others to report a worsening of their emotional state (Brill and Christie, 1974). Other college studies found cannabis users to be more alienated, less well-adjusted academically, more impulsive and rebellious, or more cynical, moody, and bored (Robbins et al., 1970). Heavy drug users in general tend to show more depression, personality disorders, and poor social adjustment.

In the case of marihuana, at any rate, excessive use of the drug seems to be symptomatic rather than causative. The personality characteristics associated with marihuana in these studies are partly psychological problems or conditions that existed before the marihuana use began. People who are depressed or coping poorly are more likely to take to heavy drug use. Several studies of heavy tobacco smokers suggest that all the psychiatric labels applied to heavy marihuana users can be applied to them as well: weak basic personality, asocial, introspective, inhibited, lack of purpose and values (Grinspoon, 1971, pp. 286–287)—yet no one has suggested that cigarette smoking *causes* the psychopathology revealed in these studies, and this assumption is no more plausible in the case of marihuana.

But as the Jamaican study reveals, it is not even the case that heavy cannabis use must be associated with prior psychopathology; that depends more on the social role played by the drug and general attitudes toward it than on any characteristic of either the drug or its users. In other words, the personality characteristics associated with marihuana in recent American studies are largely a product of its social status and will probably change as that social status changes. So long as use of marihuana is illegal and heavily stigmatized, those who turn to it are more likely to be different in various ways from more conventional people—either more moody, restless, hostile, bored, and dissatisfied with their lives or simply more self-critical, adventurous, and open to experience and therefore more willing to describe themselves in ways that might seem unflattering from a conventional point of view. As Kenneth Keniston has remarked, they may question the assumptions on which the questionnaire measures of good mental health are based and consider it desirable not to defend themselves against feelings of inadequacy. Once marihuana use has begun, the reaction of society further shapes users' attitudes. Norman Zinberg and Andrew Weil studied a group of chronic marihuana users who had begun to take the drug before 1965, at a time when they were likely to be identified as psychologically aberrant or as criminals, rebels, heroes, or prophets. They were all bitter about the attitudes of the conventional world and hostile toward and fearful of its authority; all described how these feelings were reinforced as they sought out others who used marihuana and therefore felt the same fears and bitterness. In the same study, Zinberg and Weil found that people who had begun to use marihuana after 1966 were much less rebellious and distinctive in their attitudes (Zinberg and Weil, 1970).

Personality has been defined in a multitude of ways. A psychodynamic approach sees personality as evolving over time and within the limits of genetic potentials through a prolonged series of stages of social experiencing into a system of more or less enduring and consistent attitudes, beliefs, desires, capacities for affective expression, and patterns of adaptation, which make each individual unique. The distinctive whole formed by these relatively permanent patterns and tendencies of a given person is spoken of as his personality. Once it is fully formed it is rather resistant to change; even a profound experience like psychoanalysis often has only a limited and subtle effect on it, and it is doubtful that use of marihuana could have more. The "hippie" syndrome of apparent slovenliness, indolence, and passivity once associated in the public mind with marihuana, to the extent that it was more than a construction out of prejudice and misinformation, probably manifested not a deep personality change but a more or less purposeful transformation in ideology, goals, and habits. Like a girl entering a convent, the hippie takes on a new dress and demeanor, new personal habits (including use of illicit drugs), and new expressed values; and like her usually remains the same person underneath. Now that certain hippie attitudes and styles have become more popular, it is obvious that they never did imply a decisive change in personality; in particular, now that marihuana use has separated itself from other elements of this cultural pattern and is becoming increasingly common among people who otherwise lead conventional lives, it is clear that the drug does not have the capacity to alter personality once hopefully attributed to it by its friends and fearfully by its enemies. Soon we may arrive at the situation described in Rubin and Comitas' study of Jamaica, where it is hard to find any significant differences in personality between those who use cannabis and those who do not.

Chronic Physiological Effects

Most of the recent research on medical hazards of marihuana has concentrated on physical disease and organic pathology, partly because psychiatric research produced few results and partly because new experimental techniques have become available for investigating things like chromosome breaks, immune response, and brain damage. Before reviewing some of this often highly technical work, we would like to point out that clinical observation in marihuana-using populations generally shows no organic disease or deficiency attributable to the drug. The Indian Hemp Drugs Commission reported that "Large numbers of practitioners of long experience have seen no evidence of any connection between the moderate use of hemp drugs and disease" (Grinspoon, 1971, p. 277) and this conclusion has never been seriously challenged. It should be added that, as in the case of psychiatric illness, no level of use has yet been discovered that qualifies as obviously immoderate for the purposes of this judgment. The La Guardia Committee came to the same conclusion as the Indian Hemp Drugs Commission, and studies in Jamaica (Rubin and Comitas, 1975), Greece (Stefanis et al., 1976), and Costa Rica (Coggins et al., 1977) confirm the observations made in India and New York. An examination of chronic marihuana users in the United States finds no adverse effects on physical health after 2 to 17 years (Bernstein, 1974). Laboratory work on animals also indicates no serious pathological changes after chronic use (Rosenkrantz et al., 1975).

Recent investigations have concentrated on brain damage, testosterone levels, immune response, chromosome breakage, birth defects, and pulmonary function.

Brain Damage

It is convenient to dispose of the least plausible claim first. We would expect some clinical evidence of serious brain damage if it existed—for example, some effect on neurological and neuropsychological tests in the Jamaican, Greek, and other studies—but none has been found. The recent controversy about brain damage and marihuana had its source in a report by Dr. A.M.G. Campbell and his associates (1971) stating that the brains of 10 heavy marihuana smokers showed evidence of cerebral atrophy as demonstrated by air encephalography (Campbell et al., 1971). The bias of the authors is indicated by their reference to marihuana users as "addicts" and their approving citation of the dubious work by Kolansky and Moore associating cannabis use with mental illness. Even aside from this, the deficiencies of Campbell's study are crippling. All ten subjects were psychiatric patients, and no comparison was made with psychiatric patients who do not use cannabis. At least one and maybe two were epileptics, several had suffered head injuries, one was mentally retarded, and as many as five may have been schizophrenic. All had taken LSD, most had used amphetamines, and a few were heavy users of opiates, barbiturates, and tranquilizers. The possible role of alcohol, which is known to be neurotoxic, was not considered. The peculiarity of this sample and the absence of controls make Campbell's results valueless. It would be useful to have controlled prospective studies on cannabis and brain damage, but there is little reason to expect that any connection will be discovered. In a controlled retrospective study of chronic cannabis users in Greece, for example, encephalographic measurement revealed no evidence of cerebral atrophy (Stefanis et al., 1976).

Testosterone

The question of reduced testosterone levels and possible consequent impotence or sterility in men was raised in an article published by Robert C. Kolodny and his associates (1974). Kolodny found that chronic marihuana users had lower plasma testosterone levels than controls and that abstention from marihuana after chronic use produced an immediate increase in plasma testosterone. In a later study he found that testosterone began to decline in subjects hospitalized on a research ward in their fifth week of smoking a predetermined amount of marihuana (Kolodny, 1975). Other studies failed to replicate these results either in retrospective surveys or on the experimental ward (Mendelson et al., 1974; Schaefer et al., 1975), but this work may have been methodologically inadequate (Kolodny et al., 1976). Cannabis resin in the diet of young male rats at very high doses—10 mg. THC per kg. per day, the equivalent of 700 mg. in a 150-pound man—slows the development of testes, the prostate, and seminal vesicles; but it is apparently not estrogenic, since it does not accelerate uterine development in young female rats (Okey and Truant, 1975).

The significance of these findings is very difficult to determine. Testosterone levels vary considerably from day to day and even from hour to hour without clear cause or obvious effect; it takes a very large decline to affect sexual performance much; even castration has very variable effects on sexual activity in monkeys. Kolodny himself is cautious about drawing implications from his results. In a public discussion, he mentions that two of his subjects on the research ward increased their testosterone levels up to 50 per cent by lifting weights; he also admits that making a judgment about effects of testosterone depletion from a test taken once a day is like judging a person's behavior from snapshots taken once a day. Even after the reported decline, he found no testosterone levels that could be called subnormal; he concludes that the sexual effects in normal adult males would probably be negligible, but is more apprehensive about effects on prepubertal and pubertal males and on fetal sex differentiation (Kolodny, 1975). In any case, Kolodny did not control for the effects of incarceration, and locking up men apart from women for a month or more might be expected to lower their sex hormone levels whether or not they smoked marihuana. However, Kolodny also found decreases in both testosterone and luteinizing hormone as an acute effect of a single marihuana cigarette. He states that the significance of these acute changes is unclear and recommends further investigation of the endocrine effects of marihuana (Kolodny et al., 1976).

In a recent study of chronic heavy marihuana smokers in Costa Rica, W. J. Coggins and his colleagues (1977) reached reassuring conclusions about this question. They found no difference in plasma testosterone levels between cannabis-using and control groups or between heavy and light users of cannabis. The authors suggest that tolerance develops to any possible inhibitory action of marihuana on the hypothalamic-pituitary axis that controls testosterone production. They note that their subjects began using marihuana at an average age of 15.2 years (one began at the age of 9), and they conclude that any transient decrease in testosterone levels that cannabis might have produced apparently had no effect on normal masculine development.

Immune Response

The effects of marihuana smoke and cannabinoids on immunological defenses constitute an unusually difficult research issue. Neither the reliability of the available measuring techniques nor the proper way of interpreting the results is agreed upon. Procedural variations in experiments alter the results, and retrospective design makes their significance questionable. Nothing certain can be extracted from the conflicting results of various studies. However, it is not too misleading to summarize as follows: Most evidence suggesting impairment of immune response by cannabis comes from test-tube research; the impairment has not generally been confirmed by in vivo studies (Silverstein and Lessin, 1976) and as far as we now know does not increase susceptibility to infectious diseases or cancer in human marihuana users. It is not clear whether the damage to lymphocytes observed in experiments is caused by an ingredient peculiar to marihuana, as opposed to tars or other substances present in the smoked material; and the clinical significance is doubtful in any case, since the body has a great deal of reserve lymphocyte capacity. A recent review of "Marihuana and Immunity," after discussing in highly technical detail the methods used to examine cells for this purpose, concludes that nothing substantial has been proved (Munson, 1975). Further information will require prospective studies and possibly full-scale epidemiological surveys.

Chromosome Damage and Fetal Defects

Assertions like the contention that marihuana causes violence or is a stepping-stone to heroin are easy for the user to evaluate and repudiate. The suggestion that it causes chromosome damage in reproductive cells of a kind that might lead to birth defects is very different and much more frightening, because it represents the insidious unknown. So studies by Stenchever and his associates reporting chromosome breaks in leukocytes and caused by marihuana aroused great interest and apprehension (Stenchever and Allen, 1972; Stenchever et al., 1974). But closer examination of this work and further studies have revealed that marihuana users have very little reason to worry about genetic damage. A recent review of the literature by Steven S. Matsuyama concludes, "In summary, the available cytogenetic data provide no definitive evidence for chromosome damage as a result of marihuana use" (Matsuyama, 1975, p. 23). In the same symposium, Arthur Falek states, "At present, genetic findings in drugs of abuse including marihuana are open to question.... Possibly the equivocal findings are due to the relatively gross methods of analysis now employed" (Falek, 1975, p. 12). In the discussion following these papers, Stenchever himself in effect endorses these conclusions (Stenchever, 1975), which are also echoed by the Fifth Annual Report of the Secretary of Health, Education, and Welfare on *Marihuana and Health*.

Two characteristics of studies associating marihuana with genetic damage make them questionable: they are based on examination of body cells (not even reproductive cells in particular) rather than on observation of actual fetal abnormalities; and they are all retrospective, so that it is impossible to separate the effects of marihuana from other factors. The relationship between chromosome breaks in body cells, or even reproductive cells, and genetic defects is uncertain. Many chemicals besides cannabis constituents, including aspirin and diazepam (Valium), cause such breaks. Chromosome breakage in nonreproductive cells or chromosome breakage that merely creates a nonviable cell and does not lead to a rearrangement of working genetic material is clinically of little importance. But even on their own terms cell studies do not support the suggestion that cannabis causes genetic abnormalities. Although there may be methodological deficiencies in their work, Rubin and Comitas report no chromosome abnormalities in Jamaican users (Rubin and Comitas, 1975, p. 85); and recent prospective studies on both animals and human beings have shown no chromosome differences between cannabis users and controls (Nichols et al., 1974; Matsuyama, 1975). The rule here as in other areas of marihuana research seems to be that if we either analyze another culture where heavy marihuana use is not considered deviant or abandon retrospective design in studying our own culture, we find no evidence of health hazards.

Pulmonary Function

The only well-documented common adverse effects of prolonged marihuana use are attributable to residual substances in the smoke rather than to the drug itself. Rubin and Comitas found that smokers had a lower postexercise bicarbonate level and reduced lung capacity; they concluded that smoking causes a mild functional hypoxia in body tissues (Rubin and Comitas, 1975, pp. 85–101). Donald P. Tashkin and his associates (1976) found a "mild but statistically significant airway obstruction" after 47 to 59 days of heavy smoking. Eleven of his 28 subjects smoked marihuana daily before as well as during the experiment, but none reported coughs, wheezing, or chest illness. Even at the end of the experiment, pulmonary function was still in the normal range. Tobacco smoking has similar effects on the lungs; but they are probably more severe because tobacco does not dilate the bronchi as tetrahydrocannabinols do, and also because heavy tobacco users smoke much more than even the heaviest marihuana users.

There is no convincing evidence that chronic use of cannabis does serious damage to the body or the mind. Even a relatively conservative group of authorities like those who participated in the symposium headed by Jared R.

Tinklenberg on *Marihuana and Health Hazards* in 1975 had little ill to speak of it. The question remains whether some pathology has been ignored either because it is too subtle to be detected even with modern laboratory techniques or because it is too rare to be uncovered without full-scale epidemiological analysis. The samples in the Jamaican, Greek, Costa Rican, and other research, it is said, were too small to reveal the kind of association represented by the relationship of tobacco smoking to lung cancer; a prospective study on a much larger scale is needed before we can give marihuana a clean bill of health (something which no other drug or medicine has achieved). It has been estimated that this would require at least $2,000,000 and five years (Maugh, 1976).

The never-ending call for more research before making policy changes is wearily familiar to advocates of legalization. It can be answered in two ways. First, the chances are poor that we will find out something new and important. Usually a large-scale study is undertaken because some unexpected correlation has been noticed, for example between mothers' use of diethylstilbestrol (DES) during pregnancy and daughters' vaginal cancer. If marihuana had some such effect, we would probably have a hint of it by now. The search for damaging effects of marihuana has been more like a fishing expedition than an attempt to validate a causal connection with an observed clinical abnormality. No one can prove that if we search long and hard enough we will not find a relationship between marihuana use and some disease or deficiency, but there are more important uses for our medical resources, including those devoted to the study of marihuana.

The second and more important answer is that although continued research will undoubtedly be of value, the cry that we don't know enough yet should no longer be used as an excuse for delay in the matter of legalization: we *do* know enough about the disastrous effects of present policies. If we balance the concrete, immediate, and substantial harm caused by the present punitive, repressive approach to marihuana against some dubious and nebulous possible cumulative effect of legalized marihuana use, it should be obvious where the weight falls. There is a *prima facie* case against any such restrictions on liberty, and the case here is a particularly strong one. Let advocates of prohibition continue to try to prove that some effect of legalized marihuana would be worse than the effects of criminal penalties for its use, but let the burden of proof be on them. Possibly even this way of posing the question grants too much to the prohibitionists. Decriminalization has not caused any increase in the use of marihuana in Oregon, and it is doubtful that full legalization would make any more difference. So there may be nothing at all to balance against the disadvantages and injustices of prohibition.

Since legalization of marihuana would not do any obvious harm and possibly would not even affect the rate at which its use is increasing, there seems to be little reason for opposing it. But reason has had limited influence in this matter. Past crusades against marihuana were often the expression of displaced anxiety, projection, and cultural factors that had nothing to do with the effects of the drug itself (Grinspoon, 1971, pp. 331–343). In milder forms, these prejudices remain. For example, Dr. Robert L. DuPont, Director of the

National Institute on Drug Abuse, who now favors a civil fine for possession and continued criminal prosecution of bulk traffickers, is quoted in an interview in *Science* as warning that marihuana is dangerous because it represents "the leading edge of change in drug-using behavior" (Maugh, 1976, p. 648). This is either a nonsequitur stating that marihuana use should remain illegal *because* it is becoming more common; or a revival in modified form of the discredited stepping-stone hypothesis; or, more likely, simply an expression of the kind of vague anxiety that should not be influencing policy. There is also some feeling that legalization would be bad because it would imply official endorsement of marihuana use, as though, after all these years, potential marihuana users are likely to change their attitudes to conform to what they believe is official approval; if anything, it might make them suspicious. Besides, legality would not imply endorsement in the case of marihuana any more than it does in the case of tobacco or alcohol. Again, it is the emotional symbolism involved rather than any anticipated actual effects of legalization that gives this kind of argument what weight it has.

Rigorously impartial scientific investigation is important to counteract the prejudice and irrationality that have characterized much of the debate about marihuana, but this impartiality should not be allowed to degenerate into a false objectivity that declares it unscientific to make policy recommendations. We must take the scientific conclusions where they lead us as citizens, and stop the increasingly unjustifiable persecution of marihuana users.

Medical Potential of Cannabis

Cannabis derivatives have a long medical history that has been largely forgotten over the last forty years in the West. They are important in folk medicine in the West Indies, South America, the Near East, and India and were the subject of great professional interest in Europe and the United States from 1840 to 1900. Use of cannabis declined when apparently more reliable drugs were introduced, but even in 1937 there were 28 preparations containing it in the *U. S. Pharmacopeia;* it was removed in 1941, after legal difficulties imposed by the Marihuana Tax Act of 1937 made it nearly impossible to use. Memories are so short that in 1967 a *Journal of the American Medical Association* position paper could declare that "Cannabis (marihuana) has no known use in medical practice in most countries of the world, including the United States" (Grinspoon, 1971, p. 227). Now that some of the bars to clinical research are down and the past of cannabis as a medicine is being recalled, its future is very promising.

In the nineteenth century cannabis was used most often as a sedative-hypnotic and analgesic. For example, Dr. R. R. M'Meens, reporting on the findings of a Committee on Cannabis Indica to the Ohio State Medical Society in 1860, declared that it deserved a place next to opium as a hypnotic; it was less reliable and less intense in its effects, but disturbed digestion and appetite less and produced a more natural sleep (Grinspoon, 1971, p. 219). Dr.

J. R. Reynolds in 1890, summarizing 30 years of experience with cannabis, recommended it especially for senile insomnia; and in 1891 J. B. Mattison expressed his preference for it over the increasingly popular "modern mischief-maker, hypodermic morphia," as a safe hypnotic. Cannabis was also used as an analgesic in childbirth, tetanus, facial neuralgia, rheumatism, and especially migraine. Mattison calls this its most important use and states that it not only relieves the pain of migraine but prevents attacks; Sir William Osler also regarded cannabis indica as the most satisfactory remedy for migraine (Reynolds, 1890; Mattison, 1891; Osler, 1913, p. 1089). Their data and arguments are so convincing that it seems particularly unfortunate that migraine sufferers today are not permitted to use it therapeutically. A recent double-blind experiment has confirmed that smoking marihuana heightens pain tolerance (Milstein, 1975); and paraplegics in a V.A. hospital have reported some relief of phantom pain, spasticity, and headache (Dunn and Davis, 1974). Delta-l-tetrahydrocannabinol at the level of 15 mg. has been shown to relieve the pain of cancer patients, by an action that seems to be distinct from its sedative and euphoriant effects (Noyes et al., 1975). Hypodermically administered opiates and then synthetic analgesics like aspirin and hypnotics like barbiturates took the place of cannabis; now that the dangers and disadvantages of these drugs are clearer, and cannabis preparations of more consistent quality are available, consideration of cannabinoids as sedative-hypnotics and analgesics is a better idea than ever.

Cannabis has also been investigated as an antidepressant since the middle of the nineteenth century; the research, usually uncontrolled, has produced mixed results and conflicting contentions. The few controlled studies have not shown cannabis to be effective in cases of moderate to severe depression. For example, delta-l-tetrahydrocannabinol at 0.3 mg. per kg. administered twice daily to depressed patients for a week in a double-blind experiment produced no mood change (Kotin et al., 1973). But THC proved to be an effective mood elevator and tranquilizer in cancer patients receiving chemotherapy (Regelson et al., 1976).

Cannabis has been recommended for the relief of symptoms of opiate and alcohol withdrawal and as a benign alternative for alcoholics and addicts. Mattison called it the best treatment for delirium tremens and also used it as a substitute for morphine in addicts (Mattison, 1891). Drs. S. Allentuck and K. M. Bowman, in a 1942 study of 49 cases, found that cannabis alleviated opiate abstinence symptoms and enabled patients to return to work sooner; L. J. Thompson and R. C. Proctor reported similar results in 1953 from the use of a synthetic cannabinoid in treating alcohol, barbiturate, and opiate withdrawal symptoms. More recent research also indicates that marihuana may be useful in therapy for alcoholics (Rosenberg, 1975). There may be some people who cannot avoid dependence on a drug but are able to substitute one drug for another; in these cases a cannabis habit would unquestionably be preferable to an alcohol or opiate habit. It has in fact been suggested that *ganja* in Jamaica provides protection from alcoholism and its consequences (Rubin and Comitas, 1975, pp. 155–156, 163).

Cannabis has also been proposed as an adjunct to psychoanalytically oriented psychotherapy, but it is doubtful whether the patient's heightened sense of insight and communication is conveyed to the therapist. Nevertheless, the drug might be useful in promoting fluidity of associations.

The medical literature on cannabis as an anticonvulsant begins as early as O'Shaughnessy's report from Calcutta in 1839 but has been sparse since. In 1949 J. P. Davis and H. H. Ramsey, in an experiment on five institutionalized grand mal epileptic children, found that two tetrahydrocannabinol congeners were as effective in three of them as the usual treatment of phenobarbitol and phenytoin (Dilantin) and more effective in two; one became entirely free of seizures (Davis and Ramsey, 1949). A more recent clinical report describes a patient who needed marihuana as well as phenobarbital and Dilantin to control his epileptic seizures (Consroe et al., 1975). Both delta-l-tetrahydrocannabinol and cannabidiol, a nonpsychoactive constituent of cannabis, raise the threshold of convulsive reaction to electric shock in mice (Karler, 1973).

It is universally reported that cannabis stimulates appetite, so it would presumably be useful in any illness where appetite loss is a problem and especially in the symptomatic treatment of anorexia nervosa. It is disappointing, although not surprising, that psychiatrists have not yet systematically experimented with marihuana or cannabinoids in treating this syndrome; they should certainly consider it.

The subject of marihuana as a treatment for glaucoma reached the newspapers recently, when a victim of that disease petitioned for the right to smoke it after being arrested for possession; his lawyer stated that he needed it to save his sight (Johnson, 1976). Experiments show that a dose-related, clinically significant drop in intraocular pressure lasting several hours is produced by smoking marihuana and by oral or intravenous delta-l-tetrahydrocannabinol in both normal subjects and those with increased ocular tension. The effect seems to be specific to THC and other cannabis constituents rather than a consequence of general euphoria and sedation; diazepam, for example, does not produce it (Hepler and Frank, 1971; Hepler et al., 1976).

Another possible use of marihuana is suggested by its bronchodilator effect. Vachon and his associates found that smoked marihuana reversed the bronchoconstriction of asthmatic patients for hours (Vachon et al., 1973). Tashkin and his associates, in a controlled study, determined that "Inhaled delta-9-THC [delta-l-THC, in the notation we prefer] (in the form of marihuana) causes a prompt, complete, and sustained reversal of methacholine-induced bronchospasm and correction of the associated hyperinflation" in asthmatics (Tashkin et al., 1975, p. 382). They doubt its therapeutic usefulness because of the psychoactive effects and possible airway obstruction from chronic use. Aerosolized THC may be preferable to marihuana in treating asthma because it does not contain the terpenes and other irritants in marihuana smoke.

If the results of Harris and his associates in experiments on mice are confirmed, cannabinoids may even have some use in the treatment of cancer. They found that oral delta-l-THC, delta-6-THC, and cannabinol reduced the size of lung tumors and lengthened survival time by a quarter to a third. Delta-l-THC also inhibited the growth of one kind of leukemia virus. The authors conclude that cannabinoids may be antineoplastic because they preferentially inhibit RNA and DNA synthesis in tumor cells (Harris, et al., 1976).

But probably the most promising use of cannabis in cancer treatment is as an antiemetic for patients undergoing chemotherapy. In a study using placebo controls, oral delta-l-THC prevented vomiting in 14 of 20 cancer victims who were refractory to conventional antiemetics; the dose was 15 mg. every four hours (Sallan, 1975). Since cannabis also reduces pain, sedates, tranquilizes, and stimulates appetite, it might be helpful in many ways to these patients.

The greatest general advantage of cannabis as a medicine is its unusual safety for a drug with such powerful effects: no addiction, no tolerance, extraordinarily high ratio of lethal to effective dose, practically no disturbance of vegetative functions or organ toxicity. The main disadvantages are deterioration in potency over time (about 6 per cent a year), insolubility in water, and difficulty in penetrating the bloodstream from the gastrointestinal tract. It should be possible to overcome these problems by the use of suitable production and storage techniques or by producing synthetic cannabinoids; water-soluble cannabinoids that lower blood pressure have been synthesized, and other synthetic congeners may be found to serve particular medical purposes.

Recreational use of cannabis has affected physicians' opinions of its medical potential in some irrational ways. When marihuana was regarded as the drug of blacks, Mexican-Americans, and bohemians, doctors were ready to go along with the Federal Bureau of Narcotics, ignore its medical uses, and urge prohibition. The results of this alliance are incorporated in the Controlled Substances Act of 1970, which governs federal policy on psychoactive drugs; it places cannabis and its derivatives in Schedule I as drugs with a high potential for abuse and no current medical use. Now that marihuana has become so popular among middle-class youth, we are more willing to investigate its therapeutic value seriously; recreational use is now spurring medical interest instead of medical hostility. Whatever the cultural conditions that have made it possible, there is no doubt that the discussion about marihuana has become increasingly sensible. We are gradually becoming conscious of the irrationality of classifying this drug as one with a high abuse potential and no medical value. If the trend continues, it is likely that within a decade marihuana will be sold in the United States as a legal intoxicant. Even before that cannabis-derived compounds, possibly in the form of synthetic homologues of the natural cannabis constituents, will be available to physicians as prescription drugs.

References

Allentuck, S., and Bowman, K.M.: The psychiatric aspects of marihuana intoxication. Am. J. Psychiatry, 99:248–251, 1942.

Babor, T.F., Rossi, A.M., Sagotsky, G., and Meyer, R.E.: Group behavior: Problem solving efficiency. *In* Mendelson, J.H., Rossi, A.M., and Meyer, R.E. (eds.): The Use of Marihuana: A Physiological and Psychological Inquiry. New York, Plenum Publishing Corporation, 1974.

Benowitz, N.L., and Jones, R.T.: Cardiovascular effects of prolonged delta-9-tetrahydrocannabinol ingestion. Clin. Pharmacol. Ther., *18*:287–297, 1975.

Bernstein, J.G., Meyer, R.E., and Mendelson, J.H.: Physiological assessments: General medical survey. *In* Mendelson, J.H., Rossi, A.M., and Meyer, R.E. (eds.): The Use of Marihuana: A Physiological and Psychological Inquiry. New York, Plenum Publishing Corporation, 1974.

Brill, N.Q., and Christie, R.L.: Marihuana use and psychosocial adaptation: Follow-up study of a collegiate population. Arch. Gen. Psychiatry, *31*:537–541, 1974.

Bro, P., Schon, J., and Topp, G.: Cannabis poisoning with analytical verification. N. Engl. J. Med., *293*:1049–1050, 1975.

Bromberg, W.: Marihuana: A psychiatric study. J.A.M.A., *113*:4–12, 1939.

Campbell, A.M.G., Evans, M., Thomson, J.L.G., and Williams, M.J.: Cerebral atrophy in young cannabis smokers. Lancet, *2*:1219–1224, 1971.

Cappell, H., and Pliner, P.: Cannabis intoxication: the role of pharmacological and psychological variables. *In* Miller, L.L. (ed.): Marihuana: Effects on Human Behavior. New York, Academic Press, Inc., 1974.

Carlin, A.S., and Post, R.D.: Patterns of drug use among marihuana smokers, J.A.M.A., *218*: 867–868, 1971.

Coggins, W.S., Swenson, E.W., Dawson, W.W., Fernandez-Salaz, A., Hernandez-Bolanos, J., Jimenez-Antellon, E.F., Solano, J.R., Vinocour, R., and Faerron-Valdez, F.: Health status of chronic heavy cannabis users. *In* Dornbush, A.M., Freedman, A.M., and Fink, M. (eds.): Chronic Cannabis Use. Ann. N. Y. Acad. Sci., 1977, in press.

Cohen, M.J., and Rickles, W.H., Jr.: Performance on a verbal learning task by subjects of heavy past marihuana usage. Psychopharmacologia, *37*:323–330, 1974.

Consroe, P.F., Wood, G.P., and Buchsbaum, H.: Anticonvulsant nature of marihuana smoking. J.A.M.A., *234*:306–307, 1975.

Culver, C.M., and King, F. W.: Neuropsychological assessment of undergraduate marihuana and LSD users. Arch. Gen. Psychiatry, *31*:707–711, 1974.

Davis, J.P., and Ramsey, H.H.: Antiepileptic action of marijuana—active substances. Fed. Proc., *8*:284–285, 1949.

Dott, A.B.: Effect of marijuana on aggression and risk acceptance in an automotive simulator. Clin. Toxicol., *7*:289, 1974.

Dunn, M., and Davis, R.: The perceived effects of marijuana on spinal cord injured males. Paraplegia, *12*:175, 1974.

Falek, A.: Genetic studies of marijuana: Current findings and new directions. *In* Tinklenberg, J.R. (ed.): Marijuana and Health Hazards: Methodological Issues in Current Research. New York, Academic Press, Inc., 1975.

Freedman, H.L., and Rockmore, M.J.: Marihuana: A factor in personality evaluation and army maladjustment. J. Clin. Psychopathology, *7*:765–782; *8*:233, 1946.

Grinspoon, L.: Marihuana Reconsidered. Cambridge, Mass., Harvard University Press, 1971.

Halikas, J.A.: Marijuana use and psychiatric illness. *In* Miller, L.L. (ed.): Marijuana: Effects on Human Behavior, New York, Academic Press, Inc., 1974.

Harris, L.S., Munson, A.E., and Carchman, R.A.: Anti-tumor properties of cannabinoids. *In* Braude, M.C., and Szara, S. (eds.): Pharmacology of Marihuana. New York, Raven Press, 1976.

Hepler, R.S., Frank, I.M., and Petrus, R.: Ocular effects of marihuana smoking. *In* Braude, M.C., and Szara, S. (eds.): Pharmacology of Marihuana. New York, Raven Press, 1976.

Hepler, R.S., and Frank I.M.: Marihuana smoking and intraocular pressure. J.A.M.A., *217*:1392, 1971.

Hochman, J., and Brill, N.O.: Chronic marijuana use and psychosocial adaptation. Am. J. Psychiatry, *130*:132–140, 1973.

Johnson, J.: Victim of glaucoma asks to smoke pot. *Washington Post,* June 9, 1976, p. Bl.

Karler, R., Cely, W., and Turkanis, S.A.: The anticonvulsant activity of cannabinol and cannabidiol. Life Sciences, *13*:1527–1531, 1973.

Klonoff, H.: Effects of marijuana on driving in a restricted area and on city streets. *In* Miller, L.L. (ed.): Marijuana: Effects on Human Behavior. New York, Academic Press, Inc., 1974.

Klonoff, H., and Low, M.D.: Psychological and neurophysiological effects of marijuana in man: An interaction model. *In* Miller, L.L. (ed.): Marijuana: Effects on Human Behavior. New York, Academic Press, Inc., 1974.

Kolansky, H., and Moore, W.T.: Effects of marihuana on adolescents and young adults. J.A.M.A., *216*:486–492, 1971.

Kolodny, R.C.: Research issues in the study of marijuana and male reproductive physiology in humans. *In* Tinklenberg, J.R. (ed.): Marijuana and Health Hazards: Methodological Issues in Current Research. New York, Academic Press, Inc., 1975.

Kolodny, R.C., Lessin, P., Toro, G., Masters, W.H., and Cohen, S.: Depression of plasma testosterone with acute marihuana administration. *In* Braude, M.C., and Szara, S. (eds.): Pharmacology of Marihuana. New York, Raven Press, 1976.

Kolodny, R., Masters, W., Kolodner, R.M., and Toro, G.: Decreased testosterone after chronic marihuana use. N. Engl. J. Med., *290*:872–874, 1974.

Kotin, J., Post, R.M., and Goodwin, F.K.: Delta-9-tetrahydrocannabinol in depressed patients. Arch. Gen. Psychiatry, *28*:345–348, 1973.

Lessin, P.J., and Thomas, S.: Assessment of the chronic effects of marihuana on motivation and achievement: A preliminary report. *In* Braude, M.C., and Szara, S. (eds.): Pharmacology of Marihuana. New York, Raven Press, 1976.

Mandel, J.: Who says marijuana use leads to heroin addiction? J. Second. Ed. *43*:211–217, 1968.

Matsuyama, S.S.: Cytogenetic studies of marijuana. *In* Tinklenberg, J.R. (ed.): Marijuana and Health Hazards: Methodological Issues in Current Research. New York, Academic Press, Inc., 1975.

Mattison, J.B.: Cannabis indica as an anodyne and hypnotic. St. Louis Med. Surg. J., *61*:265–271, 1891.

Maugh, T.H., II: A conversation with NIDA's Robert L. Dupont. Science, *192*:647–649, 1976.

Mendelson, J.H., Kuehule, J., Ellingboe, J., and Babor, T.F.: Effects of marijuana on plasma testosterone. *In* Tinklenberg, J.R. (ed.): Marijuana and Health Hazards: Methodological Issues in Current Research. New York, Academic Press, Inc., 1975.

Meyer, R.E.: Psychiatric consequences of marijuana use: The state of the evidence. *In* Tinklenberg, J.R. (ed.): Marijuana and Health Hazards: Methodological Issues in Current Research. New York, Academic Press, Inc., 1975.

Milstein, S.: Pain tolerance and cannabis. Reported at the Collegium Internationale Neuropsychopharmacologicum Convention, Paris, 1975.

Munson, A.E.: Marijuana and immunity. *In* Tinklenberg, J.R. (ed.): Marijuana and Health Hazards: Methodological Issues in Current Research. New York, Academic Press, Inc., 1975.

Nichols, W.W., Miller, R.C., Heneen, W., Bradt, C., Hollister, L., and Kanter, S.: Cytogenetic studies on human subjects receiving marihuana and delta-9-tetrahydrocannabinol. Mutat. Res. *26*:413–417, 1974.

Noyes, R., Brunk, F., Baram, D.A., and Canter, A.: Analgesic effect of delta-9-tetrahydrocannabinol. J. Clin. Pharmacol., *15*:139–143, 1975.

Okey, A.B., and Truant, G.S.: Cannabis demasculinizes rats but is not estrogenic. Life Sci., *17*:1113–1118, 1975.

Osler, W. The Principles and Practice of Medicine. 8th ed. New York, Appleton-Century-Crofts, 1913.

Reed, H.B.C., Jr.: Cognitive effects of marihuana. *In* Mendelson, J.H., Rossi, A.M., and Meyer, R.E. (eds.): The Use of Marihuana: A Physiological and Psychological Inquiry. New York, Plenum Publishing Corporation, 1974.

Regelson, W., Butler, J.R., Schulz, J., Kirk, T., Peek, L., Green, M.L., and Zalis, M.O.: Δ-Tetrahydrocannabinol as an effective antidepressant and appetite stimulation agent in advanced cancer patient. *In* Braude, M.C., and Szara, S. (eds.): Pharmacology of Marihuana. New York, Raven Press, 1976.

Reynolds, J.R.: Therapeutic uses and toxic effects of cannabis indica. Lancet, *11*:637–638, 1890.

Robbins, E.S., Robbins, L., Frosch, W.A., and Stern, M.: College student drug use. Am. J. Psychiatry, *126*:1743–1751, 1970.

Rosenberg, C.M.: The use of marihuana in the treatment of alcoholism. Personal communication reported in Marihuana and Health: Fifth Annual Report to the U.S. Congress from the Secretary of Health, Education, and Welfare. Washington, D.C., U.S. Government Printing Office, 1975.

Rosenkrantz, H., Sprague, R.A., Fleischman, R.W., and Braude, M.C.: Oral delta-9-tetrahydrocannabinol toxicity in rats treated for periods of up to 6 months. Toxicol. Applied Pharmacol., *32*:339–417, 1975.

Rubin, V., and Comitas, L.: Ganja in Jamaica. The Hague, Mouton, 1975.

Sallan, S.E., Zinberg, N.E., and Frei, E., III: Antiemetic effect of delta-9-tetrahydrocannabinol in patients receiving cancer chemotherapy. N. Engl. J. Med., *293*:795–797, 1975.

Satz, P., Fletcher, J.M., and Sutker, L.S.: Neuropsychologic, intellectual, and personality correlates of chronic marijuana use in native Costa Ricans. *In* Dornbush, R.L., Freedman, A.M., and Fink, M. (eds.): Chronic Cannabis Use. Ann. N. Y. Acad. Sci., in press.

Schaefer, C.F., Gunn, C.S., and Dubrowski, K.M.: Normal plasma testosterone concentrations after marihuana smoking. N. Engl. J. Med., *292*:867–868, 1975.

Silberstein, M.J., and Lessin, P.J.: DNCB Skin testing in chronic marihuana users. *In* Braude, M.C., and Szara, S. (eds.): Pharmacology of Marihuana. New York, Raven Press, 1976.

Stefanis, C., Boulougouris, J., and Liakos, A.: Clinical and psychophysiological effects of cannabis in longterm users. *In* Braude, M.C., and Szara, S. (eds.): Pharmacology of Marihuana. New York, Raven Press, 1976.

Stenchever, M.A.: Observations on the cytogenetic effects of marijuana. *In* Tinklenberg, J.R. (ed.): Marijuana and Health Hazards: Methodological Issues in Current Research. New York, Academic Press, Inc., 1975.

Stenchever, M.A., and Allen, M.: The effect of delta-9-tetrahydrocannabinol on the chromosomes of human lymphocytes *in vitro*. Am. J. Obstet. Gynecol., *114*:821, 1972.

Stenchever, M.A., Kunysz, T.J., and Allen, M.A.: Chromosome breakage in users of marijuana. Am. J. Obstet. Gynecol., *118*:106–113, 1974.

Tashkin, D.P., Shapiro, B.J., Lee, Y.E., and Harper, C.E.: Effects of smoked marijuana in experimentally induced asthma. Am. Rev. Respir. Dis., *112*:377–386, 1975.

Tashkin, D.P., Shapiro, B.J., Lee, Y.E., and Harper, C.E.: Subacute effects of heavy marihuana smoking on pulmonary function in healthy men. N. Engl. J. Med., *294*:125–128, 1976.

Tennant, F.S., Jr., and Groesbeck, C.S.: Psychiatric effects of hashish. Arch. Gen. Psychiatry, *27*:133–136, 1972.

Thacore, V.R., and Shukla, S.P.R.: Cannabis psychosis and paranoid schizophrenia. Arch. Gen. Psychol., *33*:383–386, 1976.

Thompson, L.J., and Proctor, R.C.: Pyrahexyl in the treatment of alcoholic and drug withdrawal conditions. N. Carolina Med. J., *14*:520–523, 1953.

Tinklenberg, J.R.: Marijuana and human aggression. *In* Miller, L.L. (ed.): Marijuana: Effects on Human Behavior. New York, Academic Press, Inc., 1974.

Vachon, K., FitzGerald, M.X., Solliday, N.H., Gould, I.A., and Gaensler, E.A.: Single dose effect of marihuana smoke. N. Engl. J. Med., *288*:985–989, 1973.

Zinberg, N.E., and Weil, A.T.: A comparison of marijuana users and nonusers. Nature, *226*:119–123, 1970.

Comment

Drs. Grinspoon and **Bakalar** take the position that marihuana and related cannabis derivatives are remarkably safe drugs and that their continued prohibition is medically unjustified and socially counterproductive. They acknowledge that marihuana may provoke anxiety reactions and that an overdose may induce a toxic psychosis. However, they also point out that efforts to confirm the existence of a "cannabis psychosis," as has been described in a number of cultures, from the regular use of the drug have failed. In particular, they argue that if such an entity existed, it would be clearly identifiable in a convincing manner among the 13 million current regular users of marihuana in the United States. Grinspoon and Bakalar believe that the presence of psychosis in marihuana users is attributable to pre-existing disturbance or the concomitant use of other drugs. They argue that the past findings of an association between the use of marihuana and psychopathology are more likely symptomatic than causal: that is, persons who are depressed or not coping well in general are more likely to become heavy users of drugs. Furthermore, the illegality of marihuana itself has led to its greater use by rebellious and disaffected members of the culture. As the smoking of marihuana becomes decriminalized and in general more acceptable, the difference between users of the drug and the general population will diminish further. Grinspoon and Bakalar point out that prospective, experimental studies have failed to demonstrate any consistent adverse effects of the drug on neuropsychological, intellectual, or personality functioning.

In examining reports of chronic physiological effects of cannabis use, Grinspoon and Bakalar find the evidence weak, pointing out that most of the studies paid little attention to control groups, and that the magnitude of observed changes, as in the case of suppression of testosterone production, is too small to be clinically significant. Grinspoon and Bakalar conclude that there is no convincing evidence that chronic use of cannabis does serious damage to the body or the mind.

Interestingly, Grinspoon and Bakalar also invoke social and psychodynamic factors to account for society's reaction to marihuana. However, rather than cite these to account for the relative acceptance of the drugs, as by the parents of adolescent users, Grinspoon and Bakalar try to account for the continued but waning resistance by society to the recreational use of marihuana. They believe that the past association of marihuana with the less advantaged or disaffected segments of society may account in part for society's harsh evaluation of its effects. Now that the drug is becoming more widely accepted and used by persons of higher social status, attitudes toward the drug and its hazards are also changing.

Grinspoon and Bakalar call attention to the revival of interest in the therapeutic use of marihuana in medical practice. These include its use as an analgesic, sedative, anticonvulsant, and antiemetic agent and its possible use in the treatment of glaucoma. They argue that these legitimate medical uses have not been exploited and developed because of the exaggerated concern for a possible relationship between the use of the drug and physical or psychological harm on the one hand and the road to perdition on the other. It is of note that legislative approval has finally been achieved to utilize cannabis derivatives in the treatment of some medical illnesses.

Others would argue that there is a large number of reports suggesting that marihuana has deleterious effects on the immune mechanism, germ cell structure, metabolic processes, and specific organs such as the lungs. They would emphasize the effects of the drug on the psychological development of the adolescent. Some even point to the use of marihuana as the first step in a rapidly escalating commitment to addicting drugs such as heroin or the hallucinogenic agents such as LSD.

Clearly, a well-designed, large-scale, long-term prospective study of the effects of the drug could add significantly to our present knowledge. The data are not yet in, but with time may come a greater understanding of the potential hazards of this substance.

JOHN PAUL BRADY, M.D.
H. KEITH H. BRODIE, M.D.

Do Emotional Problems of the Child Always Have Their Origin in the Family?

E. JAMES ANTHONY

Washington University School of Medicine

> We have learned the answers, all the answers: It is the question that we do not know.
>
> Archibald MacLeish

Anyone who deliberately chooses (or, in this case, is deliberately chosen) to become involved in controversy must first come to terms with the residual conflict within himself before he can expose the opposing arguments without undue bias. He must also believe in the use of controversy to generate not only heat and doubt but also illumination, agreeing with Beecher that "no great advance has ever been made in science, politics, or religion, without controversy" or with Hazlitt that "when a thing ceases to be a subject of controversy, it ceases to be a subject of interest." In general, it is more usual for controversy to provide fresh questions than to furnish answers, but, in order to get at the heart and soul of controversy, we need to look at the answers from both sides and then to try to reach some seminal questions. It is the answers that provoke controversy: the questions stimulate the spirit of inquiry. I propose, therefore, in this controversial chapter, to deal first with the answers before ultimately reaching out to the questions.

There is one further general problem associated with the controversial issue at stake: one must know to some extent with whom the arguments are being raised. In a lecture hall, the matter is simple, since the opposing factions are there to see and answer back. One can begin with some common point of reference to bring the audience together before separating them into their different groups. I recall Margaret Mead, addressing a women's club in America on a controversial theme, searching in the first instance for a common denominator from which to start. She eventually became intensely aware (not surprising for an anthropologist) that all her audience wore clothes and several layers of them and that although a large number of them were of childbearing age, no babies were to be seen and no babies were being breast fed. I am in a more ambiguous state than she was. My readership will comprise both men and women with their often varying views on the individual and the group, on the subjective and the objective, and on the relative importance of inner and outer phenomena. My readership may also be composed of individual, family, or social psychopathologists with similar divergences in their basic points of view and dogmatically prepared to blame the child, the family, or society for any or every disturbance. In fact, unlike Mead, I cannot even entertain the fundamental conviction that my readership will all be fully clothed at the time of reading this contribution. However, most of them would agree, I think, that Freud opened up the province of psychopathology and made it possible not only to look at it in a meaningful way but also in a variety of different ways. I am going to assume, therefore, that all of us are at least covered with the Freudian mantle and that we can look to him, in the first place, for an answer to the question: Is child psychopathology always family psychopathology?

Is Childhood Psychopathology Always Family Psychopathology? Freud's Answer: Yes and No, Depending on the Year

It is well to remember that Freud's first theory of neurosis was external, environmental, and to a large extent familial. Children who were seduced in their homes by family members or family servants succumbed to two primary forms of neurosis: hysteria and obsessionalism. Freud accumulated a good deal of evidence around this theory and convinced himself of its truth. It seemed that the Viennese households were often haunted by pedophilics who ravished the young and induced psychopathology. The family neurosis (or degeneracy as Freud would have termed it at the time) was antecedent to the child's psychopathology (1896). A little later, when analyzing Dora, he was struck by the amount of neuropathology in the family and regarded this as a determinant of her own psychopathology. As he put it: "It follows from the nature of the facts which form the material of psychoanalysis that we are obliged to pay as much attention in our case histories to the purely human and social circumstances of our patients as to the somatic data and the symptoms of the disorder. *Above all, our interest will be directed towards their family circumstances*" (1905).

His speculations in this area may well have led him to develop a dynamic psychology and psychopathology of the family, but at this point his own internal development, monitored by an intense self-analysis, deflected his psychological interest inwardly. However, before he succumbed completely to the fascination of the intrapsychic, he formulated an intergenerational theory of family life to which there were three parts: first, that there is a sort of "family psyche" very similar to the individual psyche and making use of the same kind of psychological processes; second, that there is a continuity in emotional life from one generation to the next in much the same way as the individual's emotional life continues from one developmental stage to the next; and third, that this surprising continuity is brought about, not simply by communication and contagion but by some mysterious unconscious factor that made the inner life of one generation accessible to the next. (Later, he concluded that this mysterious unconscious transmitting factor was no other than the superego which was still to be discovered.) There is no problem in extrapolating from this intergenerational theory to the concept of a childhood psychopathology deriving from a family psychopathology (Freud, 1913).

As he continued his self-analysis, his conceptualization of the family also began to take an introverted course. In the deepest and most unconscious layers there was a latent family that only reached consciousness indirectly through dreams, fantasies, or symptoms. At the next level, the preconscious one, the imagery was more childlike, with oedipal dissatisfactions giving place to various versions of an imaginary family or "family romance." At the conscious level, there existed the family of everyday life, replete with everyday problems and causing enough trouble in the "here and now" to turn attention away from the more latent families. If Freud had continued to elaborate a dynamic theory of the family (in the way that he did with the group), he would have pointed out how difficult it was to carry three different kinds of families within oneself, each with its own wishful needs that were likely to be in conflict with one another.

Psychopathology might stem from any of these family levels and the problems of coexistence would be exacerbated by the fact that every family member would be functioning consciously, preconsciously, and unconsciously in the same way, so that incompatible intrapsychic and interpersonal fantasies were only too likely to clash. Family pathology would then emerge as a summation of the individual family psychopathologies. The direction of transmission might then be reversed according to whether the disturbance was more intrapsychic or interpersonal: with intrapsychic disturbances child psychopathology would generate family psychopathology and on the interpersonal level, family psychopathology might give rise to childhood psychopathology. Each member of the family would experience the other member throughout a wide range and depth of fantasy. A brilliant literary example of this interplay occurs in Dostoevski's *Crime and Punishment,* where he illustrates, in the case of Raskolnikov, the system of memories, reveries, dreams, imaginative reconstructions, and family interactions that acted as such a powerful determinant in the abnormal psychic life of the individual. While trying to be what he is, Raskolnikov is compelled to enact his pathological fantasied interactions with his family from which reality has been largely dissociated. French psychopathologists have referred to this meshing of neurotic fantasies originating in different family members as a "family neurosis," in which the emphasis is on a network of unconscious interrelations rather than on the actual interactions. This presupposes a complementarity in the intrapsychic as well as in the interpersonal fields of the family.

In 1917, Freud took an even bolder step in postulating a family psychology (with its implicit corollary of a family psychopathology). He introduced the construct of a "family complex" in which the intrapsychic and interpersonal reverberated together. The following elements constituted the "family complex" or family psychopathology with the nuclear or oedipal structures central to the total complex:

1. Within the family of children and parents, the oedipal conflict would have undergone different degrees of resolution and would engage with one another in different ways.
2. The oedipal conflict within any particular child and the subsequent psychopathology stemming from it could be aggravated by the seductive or aggressive behavior of the parents (Anthony, 1975a).
3. Because the siblings each had their own oedipal wishes and needs, the interaction within the family could provoke narcissistic hurts, jealousies, hostilities, bitterness, and dissatisfaction, all of which could engender variable degrees of psychopathology (Anthony, 1975a).
4. Incestuous interplay between the siblings in the form of sexual experimentation could lead to the acute discovery of sex differences with the precipitation of the castration complex.
5. The siblings could also play their part in duplicating the Oedipus complex at a more acceptable level so that young girls who have lost the interest of the father may turn to an older brother as a father substitute or to a younger sibling as the substitute of the baby that the father failed to give her. Such sibling relationships within the family can also create their own peculiar psychopathology.
6. The order of birth within the family, according to Freud, also played a decisive role in creating the family complex and in shaping subsequent psychopathology.
7. Actual experiences within the family, such as the loss of a sibling at a time when intrapsychic death wishes are predominant, could lead to abnormal personality development.

In this theory of the "family complex," Freud attempted to compound the intrapsychic and extrapsychic life of the family and suggested that such external events as parental attitudes and behavior, sibling birth and rivalry, family hierarchy, and the loss of a family member could affect the individual psychopathology.

In spite of these theoretical extensions and expansions, psychoanalysis continued to cultivate its own special garden of the intrapsyche and to feel more at home with such exotica than in the common, bread-and-butter interpersonal happenings that pervade family life. Nevertheless, analytically oriented child psychiatrists and child psychologists began to look beyond the individual to his immediate milieu and to examine more directly the actual behavior of infants and toddlers with their parents. They gradually began to realize that the environment could fail the child even when his psychological maturation was proceeding without the hindrance of some innate handicap.

Is Childhood Psychopathology Always Family Psychopathology? The Individual Psychopathologist's Answer: Almost Always No But Occasionally Yes

The new generation of analysts that followed Freud were not yet bold enough to speak openly of "the family" within the analytic framework, confining themselves mainly to such euphemisms as "environment," "mother-child relationships," "dyadic and triadic structures," etc., but they did appear to be more aware of the individual's ambience and its impingements than their predecessors. Erikson (1968), for example, complained that some analysts still continued to regard outer reality as a "conspiracy" against instinctual wishes rather than as an all-important entity in itself, and Hartmann (1964) constantly took issue with the idea of pure "intrapsychicism," conceiving of the human infant as preadapted to the average expectable environment provided by his caretakers. He expressed the strong opinion that the individual could not be considered "in splendid isolation" and that this was contrary to Freud's views as Hartmann understood them. The Freudian individual was part of a social system in which the ego met society's needs by adapting to it and society met the ego's needs by "environmental compliances." The stage was therefore set for individual psychopathologists to look analytically at the individual and his surroundings in reciprocal terms.

The third member of the trio that took the outside world into at least partial consideration was Rapaport (1967). He, too, was cognizant of Freud's dilemma. Within the short span of human creative life, there is rarely an opportunity for more than the development of one major idea and a choice, at some point or another, has to be made. If one devotes one's full attention to the creation of an intrapsychic model of human functioning, there is almost certain to be a comparative neglect of the organic factor, the role of the environment, especially the family, and the overall influence of culture and society. We know something today about "object choice," but professional choice, apart from a few scattered speculations, remains unexplored. Why does a particular psychiatrist or psychologist turn more to the inner than to the outer world? Why does he concentrate his attentions on the body rather than on the mind? Why does he wish or need to involve himself in individuals rather than in groups? Why do some remain persistently subjective and introspective and others objective and outer-directed? Rapaport was one of those complicated bifocal theorists who always insisted that the organization of the mind was co-determined by drive and environment and that it was the business of psychoanalysis to investigate the relationship between the two and to do justice to the importance of both. There were benefits to one-sidedness, but dangers as well. Freud made original and revolutionary discoveries relating to the inner drives but left psychoanalysis a legacy that more or less excluded the role of the real family in the causation of psychopathology. Rapaport stood firmly with

Hartmann and Erikson in the attempt to unify body, mind, and environment.

This brings us to two others who have continued "in the service of the ego" to include the totality of the human experience. Anna Freud's work with children has been crucial in differentiating some of her ideas, at least, from those of her father. Although she has never quoted it with approval, she would tend to agree with Winnicott that there is no such thing as a child, only a child-parent, and that this was obvious during the earliest phases of infantile helplessness. As Ackerman (1970) has reminded us, she has "pointedly indicated that the child's ego takes its cue from the social interaction processes of the family, but there she stopped, since she was not in a position to investigate these relationships." This argument, frequently repeated, has some validity: it is not within one's competence to speak with any assurance on the pathogenicity or nonpathogenicity of the family if one has never worked with or within the family. One can only make inferences and these are frequently based on little more than prejudice. Anna Freud, however, has had certain advantages: she has worked with groups of war refugees; she has supervised a wartime nursery; she has maintained day care centers for blind children; and, she has encouraged the simultaneous, if separate, treatment of the child and the mother. She has therefore not remained strictly a one-to-one individual psychopathologist, at least in her observational work. Yet she has the same reluctance as any of her colleagues in making use of the term "family" as a dynamic unity of itself. She has considered that the familial environment exercises less causal influence on the emotional illness of the child later in development and felt that there must be some point along the way when the child ceases to be considered "as a product and dependent of his family and should be given the status of a separate entity, a psychic structure in his own right." Her experience informed her that there were limits to which parents could influence the psychological processes in the child and that these influences operated nearer the surface. "Mothers cannot alter the unconscious fantasies of their children. But they can, by their actions, strengthen the healthy, conscious moves toward the next stage of development" (1967). Like a true Freudian, nevertheless, she challenged the usual assumption that parents created the child's psychopathology. There were many links, she said, in this causal process of which the parent represented only one. She warned against the danger of "environmentalism" that ignored the internal meaning of the child's translation of his perception of the environment. In spite of manifest appearances, she thought that there was no direct linear relationship between the illness in the mother and the illness in the child. The parent was not the sole pathogen for the child, nor the child for the parent. It could be said that because the child cherished the parent, he also at times identified with her pathology and could be assigned a role within it:

> Many mothers actually pass on their symptoms to their young children and subsequently act them out together with them in the form of a *folie à deux*. . . . Parents also may play a part in maintaining a child's disturbance. Some of the

phobias of childhood, food avoidances, sleeping rituals, are kept up by the child patient only in collusion with the mother. Owing to her dreading the child's anxiety attacks as much as the child does himself, the mother participates actively in keeping up defenses, precautions, etc., and thereby camouflages the child's illness. . . . Some parents for pathological reasons of their own seem to need an ill, disturbed, or infantile child and maintain the *status quo* for that purpose (1965).

The relationship between parental and childhood psychopathology is consequently not simply a matter of "contagion," although infants may become fearful kinesthetically when they are in intimate contact with fearful mothers. As the child grows in individuality and autonomy and as his psychopathology becomes increasingly internalized, the individual treatment of the parent no longer acts curatively for the child, nor does separation from the parent magically heal the child. In my own investigations on the phenomenon of *folie à deux,* the situation had to be frightening, the relationship had to be intense, the dyad had to be isolated, and even then, the psychopathology that was manifested in the child was not a mirror image of the mother's disorder or a simple reaction to it, but an elaboration that involved developmental psychological inputs (1970b). Winnicott also stated quite categorically that even in severe cases of chaotic psychosis in the mother, the child's psychopathology did not merely reflect the parental turmoil in a reactive way but was largely self-generated in accordance with the child's own inner developments.

Winnicott, also because of his experience of children and their parents, took more cognizance of environmental factors than was usual with analysts. For example, he took issue with Anna Freud's warning that the blame for infantile neurosis should not be placed on the mother's shortcomings in the oral phase, because disappointment and frustration were inevitable within the mother-child unity and could not therefore be cited as etiological factors in neurosis. He himself felt that the mother's position must be taken into account if she has failed to provide "good enough" mothering. (He could have added, but did not, "good enough" fathering, "good enough" sibling experience, and "good enough" family life as a whole.) His observations of the early environment led him to postulate a theory of environment in which he stated that in certain cases, a failure of the environment led to a basic split in the linkage between the individual and his milieu so that a false life and a false self were produced. He insisted that every diagnostician must consider the environmental factors in the etiology of any disorder, beginning with the intrauterine experience, the mother's care, and the capacity of the parental team for taking joint responsibility for the children.

Because of these "environmental impingements" on the inner life of the child, it could be said that individual child psychopathology was not always inwardly developed and not always susceptible to individual ingoing treatment. Both Anna Freud and Winnicott came to similar classifications of disorder and treatment. They each postulated:

1. An etiological group where the disorder was inwardly derived and had reached, without disturbance from the environment, a mature level of development

characterized by internalization and autonomization, so that treatment was best and most effectively carried out by intensive individual psychotherapy (classical psychoanalysis).

2. A second set of disorders where some pre-oedipal advances had been made but "wholeness" had not yet been achieved and the child was still in a state of ambivalent dependency, interacting badly with his mother and making training an exasperatingly negativistic experience. The moods generated in the child needed careful analysis, but management problems dealing with training required careful counseling. Nevertheless, analytically oriented psychotherapy could be undertaken if one bore in mind the interpersonal struggles currently in existence.

3. The disorders in this group stemmed very much from a failure of the total environment at a very early stage of development so that therapeutic management becomes the central approach to the patient. The milieu, the day-to-day routines, the attitude and behavior of the caretakers, etc., must all be carefully considered. Analytic interventions are not as helpful as they are in the second group or as effective as in the first.

If one were to summarize (and perhaps distort) the conclusions gained from these several viewpoints, and if one translated the term "environment" into the term "family," one might be able to state that high-grade disturbances were more internally derived and better internally treated, and that more low-grade disturbances were more externally derived and better externally treated. There would, of course, be exceptions to these "rules of thumb," but they would point to territories belonging to the individual and familial psychopathologist and psychotherapist.

Is Child Psychopathology Always Family Psychopathology? The Family Psychopathologist's Answer: Yes, But Sometimes No, Depending on Initial Orientation

We come now to a different and new perspective, which is that of the family psychopathologist. This encompasses a history that hardly goes back more than 25 years and has been prominent only in the past 15 years. The family psychopathologist looks at the family both directly and totally. The model employed is a transactional one stressing family interaction together with change and growth in the relationship of the family members. It attempts to look at the individual in the context of his natural environment, linking his psychological disorders with the family pathology. The intense scrutiny focused by the individual psychopathologist on the individual detracts from an understanding of what is taking place in and between the others. To quote Bell (1970):

> I had to wipe clean the blackboard of my mind and find a fresh piece of chalk to write large: "The family is the problem." I learned to reject the notion that the child who brought the family to treatment presented the family with which I was to work; the child might be *a* problem, his behavior having provided the occasion for starting the treatment, but I learned that I must not regard him as *the* problem for therapy, not even at the moment of beginning the therapy. *The problem is the family.* Here was the crux of the matter. Here was the transition and thought that I

must make. This is the new idea, seemingly so small, but actually so major. "The family is the problem!"

Once this apparently central concept is assimilated, according to Bell, it becomes dominant in the mind of the clinician and he then substitutes a social psychological orientation for a clinical psychological one and no longer thinks etiologically in terms of the individual. Furthermore, when he thinks of therapeutic change, he no longer conceives of it as change in the psychopathology of the individual but of the group. The family, rather than the individual, becomes the unit of health and illness. The family is the measure of all things, including psychopathology. What the individual approach fails to note, because of submersion in the intrapsyche, is the continuous interchange between mind and mind, between internal and external, between one set of consciousness and another, between one group of fantasies and another, and between one individual's reality and another's. This means, says Ackerman (1970), that a large number of causal elements, specific and nonspecific, inner and outer, generic and contemporary, must somehow be integrated within a single theoretical system. It should be understood, in order to clarify theoretical issues, that the family psychopathologist who originated as an individual psychopathologist, like Ackerman, tends to have a different point of view from that of the family psychopathologist who has never been anything else but that, for example, like Haley (1976).

The first type continues to believe that the past sources of pathogenesis continue into the present conflicts but are somewhat differently organized. He assumes "that the forces of the individual and the forces of the family are interdependent and interpenetrating, that these relations are relative to causation, course and outcome of illness and response to therapy" (Ackerman, 1970). Here again, we have an interlocking and reciprocal model of etiology: child psychopathology is part of family psychopathology and family psychopathology grows out of child psychopathology. The child is father to the family and the psychopathology of the family begins in the childhood of its members. This can also mean that children can be disturbed in their own right (as in the classical viewpoint) and subsequently, as they respond increasingly to developmental stresses, generate disturbances in the parent, all of which is reminiscent of the old genetic joke: "Insanity is inherited; parents get it from their children!"

For those family psychopathologists who are more exclusively systems-oriented, the individual as an individual is treated with comparative benign neglect. Their view of the family process is radically different because it is the family as a totality that occupies the stage to the exclusion of the various members. Thus, while the family psychopathologist who is an ex-individual psychopathologist continues to pay attention to the emotional content of what the individual members of the family say to one another and how they relate to one another, the systems psychopathologist observes the process, the problem solving, the negotiations, the transactional sequences, the praising and blaming interactions, the forming of alliances, and the invalidating of another's perceptions: all these processes remain largely unresolved and somewhere along the line, the child's psychopathology begins to take shape in the form of symptoms. Unhappy families repeat these unsatisfactory transactions endlessly and automatically whenever they get together. For the Bateson school (1956), the double-bind communication is the main etiological factor at work. The parents leave ambiguous signals or "meta-messages" from which the child is unable to infer whether they are to be taken seriously, playfully, imaginatively, literally, ironically, sarcastically, realistically, or metaphorically. In fact, all communications are treated as if they had the same value, the same significance, and the same bearing on the problems under discussion. Since the child accepts the contradictory messages as noncontradictory, he is fundamentally perplexed and unable to act logically. His psychopathology has its roots in this "dysfunctional relationship."

While the individual psychopathologist looks back in time to what created the first ambivalences, the family psychopathologist shifts the emphasis from past to present, from inner dynamics to communication, and from pathology to a peculiar sort of adaptation overlying power struggles. The individual psychopathologist remains content-oriented, while the family psychopathologist has become "context-oriented" and is prone to think not etiologically but ecologically, as Bateson put it, in terms of patterns and relationships rather than in terms of cause and effect, individual versus environment, past versus present, or inside versus outside. In general, family psychopathologists of the systems type appear to have an innate mistrust of etiological or explanatory concepts. If there is any etiology at all within the systems theory, it links the emergence of symptoms or disturbances to a faulty regulation of the homeostatic mechanisms within the family. Symptoms are then seen to be system-maintaining devices. (Some family psychopathologists who are ex-individual psychopathologists will allow that a symptom may arise because of the individual's particular life circumstances but that it is always supported from then on by the system. Even though the symptom may have begun individually and earlier, the origin is generally trivial but gains in seriousness as it is elaborated within the system of the family.)*

I had earlier discussed the fact that individual psychopathologists, working within psychoanalytic theory, have lately set limits to what is possible to accomplish with classical psychoanalysis. Internalizing disorders, they feel, fall within the province of analytic therapy, whereas externalizing disorders require external interventions or, in Winnicott's term, management. It is of interest that family psychopathologists, operating within a different context, have come to fairly similar conclusions as to what can be properly treated by family interventions as opposed to individual treatment. For example, adolescence, which is the prime time for acting out, is also the prime time for family therapy. A number of externalizing

*"To understand a symptom, the family system of the symptom bearer must be understood.... The main premise underlying the idea that symptoms are a family production is the notion that all families operate as systems. . . . From this point of view, the behavior of any member is entirely appropriate and understandable in terms of his family system" (Satir, 1971).

disorders are considered to be born within the family and to be best treated by the family. These include conflicts with authority, destructiveness and disruptiveness at home and in school, assaultive behavior, truancies, stealing, running away, promiscuity, poor performance at school, and suicidal attempts. Lyman Wynne (1965) would include certain types of psychopathology as belonging to the family context, such as identity crises, rebelliousness, symbiotic dependencies and, in fact, the whole class of patients who tend to "externalize" or make use of "projective identification" as part of a character disorder. Such patients do not perceive themselves as having any intrapsychic problems, but they are disturbing to live with and their abnormal attitudes and behavior make for many repercussions on other family members. They are not usually brought to or bring themselves to individual therapy or psychoanalysis, but if by chance they do show up, they present extraordinary challenges to the individual psychotherapist. Family psychopathologists have not made it clear whether they consider that externalizing disorders stem from family psychopathology or whether, because they are disturbing to the family life as a whole, they are best treated within the family. The same is true for patients with difficulties in communication and closeness because, on closer inspection of the family situation, the problem does appear to be a collective one in that intimacy and affection are singularly absent from all family transactions. Nevertheless, it is debatable whether the schizoid tendency stems from a common genetic disposition, whether schizoid parents induce withdrawal reactions in the children, or whether "unforthcomingness" is part of a peculiar cultural milieu such as occurs in isolated communities.

There is no doubt, and this has been frequently verified, that disturbed parents such as psychotics, alcoholics, drug abusers, child abusers, etc., have children who show an increased risk for psychopathology, but in these very same families there are also children who seem practically immune and invulnerable. Can one doubt that irrationality and abusiveness as a chronic element of the milieu may not in time exercise a pathogenic influence, especially if there is some in-built susceptibility. In my own work, for instance, I have found that observers who have been sent to live with families where there was a psychotic parent, began, within a week, to manifest clinical reactions, symptoms, nightmares, anxieties, depressions, and catastrophic responses that were not too dissimilar from those shown by children brought up in the same setting. The psychopathology in the observers was generally short-lived and less manifest among the more stable personalities. I have also described a number of children of psychotic parents who have displayed *folie à deux* and even, more rarely, evidence of hysterical "Ganserism" where removal from the family had led to a cessation of the "contact" disorder (1970b).

It would seem, judging from these experiences, that we still have a great deal to learn about the pathogenicity of different family environments and about the time that it takes for abnormal "free-floating" affects to be assimilated by the individual and eventually becoming part of his psychic structure. Family psychopathologists have often accused individual psychopathologists of living in an unreal world divorced from the natural environment of the child and have suggested that a little firsthand experience with the family would cure the individual psychopathologist of many of his etiological illusions. Many family psychopathologists have reported such "conversions" in themselves as a result of shifting from individual to family work.

Is Child Psychopathology Always Family Psychopathology? The Laingian Rejoinder: Neither Yes or No: The Question Is Irrelevant

According to Laing and his colleagues, the concept of family pathology is a confused one, and they have attempted to put sense into nonsensical family theory by borrowing heavily on the ideas of the existentialist, Sartre (1960).

Jean Paul Sartre, who does not pretend to be a psychiatrist, a psychologist, or a psychotherapist, has postulated that the relationship between persons and the group that they comprise can best be understood in terms of three basic concepts: *praxis* (which implies that someone in the group is doing something to someone else in the group), *process* (which means that something is happening in the group but cannot be attributable to any particular member), and *intelligibility* (which links together in a meaningful way what is happening in the group and who is bringing this about). If one keeps this simple formulation in mind, one gets an immediate feel for the phenomenology of the family and that once this is obtained and mystification has been resolved, the question of etiology becomes insignificant. There is no need to blame anyone since everyone is in the "same boat."

Laing goes even further. He points out that the family group may be even more confused by the concept of family psychopathology than by the concept of individual psychopathology and by the fact that the family, not the individual, is the unit of illness and that the family, not the individual needs to be cured. This makes the family, as he says, "a sort of hyperorganism with a physiology and pathology that can be well or ill. One arrives at a panclinicism that is more a system of values than instrument of knowledge." He thus accuses the present-day family psychopathologists of resurrecting the old mystique of the family organism.

Having beaten the family psychopathologist sharply over the knuckles, Laing then proceeds to castigate the individual psychopathologist who,

> adopting his clinical stance in the presence of the pre-diagnosed person, whom he is already looking at and listening to as a patient, has too often come to believe that he is in the presence of "fact" of "schizophrenia." He acts "as if" its existence were an established fact. He then has to discover its "cause" or multiple "etiological factors," to assess its "prognosis," and to treat its course. The heart of the "illness," all that is the outcome of process, then resides outside the agency of the person. That is, the illness or process, is taken to be a "fact" that the person is subject to, or undergoes, whether it is supposed to be genetic, constitutional, endogenous, exogenous, organic or psychological, or some mixture of them all. *This, we submit, is a mistaken starting point* (1964).

Here Laing is throwing the medical model out along with all its paraphernalia of etiology, diagnosis, prognosis, treatment, and course. All this is merely nonsense and exists for the most part in the feverish imaginations of the individual and family psychopathologists. It is not what is there, because what is there can only be experienced phenomenologically without any requirement to speculate about organic, individual psychopathological or family psychopathological etiology. Such issues must simply be "bracketed off" and put into cold storage.

Although Laing is contemptuous of psychiatric parlance, he gives every indication of seeing the family as the primary etiological agent of every kind of psychopathology besetting mankind, including, of course, schizophrenia. The family is very much central to this antipsychiatric or existential theory that maintains the extraordinary notion that mental illness is in fact a sane, self-preserving response to the conflict and confusion within the family, and that psychopathology, even in its grossest form, represents an individual's "true self" breaking through the "false self" manufactured on demand from the family. This radical image of the family as a pathogenic agent maintains that it puts taboos on tenderness, trust, solitude, and sexuality; that what passes for love within it is actually disguised violence; and that it pervades our inner and outer lives like the ultimately perfected mass medium that never leaves us alone and that mutilates our consciousness. By giving each member a role to play such as mother, father, brother, and sister, it teaches us to live behind the label and to live only relative to others rather than for ourselves alone. It not only mutilates individual potential, but it forces the entrapped member to develop psychopathological behavior as a meaningful defense against its destructive inroads. In brief, we have, as a society, the duty to destroy the family in order to become ourselves and free from the necessity of using abnormality.

Laing's family circle is less mechanistic than Haley's and has an other-worldly quality that gives it its power for evil. It is made up of a system of persons where each person is an object in the world of the other and occupies a position in space and time from which he experiences, constitutes, and acts in his own particular world of which he is the center. The collision between these separate worlds becomes the starting point of the Laingian inquiry of the family nexus. Laing therefore shares with the family psychopathologist, who is an ex-individual psychopathologist, the need to keep the individual in the forefront. In fact, his main wish is to preserve the individual and his individuality against the "hyperorganism" of the family.

When the clinician restricts himself to the phenomenological and existential point of view, he finds manifest contradictions affecting family life that need to be dealt with without necessarily exploring the underlying factors that may be supposed to produce and maintain them. Since they have come into the clinical picture somewhat late, when psychopathology has already developed, they make no attempt to trace the origins of symptomatic behavior but rather to make it intelligible within the totality of the family. What matters is not an etiology but intelligibility, not connections but experience. From this phenomenological point of view, etiology is nothing but a wild goose chase that serves no purpose but to satisfy the inquisitiveness of the psychopathologist. So to the question: Is child psychopathology always family psychopathology? the Laingian response is: Does it matter? Is it relevant to the survival of the individual within the destructive milieu of the family? Does it help to demystify the categorized, conforming, falsely-living individual in search of his true self? Such exaggerated notions stand at the other etiological extreme to the one with which we started.

Conclusion

Individual and family psychopathologists have their own variable responses to the question of etiology and the answers we have been considering have, as we expected, added more heat than light to the situation. The individual psychopathologist, in his constant search for primitive etiological factors, tends to regard "here-and-now" etiologies not based on transference as proverbial red herrings having much to do with reaction and interaction but little to do with causality. The family psychopathologist, on the other hand, sees this individual form of etiology not only as lost in the mists of time but also shorn of an etiological vitality that they may have once possessed. It is the interpersonal factors that preserve their strength for positive and negative influence at all stages of life. What is buried within the intrapsyche is as good as dead in comparison with the current disturbances and distortions that frequently overwhelm the family and bring about a chronic disequilibrium. Even transient situational disorders are no longer considered as a child's idiosyncratic response to stress. To quote Sobel (1967):

> Recent work in the field of family therapy has brought to light the role of the entire family, particularly that of fathers, in the genesis of these disorders. It is possible in the case of separation that the child may be more disturbed by the father's anxieties and their effect on the mother than by the loss of dependency on the mother herself. . . . Every adjustment reaction, whether in infancy or childhood or adolescence, involves a disturbance of interaction between the child and his environment, particularly the significant adults. More often than not, the child's disturbed behavior serves as a loudspeaker for a larger family disturbance. It may also serve as a tension-releasing device in the family, a system of emotional checks and balances as in the case of scapegoating.

The individual psychopathologist has reacted, almost mournfully, to the loss of the child's individuality within the organism of the family, reacting to the notion that the child is little more than an "expresser" of the family's disturbance, a representative of the family's psychopathology, a symptom of the family's conflict, a scapegoat of the family's tensions, and a cog in the homeostatic machine.

Other disorders, such as psychophysiological ones (ulcerative colitis, asthma, anorexia nervosa, etc.) that used to have a comfortable etiological niche within the individual or, at most, within the mother-child relationship, are now well and truly ensconced within the family and its psychopathology. This is also becoming true of learning disabilities where the attitudes and behavior are not only given reactive significance but also etiological prominence. Drug addiction equally is said to emerge from families where the organization has broken down, where family problems are massive, and where interrelations may oscillate pathologically between seductiveness and vindictiveness. The field of individual psychopathology is therefore constantly being encroached upon by the family psychopathologist.

The two approaches, individual and familial, seem to have set up their own etiological frameworks. The one is intrapsychic and the other interpersonal and transactional; the one is located primitively in time while the other is contemporary; the one is incorporated into a postulated structure of the mind whereas the other apparently has no structural theories; the one seems to deal mainly with internalizing psychopathology whereas the other confines its etiological interests to the externalizing psychopathologies.

The basic premise of family theory (and one needs to remember that there are several not very clearly delineated theories) is that the family is the fundamental unit of conceptualization and that patients within the family externalize through their symptoms an illness that is inherent in the family itself. They are analogous to dysfunctional organs in a diseased organism. To account for etiology adequately, one needs an adequate theory, and family theory is still far from adequate for this crucial task. Simply to describe family processes is not enough: to formulate theory, one needs different levels of analyses—behavioral, transactional, and emotional. There are other requirements for theory making, and Meissner (1970) has expressed these very clearly:

> There is a stage in the family process in which the emotionally involved family members are all more or less susceptible of becoming "the patient." It is essential, therefore, that the family theory express and explain this undifferentiated equipotentiality; that it articulate a concept which represents the functional unity of the family system. It can be questioned whether any of the transactional theories of family functioning achieve this purpose. It can be questioned, for example, whether the transactional system is so linked to the patterns of interpersonal action and reaction that it must by its nature remain a composite concept whose meaning can be spelled out only by reductive explicitation of its component interpersonal interactions. Or, putting it another way, is the transactional concept so closely tied to the level of individual interaction that it cannot be effectively raised to the more comprehensive level of the family as a unit? . . . At the present time, there are no clear-cut indicators as to where in the various levels of family functioning and analysis the significant etiological and pathogenic variables are to be located. This is an important question because it is the identification of such variables which determines the link between theory and therapy.

Meissner's argument would imply that we need to wait on a fuller and more comprehensive family theory before we can link psychopathology in the child etiologically to psychopathology in the family. Family research done so far is suggestive but not convincing. There is no question that a high degree of association has been found between parental pathology and child pathology, between pathology in one parent and pathology in the other, and between changes in the pathology of one family member with changes in the functioning of other members. For instance, when one member of a family becomes psychotic, the others appear to undergo a kind of family decompensation. Family research is also bringing into sharper relief and reciprocity the older and vaguer patterns of pathology discovered by the individual psychopathologist such as the pathogenic influence of such traits as overprotectiveness, domineeringness, maturity, remoteness, etc.

In a decade or two, the competitiveness between the individual and family systems will have passed away and both will have combined to produce better etiological connections. Individual psychopathologists must relinquish some of their prejudice and add their knowledge to that of the family pathologist to provide a better clinical opportunity for patients. In 1958, Talcott Parsons, in discussing the relationship of psychoanalysis to the social structure, had this to say:

> The sociological aspects of the family as a social system have understandably not been explicitly considered by psychoanalysts because they have concentrated on the particular relations of each patient to each of the members of his family in turn. There has been little occasion to consider the total family as a social system, though this might well yield insights not derivable from the "atomistic" treatment of each relationship in turn.

When such a desirable state of affairs has been reached, etiology itself will no longer be treated "atomistically" but in the total context of both the individual and the family.

To sum up, the individual psychopathologist of the analytic persuasion has an in-built structural system postulated in the mind into which events, either normal or abnormal, can be incorporated gradually as the process of internalization takes over during childhood (any time between four and seven years, according to Freud and Piaget). As this internalization increases, so does the child's autonomy and individuality. He becomes more concerned with the outside world, more of an extramural family member, more often in the company of peers and less dependent on the family for emotional and cognitive supplies, and altogether less caught up in family conflict. To the clinician who sees him at this time, the family that seems to participate etiologically in his psychopathology is the unconscious, latent, and fantasied family, whereas later, in adolescence, the irritating, exasperating internal family has manifestly more etiological significance.

An ex-individual psychopathologist who is now a practicing family psychopathologist has an interesting comment to make on the introjective-projective mechanisms that make it so hard to pin down the factor of etiology.

> There is clinical evidence that in the psychopathology of a child a determining factor is hypercathexis of the child as a drive object both internally and in reality by the parents, especially but not exclusively by the mother. Instinctualized impulses which cannot be contained or gratified within the marital relationship are displaced onto the child. The child's behavioral response to these stimuli become part of a mutually reciprocal projection system between the child and the parents within

which continuous mutual gratification becomes self-perpetuating. There is a corresponding hypercathexis of the parent as an object by the child. Persistent instinctual discharge interferes with development of the child's ego and superego structure so that the child remains "open" and responsive to parental impulses. Constant impingement of libidinized and aggressivized stimuli from the environment maintains regression and regressive behavior. Once an instinctualized transactional pattern becomes fixed between two people *it is for the time being not pertinent who started it.* Both are contributing to maintenance of the pathological relationship and either one is theoretically able to interrupt the vicious cycle. This projection system frequently originates from the prolonged displacement of inter-spouse conflicts, parental guilt, blame, anxiety, and inadequacy into the parent's relationships with the child. Interpersonal marital conflict as well as internalized conflict within both parents is kept relatively out of their awareness and thus produce less discomfort for the parents through their preoccupation with the child. When parents devote much of their time, attention, and psychic energy to trying to change the child's behavior, their own functioning may be stabilized (Kramer, unpublished).

One can therefore answer the question: Is child psychopathology family psychopathology? by stating that externalized but not internalized psychopathology is family psychopathology; that family psychopathology is concerned with acting out disorders, outer-directed reactions and problems of shame, whereas internalized psychopathology has more to do with psychoneurotic reactions and problems of guilt.

The old therapeutic test, belonging to medicine, may not work with multidetermined psychological situations. If individual or family psychotherapy is effective it would not necessarily mean that the etiology lies with the individual or with the family. For example, it may begin subclinically in the individual and be exacerbated by the family. Therapeutically, this may be relieved by family therapy but a relapse may occur in the individual that then responds to individual therapy; or it may work the other way around.

If one observes a family together, one immediately becomes conscious of the generational and gender differences that govern the interchanges. Role theory has scrutinized the family with respect to manifest functions, but developmental roles imposed by psychosexual status have received scant attention. This is because family theorists have generally not received any intensive training in child development, while child psychiatrists and child psychologists are usually woefully untrained in transactional dynamics. The bringing together of the developmental and transactional within a single model should certainly provide a fuller understanding of family life.

We can look at the family in several different developmental-transactional ways. Cognitively, within the framework of Piaget, it may represent a very heterogeneous group with members at the sensorimotor, the symbolic, the intuitive-representational, the concrete operational, and the formal operational levels, each one of which implies a radically different way of thinking and communicating. It should not be surprising, therefore, to find that transactions are at times confused and that members may fail to get through to one another. There is no doubt that a great deal of incomprehensibility is taken for granted in family living. The communications that do penetrate may be grossly distorted by the inadequacies and immaturities of the cognitive apparatus. Vocabulary in itself sets limits to understanding for different members. To some extent, this inherent problem is overcome by the fabrication of a basic family language which, like Esperanto, serves the purpose of everyday life by the use of simple concrete expressions and neologisms that have been manufactured for private family use.

On a psychosexual scale, the oral, the anal, the phallic, and the genital members may have basic difficulties in understanding or empathizing with one another. For example, the child who has put the anal phase for the most part behind him may behave unsympathetically and even punitively with the child still in the throes of this particular period. Older children may react with repugnance to the coprophilic interests of the toddler or the gluttonous preoccupations of the infant. A great many children, of course, pass through childhood trailing unresolved conflicts behind, and these are the ones that resonate to all the developmental conflicts occurring within a family at any given time. The adolescent, struggling with the reactivation of early conflicts within him, may display extreme intolerance to all the younger children in the family. To a certain degree, being in a certain developmental phase offers the child some immunity from the stimulations and provocations of other developmental phases, and, for the same reason, he has also some protection from traumata that is not phase-specific.

On a psychosocial scale, while younger members may be struggling to assert their autonomy, to carry out serious and satisfying work, and to achieve clear-cut roles and identities for themselves, the older members of the family may feel themselves in a rut and isolated from each other. So engrossing are these crises that the different members may find it hard to help one another with their own past experience (Anthony, 1973).

It is obvious that we have many answers, not all of them satisfying, but the questions are still increasing and multiplying.

References

Ackerman, N. W.: Family psychopathology and psychoanalysis—Implications of differences. *In* Ackerman, N. W. (Ed.): Family Process. New York, Basic Books, Inc., Publishers, 1970.

Anthony, E. J.: The reactions of parents to the oedipal child. *In* Anthony, E. J., and Benedek, T. (eds.): Parenthood. Boston, Little, Brown & Company, 1970a.

Anthony, E. J.: The influence of maternal psychosis on children—Folie à deux. *In* Anthony, E. J., and Benedek, T. (eds.): Parenthood. Boston, Little, Brown & Company, 1970b.

Anthony, E. J.: A working model for family studies. *In* Anthony, E. J., and Koupernik, C. (eds.): The Child in His Family: The Impact of Disease and Death, Vol. 2. New York, John Wiley & Sons, Inc., 1973.

Bateson, G., Jackson, D., Haley, J., and Weakland, J.: Toward a theory of schizophrenia. Behav. Sci., *1*:251–264, 1956.

Bell, J. B.: A theoretical position for family group therapy. *In* Ackerman, N. W. (ed.): Family Process. New York, Basic Books, Inc., Publishers, 1970.

Dostoyevsky, F.: Crime and Punishment. Trans. C. Garnett. New York, E. P. Dutton & Co., Inc., 1955.

Erikson, E. H.: Youth and Crisis. London, W. W. Norton, 1968.

Freud, A.: Normality and Pathology in Childhood. New York, International Universities Press, 1965.

Freud, A.: Some aspects of the relation between neurotic pathology in childhood and in adult life. Bull. Phila. Assoc. Psychoanal., *17*:111–114, 1967.

Freud, S.: Fragment of an analysis of a case of hysteria (1905): *In* Standard Edition, vol. 7, London, Hogarth Press, 1953.

Freud, S.: Totem and taboo (1913). *In* Standard Edition, vol. 13. London, Hogarth Press, 1953.

Freud, S.: Introductory lecture on psychoanalysis: Part III. General theory of the neuroses (1917). *In* Standard Edition, vol. 16. London, Hogarth Press, 1953.

Haley, J., and Hoffman, L.: Technique of Family Therapy. New York, Basic Books, Inc., Publishers, 1974.

Hartmann, H.: On the reality principle. *In* Essays on Ego Psychology. New York, International Universities Press, 1964.

Kramer, C. H.: The Relationship between Child and Family Psychopathology. Unpublished paper. Obtainable from The Family Institute of Chicago.

Laing, R. D., and Esterson, A.: Sanity, Madness and the Family. London, Tavistock, 1964.

Meissner, W. W.: Thinking about the family—Psychiatric aspects. *In* Ackerman, N. W. (ed.): Family Process. New York, Basic Books, Inc., Publishers, 1970.
Parsons, T.: Social structure and the development of personality: Freud's contribution to the integration of psychology and sociology. Psychiatry, *21*:321–340, 1958.
Rapaport, D.: Dynamic psychology and kantian epistomology. *In* Gill, M. M. (ed.): Collected Papers. New York, Basic Books, Inc., Publishers, 1967.
Satir, V.: Symptomatology: A family production. *In* Howells, J. G. (ed.): Theory and Practice of Family Psychiatry. New York, Brunner/Mazel, 1971.
Sartre, J. P.: Critique de la Raison Dialectique. Paris, Gallimaid, 1960.
Sobel, R.: Adjustment reactions, transient situational disturbances. *In* Freedman, A., and Kaplan, H. (eds.): Psychiatry. Baltimore, The Williams & Wilkins Company, 1967.
Winnicott, D. W.: Collected Papers. London, Tavistock, 1958.
Winnicott, D. W.: The Family and Individual Development. New York, Basic Books, Inc., Publishers, 1965.
Wynne, L.: Some indications and contraindications for exploratory family therapy. *In* Boszormeny-Nagy, I., and Framo, J. L. (eds.): Intensive Family Therapy. New York, Harper & Row, Publishers, Inc., 1965.

Comment

Anthony's chapter presents a brilliant historical review of the principal theoreticians' answer to the question posed in this chapter. He notes Freud's initial stand that childhood neurosis was external and to a large extent familial, that family pathology emerged as a summation of individual family psychopathologies producing child psychopathology. Freud later noted that with intrapsychic disturbances child psychopathology could generate family psychopathology. Ultimately, Freud evolved the concept of a "family complex" in which he compounded the intrapsychic and extrapsychic life of the family, suggesting that parental attitudes and behavior could affect the individual's psychopathology.

Anthony notes that the majority of individual psychopathologists support the concept that childhood psychopathology is almost always not family psychopathology. Therapists like Anna Freud and Winnicott, however, have observed that high-grade disturbances in children are more internally derived and that low-grade disturbances are more externally derived. Anthony feels that many family psychopathologists—Bell, Ackerman, and Haley, for example—would posit that child psychopathology is *sometimes* family psychopathology, depending on the initial orientation of the therapist. He quotes Bell as stating, "The problem is the family," and notes Ackerman's thesis that child psychopathology is part of family psychopathology which grows out of child psychopathology; thus, the psychopathology of the family begins in the chilhood of its members.

Anthony's review of Laingian theory projects mental illness as a sane, self-preserving response to the conflict and confusion within the family, which makes him believe that Laing would feel that the question addressed in this section is irrelevant.

This review presents a balanced historical analysis which most in the field would support. Anthony's emphasis on family psychopathology is most appropriate given recent observations that for many families, the individuals when evaluated seemed free of mental illness, yet when grouped together as a family unit, their interactions can be labeled psychopathological. More research and possibly a new nosology will be required to chronicle this type of interactive psychopathology.

H. KEITH H. BRODIE, M.D.

Should Psychiatric Patients Ever Be Hospitalized Involuntarily?

THOMAS S. SZASZ

State University of New York, Upstate Medical Center

My answer to this question is an emphatic and unqualified "No." Before setting forth my reasons for this answer, I should like to clarify and comment on the key terms used in the question that makes up the title of this chapter.

Who is a psychiatric patient? Ostensibly, it is someone suffering from a mental disease. This presents an immediate obstacle for anyone who believes, as I do, that there are no mental diseases. It also presents an immediate opportunity for demystifying a persistent psychiatric problem. I maintain that being a psychiatric patient has, in fact, nothing to do with having a mental illness. Instead, it has to do with defining oneself, or being defined by someone else, as needing the professional services of a psychiatrist; and with assuming the patient role, or being cast into it, vis-à-vis a psychiatrist (or other mental health professional) (Szasz, 1961).

The issue of consent—that is, of the voluntariness or involuntariness of the patient's relationship to the psychiatrist—thus arises prior to mental hospitalization. It does so with an antecedent question that might be framed as follows: "Should or should not a particular person be regarded and treated as a psychiatric patient?" I contend that in a free society no one should be cast into the role of mental patient against his will (Szasz, 1963). If this premise is granted, the problem of involuntary mental hospitalization is, as it were, aborted: it is "solved" because it cannot come into being. If all psychiatric patients are voluntary, there can be no involuntary

*Portions of this essay have appeared previously in Ideology and Insanity: Essays on the Psychiatric Dehumanization of Man. Garden City, N. Y., Doubleday Co., Inc., 1970, pp. 113–139. Copyright 1970 by Thomas S. Szasz; reprinted by permission of Doubleday & Company.

psychiatry—just as if all workers are voluntary there can be no involuntary servitude.*

The second key term in the title is "hospitalized involuntarily." What is involuntary hospitalization? Ostensibly, it is placing a patient in a medical institution for the purpose of treating his illness. Actually, in the case of so-called psychiatric patients, the term is a euphemistic misnomer, and indeed doubly so: first, because the alleged patient is not sick; and second, because the so-called hospital is in fact a prison.

Much of my argument *against* coercive psychiatry, and much of the argument of those who are *for* it, thus turns on whether we regard the involuntary mental patient as an object or as an agent; on whether we treat him as an irresponsible organism or as a responsible person; and on whether we accept involuntary mental hospitalization as a helpful medical-therapeutic intervention or reject it as a harmful judicial-penal sanction.

History

Involuntary mental hospitalization—or compulsory admission to hospital, as it is called in England—has always been, and still is, the paradigmatic policy of psychiatry. Whenever and wherever psychiatry has been recognized and practiced as the medical specialty dealing with the treatment of insanity, madness, or mental disease, then and there persons have been incarcerated in insane asylums, madhouses, or mental hospitals.

The coercion and restraint of the mental patient by the psychiatrist—or, better, of the madman by the alienist, as these protagonists were first called—is thus coeval with the origin and development of psychiatry. As a discrete discipline, psychiatry began in the seventeenth century with the building of insane asylums, first in France, then throughout the civilized world. These institutions were, of course, prisons in which not only so-called madmen were confined but all of society's undesirables—abandoned children, prostitutes, incurably sick persons, the aged and indigent (Szasz, 1970, pp. 13–16).

How did people generally, and in particular those directly responsible for these confinements—the legislators and jurists, the physicians and the victims' relatives—justify such incarceration of persons not guilty of criminal offenses? The answer is: by means of the imagery and rhetoric of madness, insanity, psychosis, schizophrenia, mental illness—call it what you will—which transformed the inmate into a "patient," his prison into a

*In contemporary practice there is a grey area composed of persons who do not formally or verbally consent to being psychiatric patients but who also make no protest against being so treated. For the sake of clarity, I shall here either not consider the particular circumstances of such persons, or shall consider their cases as falling in the category of voluntary psychiatric patients. My argument is thus addressed to the involuntary hospitalization of individuals who object, verbally or behaviorally, to psychiatric confinement, and who are demonstrably restrained by legal and medical authorities.

"hospital," and his warden into a "doctor." Characteristically, the first official proposition of the Association of Medical Superintendents of American Institutions for the Insane, the organization which became, in 1921, the American Psychiatric Association, was: "Resolved, that it is the unanimous sense of this convention that the attempt to abandon entirely the use of all means of personal restraint is not sanctioned by the true interests of the insane" (Ridenour, 1961, p. 76).

Ever since then, this paternalistic justification of psychiatric coercion has been a prominent theme in psychiatry, not only in America but throughout the world. Thus, in 1967—123 years after the drafting of its first resolution—the American Psychiatric Association reaffirmed its support of psychiatric coercion and restraint. In a "Position Statement on the Question of the Adequacy of Treatment," the Association declared that "restraints may be imposed [on the patient] from within by pharmacologic means or by locking the door of a ward. Either imposition may be a legitimate component of a treatment program" (APA, 1967).

Justifications for involuntary psychiatric interventions of all kinds, and especially for involuntary mental hospitalization, similar to those accepted in the United States have, of course, been advanced, and continue to be advanced, in other countries. In short, just as, for millennia, involuntary servitude had been accepted as a proper economic and social arrangement, so for centuries, involuntary psychiatry has been accepted as a proper medical and therapeutic arrangement.

It is this entire system of interlocking psychiatric ideas and institutions, justifications and practices, which—beginning some twenty years ago, first in a series of articles, and then in a series of books—I have analyzed and attacked. In these publications I describe and document the precise legal status of the mental hospital patient—as an innocent person incarcerated in a psychiatric prison; articulate my objections to institutional psychiatry—as an extra-legal system of penology and punishments; and demonstrate what seems to me, in a free society, our only morally proper option with respect to the problem of so-called psychiatric abuses—namely, the complete abolition of all involuntary psychiatric interventions (Szasz, 1961, 1963, 1970, 1977).

Evidence Against Involuntary Hospitalization

Let me now consider the evidence that supports my contention that involuntary mental hospitalization does not serve the purpose of helping or treating so-called mentally ill persons; and that, regardless of its avowed or actual purposes, involuntary psychiatry, like involuntary servitude, is incompatible with the moral principles and legal procedures of a free society.

The medical evidence. Mental illness is a metaphor. If by "disease" we mean a disorder of the physicochemical machinery of the human body, then it is clear that what we call functional mental diseases are not diseases at all. Persons said to be suffering from such disorders are socially deviant or inept, or in conflict with individuals, groups, or institutions. Since they do not suffer from disease, it is impossible to "treat" them for any sickness.

Although the term "mentally ill" is usually applied to persons who do not suffer from bodily disease, it is sometimes applied also to persons who do—for example, to individuals intoxicated with alcohol or other drugs, or to elderly people suffering from degenerative disease of the brain. When such persons are hospitalized involuntarily, the primary purpose is to exercise social control over their behavior; treatment of the disease is, at best, a secondary consideration. Frequently, therapy is nonexistent, and custodial care is dubbed "treatment."

In short, the commitment of persons suffering from "functional psychoses" serves moral and social, rather than medical and therapeutic, purposes. Hence, even if, as a result of future research, certain conditions now believed to be "functional" mental illnesses were to be shown to be "organic," my argument against involuntary mental hospitalization would remain unaffected.

The moral evidence. In free societies, the relationship between physician and patient is predicated on the legal presumption that the individual "owns" his body and his personality. The physician can examine and treat a patient only with his consent; the latter is free to reject treatment—for example, an operation for cancer. As John Stuart Mill put it, ". . . each person is the proper guardian of his own health, whether bodily, or mental and spiritual" (Mill, 1859). Commitment is incompatible with this moral principle.

This historical evidence. Commitment practices flourished long before there were any mental or psychiatric "treatments" of "mental diseases." Indeed, madness or mental illness was not always a necessary condition for commitment. For example, in the seventeenth century, "children of artisans and other poor inhabitants of Paris up to the age of 25, . . . girls who were debauched or in evident danger of being debauched," and other "miserables" of the community, such as epileptics, people with venereal diseases, and poor people with chronic diseases of all sorts, were all considered fit subjects for confinement in the Hôpital Général (Rosen, 1963). In 1860, when Mrs. Packard was incarcerated for disagreeing with her minister-husband, the commitment laws of the State of Illinois explicitly proclaimed that "married women . . . may be entered or detained in the hospital at the request of the husband of the woman or guardian . . . without the evidence of insanity required in other cases" (Szasz, 1970, p. 307).

The literary evidence. Involuntary mental hospitalization plays a significant part in numerous short stories and novels from many countries. In none that I have encountered is commitment portrayed as helpful to the hospitalized person; instead, it is always depicted as an arrangement serving interests antagonistic to those of the so-called patient.

In short, I am suggesting that commitment constitutes a social arrangement whereby one part of society secures certain advantages for itself at the expense of another part. To do so, the oppressors must possess an ideology to justify their aims and actions; and they must be able to enlist the police power of the state to impose their will on the oppressed members. What makes such an arrangement morally legitimate or illegitimate? If the use of state power to punish lawbreakers is legitimate, why is its use to commit the insane not also legitimate?

In the first place, the difference between committing the "insane" and imprisoning the "criminal" is essentially the same as the difference between the rule of man and the rule of law: whereas the "insane" are subjected to the coercive controls of the state because persons more powerful than they have labeled them as "psychotic," "criminals" are subjected to such controls because they have violated legal rules applicable equally to all.

The second difference between these two proceedings lies in their professed aims. The principal purpose of imprisoning criminals is to protect the liberties of the law-abiding members of society. Since the individual subject to commitment is not considered a threat to liberty in the same way as the accused criminal is—if he were, he would be prosecuted—his removal from society cannot be justified on the same grounds. Justification for commitment must thus rest on its therapeutic promise and potential: it will help restore the "patients" to "mental health." But if this can be accomplished only at the cost of robbing the individual of liberty, involuntary mental hospitalization becomes only a verbal camouflage for what is, in effect, punishment. Such "therapeutic" punishment differs, however, from traditional judicial punishment, in that the accused criminal enjoys a rich panoply of constitutional protections against false accusation and illegal prosecution, whereas the accused mental patient is deprived of these protections.

To lend further support to my argument against involuntary mental hospitalization, I shall now briefly review the similarities between chattel slavery and involuntary psychiatry.

Involuntary Psychiatry and Slavery

Suppose that a person wished to study slavery. How would he go about doing so? First, he might study slaves. He would then find that such persons are generally brutish, poor, and uneducated, and he might accordingly conclude that slavery is their "natural" or appropriate social state. Such, indeed, have been the methods and conclusions of innumerable men throughout the ages. Even the great Aristotle held that slaves were "naturally" inferior and were hence justly subdued. "From the hour of their birth," he asserted, "some are marked for subjection, others for rule" (Davis, 1966, p. 70). This view is similar to the modern concept of "schizophrenia" as a genetically caused disease.

Another student, "biased" by contempt for the institution of slavery, might proceed differently. He would maintain that there can be no slave without a master holding him in bondage. Accordingly, he would consider slavery a type of human relationship and, more generally, a social institution, supported by custom, law, religion, and force. From this point of view, the study of masters is at least as relevant to the study of slavery as is the study of slaves.

The latter point of view is generally accepted today with regard to involuntary servitude, but not with regard to involuntary psychiatry. "Mental illness" of the type found in psychiatric hospitals has been investigated for centuries, and continues to be investigated today, in much the same ways as slaves had been studied in the antebellum South and before. Then, the "existence" of slaves was taken for granted; their biological and social characteristics were accordingly noted and catalogued. Today, the "existence" of "mental patients" is taken for granted; their biological and social characteristics are accordingly noted and catalogued. The fundamental parallel between master and slave on the one hand, and institutional psychiatrist and involuntarily hospitalized patient on the other, thus lies in this: in each instance, the former member of the pair *defines* the social role of the latter, and *casts* him in that role by force (Szasz, 1977).

Wherever there is slavery, there must be criteria for who may and who may not be enslaved. In ancient times, any people could be enslaved. Bondage was the usual consequence of military defeat. After the advent of Christianity, although the people of Europe continued to make war upon each other, they ceased enslaving prisoners who were Christians. According to Dwight Dumond, ". . . the theory that a Christian could not be enslaved soon gained such wide endorsement as to be considered a point of international law" (Dumond, 1961, p. 4). By the time of the colonization of America, the people of the Western world considered only black persons appropriate subjects for slave trade.

The criteria for distinguishing between those who may be incarcerated in mental hospitals and those who may not be has had a similar history and evolution. At first—300 years ago—virtually anyone could be; later—in the nineteenth century—only madmen and madwomen could be; now only "mental patients" who are "dangerous to themselves or others" can be. It is significant that in each case narrowing the criteria—for enslavement in the one, for commitment in the other—has greatly strengthened the moral legitimacy of a fundamentally immoral practice.

A basic assumption of American slavery was that the Negro was racially inferior to the Caucasian. Similarly, the basic assumption of institutional psychiatry is that the mentally ill person is psychiatrically inferior to the mentally healthy. Like the black slave, the mental patient is like a child: he does not know what is in his best interest and therefore needs others to control and protect him. Psychiatrists often care deeply for their involuntary patients, whom they consider—in contrast with the merely "neurotic" persons—"psychotic," which is to say, "very sick." Hence, such patients must be cared for as the "irresponsible children" they are considered to be.

This perspective of paternalism has played an exceedingly important part in justifying both slavery and involuntary hospitalization. Aristotle defined slavery as "an essentially domestic relationship"; in so doing, writes Davis, he "endowed it with the sanction of paternal authority, and helped to establish a precedent that would govern discussions of political philosophers as late as the eighteenth century" (Davis, 1966, p. 69). The relationship between psychiatrists and mental patients has been, and continues to be, viewed in the same way. "If a man brings his daughter to me from California," declares Braceland, "because she is in manifest danger of falling into vice or in some way disgracing herself, he doesn't expect me to let her loose in my hometown for that same thing to happen" (Braceland, 1961, p. 71). Almost any article or book dealing with the "care" of involuntary mental patients may be cited to illustrate the contention that physicians fall back on paternalism to justify their coercive control over the uncooperative patient. "Certain cases," writes Solomon in an article on suicide, " . . . must be considered irresponsible, not only with respect to violent impulses, but also in all medical matters." In this class, which he labels "The Irresponsible," he places "Children," "The Mentally Retarded," "The Psychotic," and "The Severely or Terminally Ill." Solomon's conclusion is that "Repugnant though it may be, he [the physician] may have to act against the patient's wishes in order to protect the patient's life and that of others" (Solomon, 1967). The fact that, as in the case of slavery, the physician needs the police power of the state to maintain his relationship with his involuntary patient does not seem to affect this self-serving image of institutional psychiatry.

Paternalism is the crucial explanation for the stubborn contradiction and conflict about whether the practices employed by slaveholders and institutional psychiatrists are "therapeutic" or "noxious." Masters and mad-doctors profess their benevolence; their slaves and captives protest against their malevolence. In *Ward 7,* Valeriy Tarsis presents the following dialogue between his protagonist-patient and the mental hospital physician: "This is the position. I don't regard you as a doctor. You call this a hospital. I call it a prison. . . . So now, let's get everything straight. I am your prisoner, you are my jailer, and there isn't going to be any nonsense about my health . . . or treatment" (Tarsis, 1965, p. 62).

This is the monotonous dialogue between oppressors and oppressed. The ruler looks in the mirror and sees a liberator; the ruled looks at the ruler and sees a tyrant. If the physican has the power to incarcerate the patient and uses it, their relationship will inevitably fit into this mold. If one cannot ask the subject whether he likes being enslaved or committed, whipped or electroshocked—because he is not a fit judge of his own "best interests"—then one is left with the contending opinions of the practitioners and their critics. The practitioners insist that their coercive measures are beneficial; the critics, that they are harmful.

The defenders of slavery thus claimed that the Negro "is happier . . . as a slave, than he could be as a free man; this is the result of the peculiarities of his character" (Elkins, 1959, p. 190); that "it was actually an act of liberation to remove Negroes from their harsh world of sin and dark superstition"; and that "Negroes were better off in a Christian land, even as slaves, than living like beasts in Africa" (Davis, 1966, pp. 186, 190).

Similarly, the defenders of involuntary mental hospitalization claim that the mental patient is healthier—the twentieth century synonym for the nineteenth-century term "happier"—as a psychiatric prisoner than he would be as a free citizen; that "[t]he basic purpose of commitment is to make sure that sick human beings get the care that is appropriate to their needs . . ." (Ewalt, 1961, p. 75); and that "[i]t is a feature of some illnesses that people do not have insight into the fact that they are sick. In short, sometimes it is necessary to protect them [the mentally ill] for a while from themselves . . . " (Braceland, 1961, p. 64). It requires no great feat of imagination to see how comforting—indeed, how absolutely necessary—these views were to the advocates of involuntary servitude, and are now to the advocates of involuntary psychiatry.

The Master-Subject Relationship

There are essential similarities in all relationships between masters and subjects—whether they be between plantation owners and Negro slaves, or institutional psychiatrists and committed mental patients.

To maintain a relationship of personal or class superiority, it is necessary, as a rule, that the oppressor keep the oppressed uninformed, especially about matters pertinent to their relationship. In America the history of the systematic efforts by the whites to keep the Negro ignorant is well known. A dramatic example is the law passed in 1824 by the Virginia Assembly that provided a $50 fine and two months' imprisonment for teaching *free* Negroes to read and write (Dumond, 1961, p. 11).

A similar effort educationally to degrade and psychologically to impoverish their charges characterizes the acts of the managers of madhouses. In most prisons in the United States, it is possible for a convict to obtain a high-school diploma, to learn a trade, to become an amateur lawyer, or to write a book. None of these things is possible in a mental hospital. The principal requirement for an inmate of such an institution is to accept the psychiatric ideology of his "illness" and the things he must do to "recover" from it. The committed patient must thus accept the view that he is "sick" and that his captors are "well"; that his own view of himself is false and that of his captors true; and that to effect any change in his social situation he must relinquish his "sick" views and adopt the "healthy" views of those who have power over him. By accepting himself as "sick," and his institutional environment and the various manipulations imposed on him by the staff as "treatment," the mental patient is compelled to authenticate the psychiatrist's role as that of a benevolent physician curing mental illness. The mental patient who maintains the forbidden image of reality that the institutional psychiatrist is a jailer is considered paranoid. Moreover, since most patients—as do oppressed people generally—sooner or later accept the ideas imposed on them by their superiors, hospital psychiatrists are constantly immersed in an environment where their identity as "doctors" is affirmed. The moral superiority of white men over black was similarly authenticated and affirmed through the association between slaveowners and slaves.

In both situations, the oppressor first subjugates his adversary and then cites his oppressed status as proof of his inferiority. Once this process is set in motion, it develops its own momentum and psychological logic.

Looking at the relationship, the oppressor will see his superiority and hence his well-deserved dominance, and the oppressed will see his inferiority and hence his well-deserved submission. In race relations in the United States, we continue to reap the bitter results of this philosophy, while in psychiatry we are even now sowing the seeds of this poisonous fruit whose eventual harvest may be equally bitter and long.

Oppression and degradation are unpleasant to behold and are, therefore, frequently disguised or concealed. One method for doing so is to segregate—in special areas, as in camps or "hospitals"—the degraded human beings. Another is to conceal the social realities behind the fictional facade of our "language games." While psychiatric language games may seem fanciful, the psychiatric idiom is actually only a dialect of the common language of oppressors. Slaveholders called the slaves "livestock," mothers "breeders," their children "increase," and gave the term "drivers" to the men set over them at work (Dumond, 1961, p. 251). The defenders of psychiatric imprisonment call their institutions "hospitals," the inmates "patients," and the keepers "doctors"; they refer to the sentence as "treatment," and to the deprivation of liberty as "protection of the patient's best interests."

In both cases, the semantic deceptions are supplemented by appeals to tradition, to morality, and to social necessity. The proslavery forces in America argued that the abolitionists were wrong because "they were seeking to overthrow an ancient institution, one which was recognized by the Scriptures, recognized by the Constitution, and imbedded in the structure of southern society" (Dumond, 1961, p. 233). Thus, an editorial in the Washington Telegraph in 1837 asserted, "As a man, a Christian, and a citizen, we believe that slavery is right; that the condition of the slave, as it now exists in slaveholding states, is the best existing organization of civil society"; while another pro-slavery author, writing in 1862, defended the institution on mainly religious grounds: "Slavery, authorized by God, permitted by Jesus Christ, sanctioned by the apostles, maintained by good men of all ages, is still existing in a portion of our beloved country" (Elkins, 1959, p. 36). One has only to scan present-day psychiatric journals, popular magazines, or daily newspapers to find involuntary mental hospitalization similarly extolled and defended.

The contemporary reader may find it difficult to believe how unquestioningly slavery was accepted as a natural and beneficial social arrangement. Even as great a liberal thinker as John Locke did not advocate its abolition. Moreover, protests against the slave trade would have provoked the hostility of powerful religious and economic interests. Opposition to it, as Davis observes, would therefore have required "considerable independence of mind, since the Portuguese slave posts were closely connected with missionary establishments and criticism of the African slave trade might challenge the very ideal of spreading the faith" (Davis, 1966, p. 187).

Indeed, the would-be critic or opponent of slavery would have found himself at odds with all the tradition and wisdom of Western civilization. ". . . [O]ne could not lightly challenge," writes Davis, "an institution approved not only by the Fathers and canons of the Church, but by the most illustrious writers of antiquity. . . . [T]he revival of classical learning, which may have helped to liberate the mind of Europe from bondage to ignorance and superstition, only reinforced the traditional justification for human slavery. . . . [H]ow could an institution supported by so many authorities and sanctioned by the general custom of nations be intrinsically unjust or repugnant to natural reason?" (Davis, 1966, pp. 107, 115).

In Western nations and the Soviet bloc alike, there are thus two contradictory views on commitment. According to the one, involuntary mental hospitalization is an indispensable method of medical healing and a humane type of social control; according to the other, it is a contemptible abuse of the medical relationship and a type of imprisonment without trial. We adopt the former view and consider commitment "proper" if we use it on victims of our own choosing whom we despise; we adopt the latter view and consider commitment "improper" if our enemies use it on victims of their choosing whom we esteem.

Practical Implications

The change in perspective—from seeing slavery occasioned by the "inferiority" of the Negro and commitment by the "insanity" of the patient, to seeing each occasioned by the interplay of, and especially the power relations between, the participants—has far-reaching practical implications. In the case of slavery, it meant not only that the slaves had an obligation to revolt and emancipate themselves, but also that the masters had an even greater obligation to renounce their roles as slaveholders. Naturally, a slaveholder with such ideas felt compelled to set his slaves free, at whatever cost to himself. This is precisely what some slaveowners did. Their action had profound consequences in a social system based on slavery.

For the individual slaveholder who set his slaves free, the act led invariably to his expulsion from the community—through economic pressure or personal harassment or both. Such persons usually emigrated to the North. For the nation as a whole, these acts and the abolitionist sentiments behind them symbolized a fundamental moral rift between those who regarded Negroes as objects or slaves, and those who regarded them as persons or citizens. The former could persist in regarding the slave as existing in nature, whereas the latter could not deny his own moral responsibility for creating man in the image, not of God, but of the slave-animal.

The implications of this perspective for involuntary psychiatry are equally clear. A psychiatrist who accepts as his "patient" a person who does not wish to be his patient, defines him as a "mentally ill" person, then incarcerates him in an institution, bars his escape from the institution and from the role of mental patient, and proceeds to "treat" him against his will—such a psychiatrist, I maintain, creates "mental illness" and "mental patients." He does so in exactly the same way as the white man who sailed for Africa, captured the Negro, brought him to America in shackles, and then sold him as if he were an animal, created slavery and slaves.

The parallel between involuntary servitude and involuntary psychiatry may be carried one step further: denunciation of slavery and the renouncing of slaveholding by some slaveowners led to certain social problems, such as Negro unemployment, the importation of cheap European labor, and a gradual splitting of the country into pro- and antislavery factions. Similarly, criticisms of involuntary mental hospitalization and the renouncing by some psychiatrists of relationships with involuntary mental patients have led to professional problems in the past, and are likely to do so again in the future. Psychiatrists restricting their work to psychoanalysis and psychotherapy have been accused of not being "real doctors"—as if depriving a person of his liberty required medical skills; of "shirking their responsibilities" to their colleagues and to society by accepting only the "easier cases" and refusing to treat the "seriously mentally ill" patient—as if avoiding treating persons who do not want to be treated were itself a kind of unprofessional conduct; and of undermining the profession of psychiatry—as if practicing self-control and eschewing violence were newly discovered forms of immorality.

For millennia, people did not question the social necessity, and hence the moral legitimacy, of involuntary servitude. Today, they do not generally question the social necessity, and hence the moral legitimacy, of involuntary psychiatry. There is now a massive consensus, not only in the United States but throughout the "civilized" world, that, when "properly used," involuntary mental hospitalization is socially necessary for the nonpatients outside of mental hospitals and is personally beneficial for the patients inside them. Hence it is only possible to debate *who* should be hospitalized, or *how*, or for *how long*—but not *whether anyone should* be. I submit, however, that just as it is improper to enslave anyone—whether he is black or white, Moslem or Christian—so it is improper to hospitalize anyone without his consent—whether he is depressed or paranoid, hysterical or schizophrenic.

Our unwillingness to look at this problem searchingly may be compared to the unwillingness of the South to look at slavery. ". . . [A] democratic people," writes Elkins, "no longer 'reasons' with itself when it is all of the same mind. Men will then only warn and exhort each other, that their solidarity may be yet more perfect. The South's intellectuals, after the 1830s, did really little more than this. And when the enemy's reality disappears, when his concreteness recedes, then intellect itself, with nothing more to resist it and give it reasonance, merges with the mass and stultifies, and shadows become monsters" (Elkins, 1959, p. 222).

Our growing preoccupation with the menace of mental illness may be a manifestation of just such a process—in which "concreteness recedes . . . and shadows become monsters." A democratic nation, as we have been warned by Tocqueville, is especially vulnerable to the hazards of a surfeit of agreement: "The authority of a king is physical, and controls the actions of men without subduing their will. But the majority possesses a power that is physical and moral at the same time, which acts upon the will as much as upon the actions, and represses not only all contests, but all controversy" (Tocqueville, 1835-40, Vol. I, p. 273).

The idea that a person accused of crime is innocent until proven guilty is not shared by people everywhere but is, as I need hardly belabor, characteristically English in its historical origin and singularly Anglo-American in its consistent social application. And so is its corollary, namely that an individual has an inalienable right to personal liberty unless he has been duly convicted in court of an offense punishable by imprisonment. Because this magnificent edifice of dignity and liberty has been undermined, and continues to be undermined, by psychiatry, I consider the abolition of involuntary psychiatric interventions to be an especially important link in the chain I have tried to forge for restraining this mortal enemy of individualism and self-determination. I hope that my work will help people to discriminate between two types of physicians: those who heal, not so much because they are saints, but because *that is their job*; and those who harm, not so much because they are sinners, but because *that is their job*. And if some doctors harm—torture rather than treat, murder the soul rather than minister to the body—that is, in part, because society, through the state, asks them, and pays them, to do so.

We saw it happen in Nazi Germany, and we hanged many of the doctors. We see it happen in the Soviet Union, and we denounce the doctors with righteous indignation. But when will we see that the same things are happening in the so-called free societies? When will we recognize—and publicly identify—the medical criminals among us? Or is the very possibility of perceiving many of our leading psychiatrists and psychiatric institutions in this way precluded by the fact that they represent the officially "correct" views and practices? By the fact that they have the ears of our lawyers and legislators, journalists and judges? And by the fact that they control the vast funds, collected by the state through taxing the citizens, which finance an enterprise whose basic moral legitimacy I have called into question?

References

American Psychiatric Association (APA): Position statement on the question of the adequacy of treatment. Am. J. Psychiatry, *123*:1458–1460, 1967, p. 1459.

Braceland, F.J.: *In* Constitutional Rights of the Mentally Ill. Washington, D.C., U.S. Government Printing Office, 1961, pp. 63–74.

Davis, D.B.: The Problem of Slavery in Western Culture. Ithaca, N.Y., Cornell University Press, 1966.

Dumond, D.L.: Antislavery: The Crusade for Freedom. Ann Arbor, University of Michigan Press, 1961.
Elkins, S.M.: Slavery: A Problem in American Institutional and Intellectual Life. New York, Universal Library, 1963.
Ewalt, J.: *In* Constitutional Rights of the Mentally Ill. Washington, D.C., U.S. Government Printing Office, 1961, pp. 74–89.
Mill, J.S.: On Liberty [1859]. Chicago, Henry Regnery Company, 1955, p. 18.
Ridenour, N.: Mental Health in the United States: A Fifty-Year History. Cambridge, Mass., Harvard University Press, 1961, p. 76.
Rosen, G.: Social attitudes to irrationality and madness in 17th and 18th century Europe. J. Hist. Med. Allied Sci. *18*:220–240, 1963.
Solomon, P.: The burden of responsibility in suicide. J.A.M.A., *199*:321–324, 1967.
Szasz, T.S.: The Myth of Mental Illness: Foundations of a Theory of Personal Conduct. New York, Hoeber-Harper, 1961; rev. ed., New York, Harper & Row, 1974.
Szasz, T.S.: Law, Liberty, and Psychiatry: An Inquiry into the Social Uses of Mental Health Practices. New York, Macmillan, Inc., 1963.
Szasz, T.S.: The Manufacture of Madness: A Comparative Study of the Inquisition and the Mental Health Movement. New York, Harper & Row, Publishers, 1970.
Szasz, T.S.: Psychiatric Slavery: The Dilemma of Involuntary Psychiatry as Exemplified by the Case of Kenneth Donaldson. New York, The Free Press, 1977.
Tarsis, V.: Ward 7: An Autobiographical Novel. London, Collins and Harvill, 1965.
Tocqueville, A. de: Democracy in America [1835–40]. New York, Vintage, 1945.

Comment

Few questions arouse such strong feelings among mental health professionals or the public as that of involuntary commitment for reasons of mental illness. The fields of psychiatry and the law meet (or clash!) around this issue, whose resolution entails societal values and concerns of social responsibility and individual freedom.

Dr. Szasz responds with an emphatic and unqualified "no" to the proposition of involuntary hospitalization for mental illness. Szasz argues as follows: No one in a free society should become a "patient" to a psychiatrist against his will. It is only by being so designated and cast into the role of patient that one is judged to have a "mental illness." Once so designated, Szasz argues, the next step is to be hospitalized (incarcerated) involuntarily in a "mental institution," presumably for the purpose of being treated for one's disease. However, Szasz argues that "disease" and "mental illness" are being used allegorically here, since persons with schizophrenia, manic-depressive psychosis, and related disorders are not medically ill in the sense of having demonstrable abnormalities of the functioning of the brain. Rather, they are socially deviant, inept, or in conflict with other individuals, groups, or institutions. Of course if a person breaks the law, he may properly be subject to arrest and adjudication and, with due process, may in fact be convicted of a crime and appropriately sentenced. However, to curtail his personal freedom and civil liberties by the metaphorical use of the notion of sickness, mental illness, and the like is an injustice and misuse of medical practice. Szasz believes that the whole practice of involuntary hospitalization comes about as a means by which society can remove persons with objectionable or aberrant behavior.

There are problems with the extreme philosophical position Szasz takes. Unless one adopts an all-or-nothing view of liberty in which this social value is placed over all others, most persons would agree that there are circumstances in which the freedom of a disturbed, dangerous, or self-destructive individual should be temporarily curtailed. Few would take issue with preventing a toddler from wandering out into traffic, although this is restricting the freedom of an individual. Most would assent also to restraining a person who is delusional or delirious from a brain abscess or the accidental ingestion of LSD and who is about to jump out a high window or mortally wound a person he delusionally believes is persecuting him. We certainly would not wait until such a person commits a crime before restraining him.

Most of the patients who are involuntarily committed to mental institutions suffer from schizophrenia or severe forms of manic-depressive psychosis.

Part of Szasz's arguments rests on the thesis that these are not real illnesses. Recent research strongly indicates that these disorders are in fact biologically based medical diseases, at least in part. Patients with these conditions are not simply socially deviant out of choice. They are medically ill in the same sense as a person with acute bacterial pneumonia (who may also be delirious and irrational because of toxins and high fever).

In arguing his case, Szasz relies heavily upon the analogy between chattel slavery and involuntary psychiatry; that is, an analogy between the slave owner and the slave on the one hand and the psychiatrist and his involuntary mental patient on the other. Many will find such an analogy outrageous and dismiss the argument out of hand. However, the fact that Szasz commands the attention of a large audience suggests some substance to his ideas or at least that his arguments arouse a sensitivity we all share in matters of personal freedom.

The question posed in this chapter will probably never have a completely satisfactory answer. It is the inherent conflict between individual freedom and liberty on the one hand and concerns for the protection of society and the compassionate treatment of the mentally deranged on the other. It is the conflict between the reliance on an adversarial and rule-oriented system on the one hand and the reliance on sound, informed, but potentially paternalistic judgments on the other. The manner in which a society answers this question at any point in its history doubtless depends upon the current needs of that society, the dangers it perceives, and the values it treasures the most.

JOHN PAUL BRADY, M.D.

Should Homosexuals Adopt Children?

RICHARD GREEN

State University of New York at Stony Brook

General issues

What might appear at first to be a simple, easily ansered "yes" or "no" question is, in fact, highly complex. The more I contemplated the reply, the more I became entangled by the myriad issues.

Some questions which came to mind: Is there evidence that homosexually oriented persons are better or worse at parenting? What effects might parental sexual orientation have on the psychosexual development of the child? Is the prospective adoptive parent a single male or a coupled male, a single or a coupled female? How old is the child? What is the sex of the child? Does the potential family live in an urban or rural, conservative or liberal area? To what degree will the child be stigmatized? Does the friendship network of the prospective parent(s) include persons of both sexes and of both homosexual and heterosexual orientation? What is the degree of commitment of the prospective parent toward encouraging a homosexual or heterosexual orientation for the child? How explicit would the prospective parent be regarding interpersonal adult sexuality in the presence of the child?

The most compelling argument for not responding to the editors' invitation to write this chapter is the considerable degree of speculation required in its construction. If I had a harder data base from which to generate a response, I would feel considerably more comfortable. Then I could be on relatively firm empirical ground before responding to an exceptionally controversial question. Indeed, it has been a historical mistake of psychiatry to speak beyond its data base. My concern is that I will contribute further to this mistake. On the other hand, the question is topical, currently engaging courts of law, and to ignore it might be an equal disservice. The pages which follow, in conjunction with the viewpoints of others, will, it is hoped, provide a forum for evaluating the many considerations required to answer this question.

Undoubtedly, there is something unique about the question "should *homosexuals* be allowed to adopt children?" People do not ask "should *heterosexuals* be allowed to adopt children?" When they raise questions about a prospective heterosexual parent, they are merely reflecting on specific characteristics of *that* heterosexual. Thus, there is an implied assumption that homosexuality *per se* might well overrule and supersede all other qualities of the individual such that the question may be simply answered "no," based solely on the prospective parent's sexual orientation.

Why should this be the case? Is there something inherently defective in the personality structure of a homosexually oriented person to render that male or female incapable of effective parenthood? Effective adoptive parenthood requires genuine commitment to the well-being and welfare of a child and promotion of that child's development to its full potential. Is there evidence of some general defect in the character of the homosexually oriented individual which demonstrates an inability to make that commitment?

Many persons, with greater or lesser degrees of homosexual orientation, have functioned as parents for years. Typically, they married heterosexually, may have been consciously aware of some degree of homosexual orientation, and mothered or fathered children prior to disruption of the marriage. To date there is no evidence that these persons functioned any more or less effectively as parents than other predivorcing couples. Their status as parents after the divorce and the adoption of an open homosexual life style will be discussed in a section below.

Recent years have seen a resurgence of debate as to whether homosexuality in and of itself should be considered a mental disorder. Unquestionably, the pendulum of psychiatric opinion has swung, based on contemporary research, in the direction that homosexuality *per se* does not constitute a mental disorder. The early clinical, uncontrolled case studies reported a variety of psychologic defects in individuals homosexually oriented and in psychiatric treatment. Many researchers pointed to the fallacy of generalizing from these clinical samples to the vast nonpatient homosexual population (Hoffman, 1968; Marmor, 1972; Green, 1972). The parallel was given that it would be scientifically specious to generalize from a heterosexual clinical sample, perhaps rampant with a variety of psychological problems, to the general heterosexual population and then brand heterosexuality a mental disorder. Others, however, argue that while all patients may have problems, those of the homosexual sample are unique in terms of residual castration fear, penis envy, and lack of separation-individuation from a parenting figure (Bieber et al., 1962; Socarides, 1968). These defects may be seen as rendering a person less capable of effective parenting. However, the hard empirical data for this view have fallen considerably short of convincing the general scientific and nonpsychoanalytic psychiatric community. The most compelling evidence of the change in view of homosexuality being *sine qua non* of mental disorder is the removal of homosexuality *per se* from the American Psychiatric Association's Diagnostic and Statistical Manual of Mental Disorders. Recent research conducted on large, nonclinical samples of heterosexual and homosexual males and females will be reviewed later.

Theories of psychosexual development

HETEROSEXUALITY

Theories of psychosexual development abound. They include psychodynamic, social learning, role modeling, cognitive-developmental, and others. Psychosexual development or the development of sexual identity has several components. First, there is core morphologic identity, a person's initial self-concept of being anatomically male or female. Second, there is gender-role behavior, those behaviors which in a given culture and time are dimorphic for males and females. This is typically called "masculinity" and "femininity." Finally, there is sexual partner preference or sexual orientation (Green, 1974).

Psychodynamic models, simply described, view sexual identification as initially taking place with the same sex parent, with a subsequent transfer to the opposite sex parent. This occurs during resolution of the Oedipus complex for the male with disappearance of castration fear, and as a result of resolution of the Electra complex for the female, at about 5 or 6 years.

While earlier psychoanalytic writings stressed that core-identity evolved during resolution of the "family romance," more contemporary analytic work (Stoller, 1968; Kleeman, 1971) demonstrated that core-morphologic identity evolves during the first year or two of life. It appears to be a primary identification with one or the other parent, perhaps partly biologically determined, but probably largely socially learned (Stoller, 1968; 1975).

Gender-role behavior, which manifests during preschool years and becomes rapidly more dimorphic during early grade school, is also the subject of dispute with respect to its origins. Controversy exists as to the degree to which such behaviors are socially learned in consequence of a sex-typing culture personified by parent, school teacher, peer group, and mass media, or whether such behaviors are biologically programmed. In the latter view, some activities, such as rough-and-tumble aggressive play or doll-play, are more "physiologically available" to males or females, respectively (Ehrhardt and Baker, 1974).

Finally, the genesis of the direction of sexual-partner preference remains the greatest enigma of the three components of sexual identity. Many are not convinced by psychoanalytic theory, a theory which remains a minority viewpoint in world-wide psychiatry, and do not accept penis envy, castration fear, and oedipal theory as explanatory of later sexual partner preference. Social learning theorists who view same-sex identification by children and later sexual orientation as purely products of role-modeling, are also not completely secure within their theoretic corner. If sexual orientation were purely determined by modeling orientation of the same-sex parent, there would be few homosexuals, since the disproportionately vast majority had heterosexual parents. While it could be argued that the prehomosexual child is role-modeling the other sex parent, one would expect to see more evidence of this identification, other than sexual orientation. The great majority of homosexual males are not feminine, or "simulations" of their mothers, and the great majority of homosexual females are not masculine or "reincarnations" of their fathers.

The nuclear family has traditionally been seen as providing the "appropriate" role-models for adoption of the conventional societal representation of the husband-wife, mother-father, heterosexual dyadic couple. However, in recent years, we have witnessed a rapidly escalating divorce rate and increasing numbers of children being raised by female parents alone. There is no evidence that the upswing in the divorce rate since the end of World War II has been parallelled by an increase in the percentage of the population which is homosexually oriented. More visible, yes; more widespread, no.

During the same postwar period, the development of television as a major educator for children has significantly reduced the influence of the "real life" nuclear family in inculcating values and providing role models. Traditional cultural models are presented less often by parents than by mass media.

Hermaphrodism and Transsexualism

Considerable research points to the influence of early postnatal social experience on the establishment of some aspects of sexual identity. The sense of being male or female (core morphologic identity) appears to be largely influenced by the sex designated to infants, with dimorphic parenting reactions beginning with name selection, blue or pink blankets, dolls or trucks, etc. The degree to which this earliest self-labelling may fall under the influence of social forces is exemplified by persons born anatomically intersexed. The classic examples are those described as "matched pairs of hermaphrodites" (Money and Ehrhardt, 1972). Two children karyotypically female (44 + XX) and gonadally female (ovaries) are born with partially virilized external genitalia due to an inborn metabolic deficiency in the production of cortisol. The genitalia are sufficiently ambiguous that one child is designated male and one female. Typically, sexual identity in both will follow the sex of assignment. One child will develop a sense of being male, the other female. One will behave in a manner considered masculine; the other within the normal range for femininity. One will become erotically attracted to females, the other primarily to males.

Such classic cases have been attacked as unrepresentative of psychosexual development in the typical child. The argument is that the anatomically intersexed, by the very nature of being intersexed, are more "plastic" or amenable to environmental manipulation. A response to the criticism has been the report of a pair of genetically male twins, anatomically normal at birth, but raised in opposite sex roles. Here one male experienced traumatic loss of his penis at 6 months and was sex-reassigned female at 18 months. The twins are monozygotic. Thus, as best as possible in the human, prenatal endocrine and genetic variables are identical for the two children, with the principal differentiating (independent) variable being the sex of rearing of the twins. To date, at age 11, the children are developing as a typical brother and sister. Sexual orientation has yet to be determined (Money and Ehrhardt, 1972; Ehrhardt, 1977).

Sexual identity does not always follow sex of assignment in the anatomically normal. Consider transsexualism. Here, persons who by all current diagnostic tools are anatomically and physiologically normal, experience a strong sense of being of the other sex or a compelling desire to be of the other sex. This cross-sex identity/desire begins during childhood and may culminate in sex-reassignment surgery in adulthood (Benjamin, 1966; Green and Money, 1969; Stoller, 1968; Green, 1974). Transsexuals are erotically attracted to persons of the same anatomic sex.

The etiology of transsexualism is not clear. In the view of some, the phenomenon is biologically determined, perhaps by a deficiency of prenatal androgen (Dorner, 1976). In the view of others it is the product of a unique mother-child relationship coupled with special features of the mother-father and father-child relationship (Stoller, 1968; 1976). The parents of transsexuals are behaviorally *heterosexual*. However, their heterosexuality is not transmitted to the child as expressed in the child's sexual identity.

Based on the above developmental research, to maximize the chance of a given male infant evolving into a female-identified and homosexually oriented adult, one would have to delude the child into believing it belonged to the sex opposite to its anatomy. The male child would be given a girl's name, dressed as a girl, and introduced to adults and children as a girl. It would be told that having a penis defines one as female. The child must have no opportunity to visibly (or otherwise) repudiate that statement during the first years of life. This conspiracy would have to extend to all persons in the child's early environment. Comparable deception would have to occur for the female infant.

HOMOSEXUALITY

What do we know about the development of a homosexual life style? For those concerned that homosexual children will evolve from homosexual parent figures, this question is salient.

There is no shortage of theory. Most writings stress a unique mother-son relationship in the development of male homosexuality. Some theories point to a contribution, perhaps one of omission, from the father. "Mother-son closeness" theories have been espoused for half a century. Freud's analysis of the life of Leonardo da Vinci stressed this feature along with father absence (Freud, 1910). A more intricate triadic relationship was advanced 15 years ago in a multitherapist project headed by Bieber. Psychoanalysts rated features of the early family relationship of about 100 male homosexual patients and 100 male heterosexual patients. The recollections of the patients, as reported by their therapists, were significantly different for the two groups. The homosexuals' mother-son relationships were more often (though not exclusively) characterized as close-binding and intimate, and coexisting with a father-son relationship characterized by father absence, or father emotional distance and hostility. The presence of a physically and emotionally available father was seen as protective against the mother's "homosexualogenic" influence. This study can be criticized on several methodologic grounds, including unrepresentative patient samples, the use of distorted retrospective recall, invalid or unreliable therapist reporting, overlap of prehomosexual and preheterosexual parent-child relationships, and neglect of the child's contribution to the parent-child relationship. Efforts at "replication" have had mixed results. Evans' questionnaire study of a non-patient sample (Evans, 1969) found similar recalled patterns, while Siegelman's (1974) psychological test and questionnaire assessment did not.

Siegelman (1974) found that homosexuals described both their fathers and mothers as more rejecting and less loving and that they were less close to their fathers than the heterosexuals. However, for sub-samples of homosexuals and heterosexuals scoring low on neuroticism, no significant differences in family relations were found. Additionally, homosexuals low on femininity reported negative behavior for fathers but not for mothers. The author also noted that father vs. mother dominance did not differentiate between homosexual and heterosexual parental backgrounds. The author suggests that these results cast serious doubt on the assumption that negative parental behavior, especially of mothers, plays a critical role in differentiating the backgrounds of homosexuals and heterosexuals. The findings underscore the importance of using nonclinical samples. Furthermore, degree of neuroticism, even in *non*clinical samples, needs to be controlled to avoid biased data on parental backgrounds.

Whether the family constellation described by Bieber et al. does load in favor of a homosexual outcome, for this discussion the obvious point is that the description is of a *heterosexual* parent-child configuration promoting a *homosexual* orientation in the child. Socarides (1968) sees the son's fear of maternal engulfment and poor separation-individuation during the earliest life period as promoting a homosexual orientation:

> To the homosexual, the mother has, in infancy, been, on the one hand, dangerous and frightening, forcing separation, threatening the infant with loss of love and care; on the other hand, the mother's conscious and unconscious tendencies were felt as working against separation.
>
> It is my belief that in all homosexuals there has been an inability to make the progression from the mother-child unity of earliest infancy to individuation. As a result, there exists in homosexuals a fixation, with the concomitant tendency to regression, to the earliest mother-child relationship. This is manifested as a threat of personal annihilation, loss of ego boundaries and a sense of fragmentation.

Genetic theories of homosexuality peaked with the report of Kallman in 1952 of 100 per cent concordance for homosexuality in 37 "identical" male twin pairs. Since then, sets of monozygotic twin pairs discordant for homosexuality have also been reported.

Heston and Shields (1968) studied the Maudsley Twin Registry and found 12 male twins with a primary or secondary diagnosis of homosexuality. Two of the five monozygotic twin pairs were concordant for homosexuality. In a third pair, the co-twin had delusions of changing sex. Only one of the seven dizygotic twin pairs were concordant for homosexuality. This paper also reported a family with three monozygotic twin pairs, two concordant for homosexuality and one for heterosexuality.

The genetic field is quiescent currently, with more biologic research directed at neuroendocrine factors (which of course may be genetically induced). While few dyed-in-the-wool geneticists would argue for a purely genetic basis of sexual orientation, denying any genetic influence would fly in the face of the two larger twin series. However, whatever the degree, if any, of the contribution of genetics to homosexuality, it can hardly be mobilized to argue against the suitability of a *foster* parent.

Hormonal theories of homosexual development have enjoyed a resurgence. An avalanche of studies has appeared during the past decade. Some report homosexual males to have higher levels of testosterone than heterosexuals (Tourney and Hatfield, 1973), some to have lower (Kolodny et al., 1971), and some the same (Pillard et al., 1974). One reports higher estradiol (Doerr et al., 1973). Three suggest an alteration in the metabolism of testosterone as revealed by the urinary ratio of androsterone and etiocholanolone (Margolese, 1970; Margolese and Janiger, 1973; Evans, 1972). Another reports a difference in the degree of change in the level of plasma luteinizing hormone (LH) in response to an intravenous injection of estrogen (Dorner et al., 1975). Here, male homosexuals show a pattern of change like that of heterosexual females. Little has been done to examine the endocrine status of female homosexuals: one report of 4 subjects described a lower estrogen and a higher androgen level (Loraine et al., 1971), and another of 42 females found no difference (Eisinger et al., 1972).

These studies are provocative, but far from definitive. Those which assess basic metabolic or pituitary-hypothalamic pathways (A/E ratio, LH response) are potentially more valuable. But again, whatever the degree of contribution of neuroendocrinology, if any, to the development of homosexuality, it can hardly be mobilized to argue against the suitability of a *foster* parent.

Psychiatric health and homosexuality

Psychological health studies of homosexuals and heterosexuals have matured from rotten to passable science. The earliest, as noted, were single case or small number reports of patients consulting psychiatrists to become heterosexual. They were homosexuals experiencing conflict over being homosexual. It does not require methodological wizardry to see that patients are not representative of an entire population, and that conflicts can be induced by social pressure on a stigmatized minority group and not just by psychic defect. And where was the control group of heterosexual patients? With time, psychiatric and psychologic studies emerged which studied large, nonpatient samples, utilized control groups, and standardized interview and psychometric instruments.

A few representative studies will be cited. The first utilized a battery of tests designed to measure personality factors. Siegelman studied 307 male homosexuals and 137 male heterosexuals obtained from nonclinical sources. Most of the homosexuals could be classified as professionals and were predominantly middle-class. The 137 heterosexuals were either undergraduate or graduate students in education courses. The majority were middle-class. On the Neuroticism Scale Questionnaire (Scheier and Cattell, 1961) the homosexuals scored significantly higher on tender-mindedness, submissiveness, anxiety, and total score, and significantly lower on depression. Homosexuals had significantly higher scores than heterosexuals on goal-directedness and nurturance. There were no significant differences between the two groups on the alienation, trust, dependency, and neuroticism factors. Homosexually oriented females, compared to heterosexually oriented females, scored higher on a neuroticism scale measuring goal-directedness and self-acceptance. However, they scored lower on depression (Siegelman, 1972). Freedman (1971) studied 62 members of a female homophile group and 67 female members of a national service organization. On the Eysenck Personality Inventory and the Personal Orientation Inventory, there were no differences on the neuroticism scale and no differences in general psychologic adjustment.

While the representativeness of the samples may be questioned, what is clear is that for the homosexually oriented subjects tested, the emergent personality profile is that of a person similar to most people, with the exception of sexual partner preference. Certainly there is no emergence of the personality profile of an unfit parent.

Next, a psychiatric study. Here 89 homosexually oriented males, 87 heterosexually oriented males, 57 homosexually oriented females, and 43 heterosexually oriented females underwent intensive interviewing. The heterosexual groups were unmarried to control for marital status. The latter were recruited from a singles apartment complex, while the homosexuals were recruited from homophile organizations. For both the males and females there was essentially no difference in the incidence of neurotic or psychotic psychiatric diagnoses. The only difference which emerged was a higher incidence of problem drinking in the homosexual females. Life problems and reasons for consulting a psychiatrist (if one had been consulted) were similar for both groups (typically, breakup of a romance). The words of the authors (Saghir and Robins, 1973) best summarize their findings:

> For males: Other variables that showed no significant differences or prominent trends between homosexuals and heterosexuals include . . . ways of handling anger . . . overall prevalence of psychiatric disorders, depression and psychophysiologic illnesses, psychotic or paranoid symptoms, educational achievement and overall personal and functional disability.
>
> For females: Homosexual women, like homosexual men, usually show little impairment of function. . . . Homosexual and heterosexual women are strikingly similar . . . both groups suffer as often from neurotic and psychophysiologic disorders and premenstrual depression. . . .

Again, one might question the representativeness of the samples, particularly with the higher than expected incidence of psychiatric problems among the heterosexually oriented unmarried subjects. However, what emerges as the psychiatric portrait of the male or female homosexual is that of a person not remarkably different from most people, except for sexual partner preference. Again, what does not emerge is the psychiatric portrait of a person incapable of effective parenting.

Over a half century ago, Freud (1920) wrote "(homosexuality) is . . . found in people whose efficiency is unimpaired. . . ." Fifteen years later (1935) he wrote "homosexuality is . . . no vice, no degradation; it cannot be classified as an illness: we consider it to be a variation of the sexual functions. . . ."

Second order questions

Is the prospective adoptive parent a single or paired male? Recent years have witnessed a growing interest by males to be actively engaged in the parenting process. More fathers are seeking custody of children in divorce settlements. A shift has occurred toward more equal parental sharing of infant and early childhood care. Some single heterosexual males have applied for and received custody of foster children.

Necessary responsibilities of the male parent include adequate provision of time for the care of the child, and post–school hour companionship and supervision when the work and/or recreational schedule precludes parent-child contact. Children benefit from contact with persons of varying ages of both sexes. There is a degree of identification, role-modeling, and complementariness that occurs with adults of both sexes. The single male's social universe should include such persons. They could be female friends, relatives, or neighbors. Children of both sexes are readily available in school and in the neighborhood.

If the child is female, most of what is stated above applies. The days of mothers relentlessly teaching their daughters to cook and sew, in preparation for the wifely role, are fading. Should the child desire such experience, and the male parent is unable to provide it, the experience can come from an adult female friend, a neighbor, or in school. Thus, being a single male homosexual or heterosexual *per se* may have little bearing on the primary question.

What of the child's age? Younger children require differing amounts and types of time and attention. A male adopting an infant (or a female adopting) needs to know about formulas, diapers, infant maladies, and developmental timetables. He or she needs a high tolerance for interrupted sleep, and should be able to provide, through self or surrogate, adequate child care time. The time demands of an infant are so considerable that single parents would probably find adoption of grade school age (or older) children more compatible with their work schedule. However, if the adopting male is in a domestic life-sharing relationship with another male, opportunity exists for greater attention to both infant and occupation.

Another variable has now been introduced—two males living as a family unit. Two males (or females) in the parenting role provide an even less conventional family model. While the degree of time available to the child from two adults within a home is considerably greater, the unusual nature of the family is more visible to the child when there is a homosexual dyad. On the other hand, it is quite unlikely that the single homosexual parent's sexual orientation will remain unknown to the child.

What can be said of the impact of the adult couple on the child's psychosexual development? Here, I suggest that the quality of the relationship may supersede the anatomic sex of the individuals involved. A heterosexual couple with an alienated, perhaps violent relationship, is of dubious value in providing the climate for *e*ffective *a*ffective child growth and a positive role model for adult relationships. This holds true whether the couples are of the same or different anatomical sex.

The above section, perhaps paradoxically, has focused on adoptive male parents. It might appear more logical to commence discussion with adoptive female homosexual parents since they probably outnumber males. However, I have chosen to focus initially on the male in that the closing section of this essay deals with children *actually* being raised by homosexual females. Therefore, more attention has addressed issues of a homosexual parent in general, with specific reference to the male. Since our culture thinks of females as being more "natural" parents, all other things being equal, my approach renders the task of convincing skeptics of the wisdom of homosexuals adopting children more difficult.

Much of what was said in the discussion of prospective male parents applies to females. I will not again address the issues of availability to the child, the quality of the mother-child relationship, the availability of alternate life models and extrafamily influences, etc. A distinction which will be made concerns the sex of the adoptive child. Here we have the converse situation to that of the male adoptive parent. Most social learning theories and psychoanalytic theories stress the importance of the same sex parent on sexual identity formation, with a relatively complementary role played by the other sex parent. Thus, one might argue that, in the case of a male child, the absence of a male parent and perhaps the coexistence of two females in the home might have a "feminizing" effect. However, the escalating divorce rate in the United States has yielded a considerable population of male children being raised in homes without a male parent. Many of these children have little residual contact with their father. Here, as noted above regarding male adoptive parents, it would appear important that the female provide the opportunity for the child to interact with adult males. The potential opportunity exists via friends and neighbors, relatives, parents of the peer group, the local Big Brother society, the Boy Scouts, etc.

Stigmatization. Discussion so far has focused on the relationship between the adoptive parent and child. Reference made to the child's more extended milieu, e.g., the peer group, has presented the positive side. A more conventional social model was seen as being available to the child than that existing within the home. The alternate side of the coin, however, is the possibility of peer group stigmatization, based on the group's awareness of the atypical nature of the child's household.

Unquestionably, peer group alienation and stigmatization can represent a major social hardship for children. Regrettably, however, few children escape some degree of teasing and stigmatization. Some are teased because of racial characteristics, others for religious affiliation, others for deficiencies in academic performance or on the sports field, and others for some other physical attribute such as obesity.

The degree to which the adoptive child living in a homosexually oriented household may be subjected to peer group teasing may be dependent on several factors. First is the geographic locale in which the family lives. Some areas of the country are more accepting of alternate life styles than others. Next would be the degree to which the family members have become "public figures." By this is meant the extent to which the parents are known within the community as being homosexual, perhaps as a product of the extent to which they have been involved in homophile organizations or subjected to press publicity. Of even greater significance would be the extent to which the adults have involved the children in public political settings, raising them to "celebrity status." A mitigating factor, however, may be the presence of more than one child in the family. The solo child lacks communal support from closely aged siblings being similarly teased. Finally, it should not be forgotten that, just as with oppression of other minority groups, general public attitudes towards homosexuality are undergoing change. There is greater public acceptance or, at least, consideration of sexual life style as a private issue. Younger generations, particularly, are more accepting of alternate life styles. The answers here are not all known. However, the children described in this essay's final discussion have, so far, not been subjected to stigmatization.

Children's viewing of homosexual sexual conduct

This is practically a moot point but will be included for completeness. There are those who fear that homosexual persons are more likely than heterosexual persons to engage in overt sexual acts in the presence of children. In hundreds of interviews I have had with heterosexual parents, and in dozens with homosexual parents, I have yet to find an individual or couple who feels it appropriate for children to view explicit parental sexuality. The homosexual parents whom I have interviewed regarding physical affection expressed in the presence of their children are comparable to heterosexual parents, i.e., occasional embracing, hugging, affectionate kissing on the cheek, or hand-holding. Nongenital displays of affection such as the above, between adults, might well offer an important role model for the child with respect to affective expression, irrespective of the anatomic sex of the individuals involved. Such an environment would seem to be more conducive to a growing child's later capacity for positive affective expression than a home devoid of public, nongenital physical affection.

Proselytizing of children

Will homosexually oriented adoptive parents attempt to induce homosexuality in their children? As noted above, based on available research, maximizing the chance of a given infant evolving into a homosexually oriented adult would require a massive effort of deception regarding the child's gender. Would more subtle strategies work? Do homosexually oriented parents want their children to become homosexual? Homosexual parents, when asked the latter question, typically respond, "I want my child to be happy." When pressed as to whether they would try to proselytize their child into homosexuality, they typically respond, "I wouldn't try, and if I wanted to, I wouldn't know how." Neither does the author of this essay.

Much of the above has been the marshalling of indirect data. The argument has dealt largely in the abstract. Homosexually oriented males and females have been revealed, based on psychiatric and psychologic research, to have the potential (as do heterosexually oriented persons) for those interests and capacities needed for effective parenting. What is known regarding the genesis of homosexuality was reviewed in an effort to determine whether a child being raised by a homosexually oriented parent would more likely evolve a homosexual life style. The path found to homosexuality was one of "defects" in the relationship of heterosexually oriented parents. But, this is indirect. Are there data describing children raised by parents with a same-sex partner preference? Yes.

Children raised by homosexual and transsexual parents

I have evaluated 21 children being raised by homosexual parents (all female parents) and 14 being raised by transsexual parents (half the parents had changed sex in the direction of male to female, and half female to male). Both homosexual and transsexual parents and their children will be described because both types of parent have a sexual partner preference which is the same as that of the sex in which they were born. Thus a female who is now living as a man has a sexual partner preference for females, and when the sex-change status of the parent is known to the child, a message of homosexual partner preference is being communicated.

The sexual identity of the younger children was made on parameters which best reflect emerging sexual identity. These include toy and game preferences, peer group composition, clothing preference, roles played in fantasy games, and the Draw-A-Person test (Green, 1974). These features appear to discriminate a sample of children who appear to be pretranssexual or prehomosexual. The evidence for this is both direct and indirect. Retrospective reports by nearly all adult transsexuals are replete with atypical behavioral patterns on these parameters dating back to early childhood (Benjamin, 1966; Stoller, 1968; Green and Money, 1969; Green, 1974). Thus, transsexuals recall (if male-to-female) that their "boyhood" was characterized by a preference for the toys, games, companionship, and clothes of girls and role-playing as female. The converse is true for female-to-male transsexuals.

Recent studies of homosexually oriented adults also indicate cross-sex behavior on these parameters in the majority of subjects. In the Saghir and Robins study, about two thirds of the male homosexuals reported a "girl-like syndrome" during childhood compared to less than 10 per cent of the heterosexuals. This "syndrome" is similar to that recalled by male-to-female transsexuals. More recently Whitam (1977) found a similar pattern of feminine behavior recalled by the great majority of 206 adult homosexually oriented males compared to one tenth of 78 heterosexuals. Regarding females,

Saghir and Robins found that two thirds of the prehomosexuals recalled being "tomboys" during girlhood, vs. only one fifth of the preheterosexuals. The Draw-A-Person test has also been used for two reasons. In a series of 2400 grade school children, Jolles (1952) found that 80 per cent, when told to draw a person, drew someone of their own sex first. The interpretation is that the sex first drawn is a reflection of the drawer's sexual identity. In our smaller series of over 100 feminine and/or masculine boys (feminine boys defined by the parameters above) we found that a significantly greater percentage of feminine boys drew a female first (Green et al., 1972; Green, unpublished).

Three prospective studies add further support for the association between childhood cross-gender role behavior, as expressed on the above parameters, and an adult homosexual orientation. The first is that of myself and John Money. From 1959 to 1961 we evaluated 12 boys at The Johns Hopkins Hospital showing such behavior. Of the five on whom we have follow-up data, at least four are predominantly homosexual (Green, 1974). Lebovitz (1972) reviewed records of boys seen at the University of Minnesota who had shown feminine behavior. Sixteen were reinterviewed as adults. Three were transsexual, two were homosexual, and one was transvestic. Zuger (1966) reported on six adults who were reinterviewed after being evaluated (treated?) for boyhood femininity. Three were homosexual and one possibly transsexual. Thus, 14 of 27 previously feminine male children show atypical sexuality during adulthood.

Consider first the 21 children currently being raised by their homosexual mothers. They live in eight households. All households contained two adult female homosexuals, the mother and her romantic partner, for a period of time. At evaluation two adult females continued to live in six of the eight households.

Eleven of the children are male. Their age range is 5 to 13. The number of years they have lived in the household ranges from two to six. The peer group of 10 is male. The favorite toy of seven is a traditionally masculine toy such as a truck, gun, or racing car. For four, the favorite toy is more gender-neutral, such as a board game, model animal, or kite. For none is the favorite toy feminine, such as a doll. The vocational aspiration of eight is "conventionally masculine," such as pilot, fireman, doctor, lawyer, or athlete. For three, vocational aspiration is more gender-neutral such as artist or storekeeper. For none is vocational aspiration conventionally feminine. Three related erotic fantasies or behaviors; they were of an exclusively heterosexual nature. Six drew a male first on the Draw-A-Person test, four drew a female, and one did not draw a person.

Ten of the children are female. Their age range is 5 to 14. The number of years they have lived in the household ranges from two to five. The peer group of nine is female. The favorite toy of seven is conventionally feminine (doll) and of three is gender-neutral, such as a board game. None has a conventionally masculine toy preference. The vocational aspiration of eight is conventionally feminine (usually a nurse), for none is it gender-neutral, and for two it is "conventionally masculine" (a doctor). Erotic fantasies and behaviors are reported by one female; they are exclusively heterosexual. On the Draw-A-Person test, nine drew a female first, and one drew a male.

Consider next the 14 children being raised by a transsexual parent. Seven are being raised by a "stepfather" who was born female. They live in three households. Two children are male. They are 15 and 17 years old and have lived in the transsexual household for 14 years. They have never been told of the transsexual nature of their stepfather. The two teenagers showed conventionally masculine behavior during grade school years, aspire to conventionally masculine occupations (engineer, doctor), and report an exclusively heterosexual erotic orientation.

Five of the children are female. Their age range is 13 to 20. They have lived in the transsexual household for 9 to 16 years. They know of the transsexual nature of their "father." One was a "tomboy" during her preteen years. Four aspire to conventionally feminine occupations (waitress, nurse, housewife, stewardess) and one to a conventionally more "masculine" occupation (veterinarian). All report an exclusively heterosexual orientation.

Seven are being raised by a "stepmother" who was born male. They live in three households. Four children are male. Their age range is 4 to 13. They have lived in the transsexual household for 1 to 3 years. They know of the transsexual nature of their "mother." None show "feminine" or "sissy" behavior. They aspire to conventionally masculine vocations such as policeman, doctor, film director (the four-year-old wants to be a daddy), and the two with erotic fantasies report those of an exclusively heterosexual nature.

Three children are female. Their age range is 3 to 9. They have lived in the transsexual household for 1 to 3 years. The two older children know of the transsexual nature of their "mother." One (age 3) is a "tomboy." Vocational aspirations are teacher, artist, and "mommy" (for the three-year-old). None report erotic fantasies.

What do these preliminary data tell us? Stated most timidly, it is clear that being raised by a parent with an atypical pattern of sexual identity does not necessarily result in a child's adopting an atypical sexual identity. It does not necessarily lead to atypical core morphologic identity, cross-gender behavior in childhood, or a homosexual orientation in adulthood. Stated more boldly, it does not appear that being raised by a parent with an atypical pattern of sexual identity has any major effect on the three components of sexual identity—the sense of being male or female, masculine or feminine behavior, and sexual partner preference. Stated more cautiously, it is too early to evaluate the full sexual picture of all the children in the series. Some have been in the atypical households for relatively short periods of time. Some have not evolved a pattern of erotic preference. The duration of time the children have lived in homosexual households is briefer than for the transsexual households, and the relevancy of including the transsexual might be questioned. However, as noted above, transsexuals do experience what may be considered a homosexual orientation.

The above cautions notwithstanding, the children appear to be quite typical when assessed on major dimensions of sexual identity. Why should such be the case? We can speculate. They have good relationships with their parents. They receive adequate care from their parents. Most know their parents are atypical in one feature, but have access to more conventional life style role models. How can one avoid such access? How can a child avoid being bombarded by the pattern of the conventional nuclear family, and the conventional role expectations of boys and girls, men and women? Consider the relentless message of the mass media, along with the peer group, and the peer group's families. Children who come from unconventional homes may recognize that unconventionality and opt for the more conventional models to which they are regularly exposed. It can be argued that in contemporary American society, television has replaced parents as the most significant communicator of the cultural message. The peer group, too, has a tremendous influence on adopting conventional styles of behavior.

Conclusion

This topic may be one of the remaining social frontiers in which psychiatry is called upon to provide a factual data base. The question posed by the section's title implicitly contains assumptions which address the qualities of effective parenthood, and also societal value systems regarding patterns of sexual life style. It is our responsibility to dissect out what is factually known from private, nonscientific views regarding a pattern of living, perhaps different from our own.

In reviewing literature on psychosexual development based on objective data collection, in reviewing the milieu beyond the immediate household in which the child evolves, and in reviewing the preliminary data on children being raised by homosexually oriented parents, a search was made for evidence to reply "No" to the essay's primary question. Little, if any, was found. Rather, it appears to be a matter of judging, on an individual basis, the potential home environment of a person seeking to adopt children, judging capacities and motivations for responsible parenting, and relegating sexual orientation of the potential adoptive parent to a remote arena. To me, those who would deny homosexuals adoption, based on sexual orientation, bear the burden of proving that such persons make unfit parents.

References

Benjamin, H.: The Transsexual Phenomenon. New York, Julian Press, Inc., 1966.

Bieber, I., Dain, M., Prince, P., et al.: Homosexuality: A Psychoanalytic Study. New York, Basic Books, Inc. 1962.

Doerr, P., Kockett, G., Vogt, M., et al.: Plasma testosterone, estradiol, and semen analysis in male homosexuals. Arch. Gen. Psychiatry, *29*:829–833, 1973.

Dorner, G.: International Congress of Sexology. Personal communication, 1976.

Dorner, G., Rohde, W., Stahl, F., et al.; A neuroendocrine conditioned predisposition for homosexuality in men. Arch. Sex. Behav., *4*:1–8, 1975.

Ehrhardt, A., and Baker, S.: Fetal androgens, human central nervous system differentiation, and behavior sex differences. *In* Friedman, R., Richart, R., and Van de Wiede, R. (eds.): Sex Differences in Behavior. New York, John Wiley & Sons, Inc., 1974.

Ehrhardt, A.: Personal communication, 1977.

Eisinger, A., Huntsman, R., Lord, J., et al.: Female homosexuality. Nature, *238*:106, 1972.

Evans, R.: Childhood parental relationships of homosexual men. J. Consult. Clin. Psychol., *33*:129–135, 1969.

Evans, R.: Physical and biochemical characteristics of homosexual men. J. Consult. Clin. Psychol., *39*:140–147, 1972.
Freedman, M.: Homosexuality and Psychological Functioning. Monterey, Calif., Brooks Cole Publishing Company, 1971.
Freud, S. (1910): Leonardo da Vinci and a Memory of His Childhood. Standard Edition, *11*:63–137, 1957.
Freud, S. (1935): Letter to an American mother. Am. J. Psychiatry, *107*:786–787, 1951.
Freud, S. (1920): The Psychogenesis of a Case of Homosexuality in a Woman. Standard Edition, *18*:147–172.
Green, R.: Homosexuality as a mental illness. Int. J. Psychiatry, *10*:77–98, 1972.
Green, R.: Sexual Identity Conflict in Children and Adults. New York, Basic Books, Inc., Publishers, 1974.
Green, R., Fuller, M., and Rutley, B.: It-scale for children and Draw-A-Person test: 30 feminine vs. 25 masculine boys. J. Person. Assess., *36*:349–352, 1972.
Green, R., and Money, J. (eds.): Transsexualism and Sex Reassignment. Baltimore, The Johns Hopkins University Press, 1969.
Heston, L., and Shields, J.: Homosexuality in twins. Arch. Gen. Psychiatry, *18*:149–160, 1968.
Hoffman, M.: The Gay World. New York, Basic Books, Inc., Publishers, 1968.
Jolles, I.: A study of some hypotheses for the qualitative interpretation of the H-T-P for children of elementary school age. J. Clin. Psychol., *8*:113–118, 1952.
Kallman, F.: Comparative twin study on the genetic aspects of male homosexuality. J. Nerv. Ment. Dis., *115*:283–298, 1952.
Kleeman, J.: The establishment of core gender identity in normal girls. Arch. Sex. Behav., *1*:103–129, 1971.
Kolodny, R., Master, W., Hendryx, J., et al.: Plasma testosterone and semen analysis in male homosexuals. N. Engl. J. Med., *285*:1170–1174, 1971.
Lebovitz, P.: Feminine behavior in boys: Aspects of its outcome. Am. J. Psychiatry, *128*:1283–1289, 1972.
Loraine, J. D., Adamopoulos, K., et al.: Patterns of hormone excretion in male and female homosexuals. Nature, *234*:552–555, 1971.
Margolese, S.: Homosexuality: A new endocrine correlate. Horm. Behav., *1*:151–155, 1970.
Margolese, S., and Janiger, O.: Androsterone-etiocholanolone ratios in male homosexuals. Br. Med. J., *2*:207–210, 1973.
Marmor, J.: A symposium: Should homosexuality be in the APA nomenclature? Am. J. Psychiatry, *130*:1207–1216, 1973.
Money, J., and Ehrhardt, A.: Man and Woman; Boy and Girl. Baltimore, The Johns Hopkins University Press, 1972.
Pillard, R., Rose, R., and Sherwood, M.: Plasma testosterone levels in homosexual men. Arch. Sex. Behav., *3*:453–458, 1974.
Saghir, M., and Robins, E.: Male and Female Homosexuality. Baltimore, The Williams & Wilkins Company, 1973.
Scheir, I., and Cattell, R.: The Neuroticism Scale Questionnaire. Champaign, Ill., Institute for Personality and Ability Testing, 1961.
Siegelman, M.: Adjustment of male homosexuals and heterosexuals. Arch. Sex. Behav., *2*:9–26, 1972.
Siegelman, M.: Parental background of male homosexuals and heterosexuals. Arch. Sex. Behav., *3*:3–18, 1974.
Socarides, C.: The Overt Homosexual. New York, Grune and Stratton, Inc., 1968.
Stoller, R.J.: Sex and Gender. New York, Science House, 1968.
Stoller, R.J.: The Transsexual Experiment. London, Hogarth, 1975.
Tourney, G., and Hatfield, L.: Androgen metabolism in schizophrenics, homosexuals and controls. Biol. Psychiatry, *6*:23–36, 1973.
Whitam, F.: Childhood indicators of male homosexuality. Arch. Sex. Behav., *6*:89–96, 1977.
Zuger, B.: Effeminate behavior present in boys from early childhood. J. Pediatr., *69*:1098–1107, 1966.

Comment

There is still much disagreement among psychiatrists, psychologists, and behavioral scientists concerning the nature of homosexuality. Some regard it as an emotional disorder and others see it as simply a variant of normal sexual behavior. The preponderant view among American psychiatrists is that persistent and exclusive homosexuality is an abnormal (psychopathological) state, arising out of unconscious wishes and unresolved conflicts over separation, dependency, and related developmental tasks. Many psychiatrists would argue that such psychologically defective persons would be seriously impaired in the parental role of helping a child develop a sense of individuality and establishing a firm sense of masculinity or femininity.

Dr. Green questions the assumption that a homosexual orientation is in itself a mental disorder or a sufficient condition for concluding that a mental disorder exists. He also questions whether there is something inherently defective in the personality structure of homosexually oriented persons to make them incapable of effective parenthood. Green points out that generalizing about the personality structure and psychiatric status of homosexually oriented persons in general from the study of homosexual patient samples is invalid. While not drawing a firm conclusion on either issue, he points out that the psychological and psychometric evaluation of nonclinical samples of homosexuals has found them to be more or less like the heterosexual control groups assessed. No personality profile suggestive of unfit parenthood has emerged.

Most developmental theories regarding the origin of homosexuality account for the condition arising in families with heterosexually oriented parents. Thus arguments from these theories on the sexual orientation of children reared by parents with a same-sex partner preference are quite indirect. However, Green has more direct evidence on this issue from his own studies of 21 children raised by homosexual parents and 14 raised by transsexual parents. Although the latter parents exhibit different gender role behavior, of course they are biologically of the same sex and in this sense similar to homosexual parents. Although the sample is small and selective, and most of the children are still in their formative years, no clear disturbances in sexual identity have been identified. Although being raised by parents with atypical patterns of sexual identity, these children show no major effect in the three components of sexual identity: the sense of being male or female, masculine or feminine behavior patterns, and sexual partner preference. Green concludes, given the present state of knowledge, that the question should be answered on an individual basis, taking into account potential home environment, the capacities and motivations of the prospective adopting parents, and other factors. He believes that those who would deny homosexuals the adoption of children based on their sexual orientation bear the burden of proving that such persons make unfit parents.

The issue of whether homosexuals should adopt children illustrates a common dilemma in psychiatry—the press to provide expert opinion in an area which is poorly understood. The question is important and one of increasing relevance as homosexual individuals rightfully press for the civil rights and opportunities enjoyed by other citizens. Obviously the rights of the prospective adopted children need to be considered as well. Although theories abound in this area, they are no substitute for hard data. The latter are scant but beginning to be collected. One hopes that as the data base increases and more systematic evaluative studies are carried out, more informed opinions can be formulated and wise counsel offered.

JOHN PAUL BRADY, M.D.

When (If Ever) Should Sex-Change Operations Be Performed?

JOHN MONEY AND RICHARD AMBINDER

The Johns Hopkins University and Hospital

In the Middle Ages anomalies of sexual behavior, including transvestism and transexualism, were considered to be manifestations of demonic possession, and those who exhibited such anomalies were subject to torture and imprisonment. Unusual sexual behavior was generally considered to be outside the realm of medicine, for since antiquity the boundaries of medicine had been defined in terms of the complaints of pain and suffering which patients brought to physicians. Transvestism and transexualism may bring secondary pain and suffering whereas, primarily, in and of themselves alone they are pain relievers.

After the Middle Ages the notion of disease expanded to include much of what had previously been regarded as demonic possession and sin. In the late 1700's modern psychiatry was born with the reclassification of certain of the behavioral anomalies as mental illness. By the twentieth century, the sexual behavioral anomalies were among those so reclassified.

As the definition and etiology of disease were being broadened in the nineteenth century, the role of the physician underwent profound change. A growing knowledge of germ theory and the spread of disease served as the impetus for society to mandate medical treatment in the interests of public health. In many instances, the prerogative for the initiation of medical treatment shifted from patient to physician, government official, or lawmaker. This shift underscored a discrepancy of therapeutic goal between patient and physician, especially with respect to enforced quarantine or immunization against infection. Eventually the same discrepancy affected gender identity transpositions. Psychiatrists defined these transposi-

*Supported by USPHS #HD-00325 and by funds from The Grant Foundation, Inc., New York, New York 10022.

tions—homosexualism, bisexualism, transvestism, and transexualism—not as demonic possessions, sins, or crimes, as had formerly been the case, but as diseases. In the interest of public social health, they required treatment—treatment aimed at altering gender identity so as to match the genitalia. Viewing such therapy as a threat to their personal identity and possibly destructive of their sexual pleasure, patients who were coerced or cajoled into treatment often covertly protested, but they did not find the voice of overt political protest until very recently.

With the advent of modern plastic surgery, and the synthesis and commercial manufacture of sex hormones, in the first half of the twentieth century, persons with extreme gender identity transposition increasingly made their demands known to the medical profession. They sought surgical and hormonal alteration of their genitalia and secondary sex characteristics so as to give them the somatic appearance of the opposite sex. These people, with a conviction of belonging to the opposite sex and a compulsion to have their bodies changed, have since come to be known as transexuals.

Despite the failure of conventional psychotherapy in the treatment of transexualism, many physicians feared that honoring the request of self-proclaimed transexuals for genital surgery was little more than playing along with a psychosis, analagous to amputating the limbs or enucleating the eyes at a patient's request. However, some gave consideration to the alternative view that the wisdom of the body is such that the organism tries to heal its own prior injuries and traumas, psychic or somatic, and that there are occasions when medicine does best to respect that wisdom.

The proponents of this point of view hypothesized that by bringing about a resolution of the disparity between the mind of the transexual and his or her body and public image, hormonal and surgical sex reassignment would ameliorate the plight of the transexual. This rationale is analogous to that for the cosmetic surgical reconstruction of the breasts, nose, or face, or congenital or traumatic deformity. In all such instances, one recognizes the importance of the body image in promoting personal and social well-being, and undertakes rehabilitative therapy accordingly. Since the 1960's, the worldwide census of sex reassignments numbers in the thousands. Some few follow-up data have been published, but extensive follow-up has been prevented by the widespread disapproval of requests for the funding of any type of research pertaining to sexuality in human beings. The available evidence indicates that in authentic cases, sex reassignment does indeed prove to be rehabilitative.

Etiology

In the final analysis, the etiology of transexualism and related gender identity transpositions is unknown. However, a brief outline of the process of gender identity and gender role differentiation provides some insights into possible etiology. Chromosomes begin the process of gender differentiation, but do not preordain the end result. Their effects must be mediated by prenatal hormones, the effects of which in turn are mediated by cellular receptors. When these receptors are nonfunctional, as in the androgen insensitivity syndrome, it is possible for a normal female external physique and subsequently a normal female gender identity to differentiate in a body that chromosomally would otherwise have been male.

The prenatal hormones are known to influence the central nervous system (CNS), as well as the rest of the body. Animal researchers have demonstrated that the sex hormones control the differentiation of sex-dimorphic neural pathways in the hypothalamus. Research in humans is constrained by ethical considerations. Clinical studies do, however, permit one to infer similar CNS effects. Particularly instructive are cases of prenatal androgenization. In an earlier era, a few cases of prenatal androgenization occurred when a synthetic progestin, now known to be metabolized to an androgen, was administered to women in hopes of preserving an endangered pregnancy. More frequently, prenatal androgenization results from an adrenocortical metabolic error which leads to the endogenous production of excess androgen (the adrenogenital syndrome).

Girls thus androgenized *in utero* are more likely than their female age mates to spurn doll play, cosmetics, and jewelry in favor of vigorous outdoor athletic activity. They have a tendency to be competitive, and in later life are likely to give higher priority to career than to family. Such personality traits, although shared to a greater or lesser extent by members of both sexes, have traditionally been regarded as sex different.

It is still speculative that an unusual prenatal hormonal history makes one especially variable with respect to the differentiation of the erotic aspect of gender identity. None of the androgenized girls has ever evidenced desire for sex reassignment, though a large proportion is bisexual in fantasy or, less so, in practice.

The importance of the postnatal determinants of gender identity is indicated by studies of children matched for various characteristics, but differing in sex of rearing. Pairs of infants born with ambiguous genitalia and matched for karyotype and clinical diagnosis have been raised as members of opposite sexes and followed into adulthood. In virtually all of these cases romantic and sexual interests as well as general behavior patterns have differentiated predominantly in accord with assigned sex. This finding suggests that gender identity is in large part differentiated postnatally and is subject, like native language, to social learning.

The sort of learning which takes place is in many ways akin to the learning of language: tenacious and largely irreversible. And like the acquisition of language, the acquisition of gender identity and gender role are facilitated during a critical period which begins at about 18 months of age. While further learning can occur in later life, the critical period experience will continue to exert a strong influence. Just as an accent is a linguistic manifestation of critical-period learning, sexual idiosyncrasies may be the manifestations of critical-period, gender-identity learning.

The child differentiating gender role and identity mentally codes behavior as being masculine or feminine. This coding is a product of identification, that is of imitating or copying the behavior of one sex, and of complementation to the behavior of the other sex. Similarly, the natively bilingual child encodes words and other utterances as belonging to one language or another. In the same way that a bilingual child may have difficulty learning to speak when one speaker uses two languages, so too gender identity confusion may result when the gender-dimorphic expectancies of the parents and other important models are ambiguous and inconsistent.

Confusion may also develop when the distinctions between the sexes are clear enough, but the brain mechanism serving to differentiate the identification schema from the complementation schema becomes impaired. Just as in senility a more recently learned language may give way to the language of childhood, so too senile men and women may show traits formerly coded as belonging exclusively to the opposite sex. In some cases a brain lesion may result in a loosening of differentiation. Thus, extremely rare cases of temporal lobe epilepsy have been reported in which the epileptic focus induced not only seizures, but compulsive transvestism as well. Both the seizures and the transvestism remitted following successful neurosurgery. A similar but currently undetectable neural phenomenon may be associated with many of the gender identity transpositions.

Developmental factors in the etiology of gender identity transpositions range from covert and unidentified genetic programing, to possible effects of hormones, drugs, foodstuffs, and infections, to neonatal trauma, to inconsistencies and ambiguities in the child's social experience of gender, to gender-unrelated traumas which impair the differential coding of sex signals and/or retrieval of sexual behavior patterns.

Diagnostic Procedures

The physical examination is typically contributory only insofar as it may reveal unrelated pathology contraindicating surgery. In rare instances an EEG may indicate, in association with transexualism, temporal lobe epilepsy subject to pharmacological or neurosurgical control.

Psychologic tests may reveal associated syndromes, such as depression, schizophrenia, or character disorder (psychopathic delinquency with lying and stealing). Though they do not rule out the possibility of rehabilitation through sex reassignment, these syndromes are not relieved by sex reassignment per se.

The primary source of initial diagnostic information is the standardized, objective interview with the patient, augmented by interviews with close kin. In order to insure that all pertinent topics are discussed a standard schedule of inquiry is imperative (Money and Primrose, 1969). Tape recording and transcription of the interviews insures an accurate record and facilitates the cross checking of information with family members and others necessary to minimize the patient's editing and/or misrepresentation, deliberate or otherwise, of his or her own history.

No diagnostic test that can be carried out within a hospital clinic or physician's office substitutes for the two-year, real-life test prior to the final and irreversible step of surgical sex-reassignment. This is a difficult test. It requires that the patient become socially, vocationally, economically, and emotionally rehabilitated in the sex of reassignment prior to surgical change of the genital anatomy. During the two-year test, hormonal reassignment is permitted, for its effects can be reversed, even in the most difficult instance of surgically reversing vocal cord masculinization in the female-to-male transexual.

The two-year, real-life test allows both the patient and the physician to monitor from waking to sleeping, week by week and month by month, the experience in the new sex status as he/she habituates his/her responses to other people. Without this test of how other people react, and how he/she reacts to other people, the patient knows only his/her private convictions and fantasies of being a member of the opposite sex.

Convictions and fantasies can be notoriously unreliable. They may include a covert and magical proposition in which the reassignment operation is equated with being born again, fully accommodated, as a member of the new sex, to the gender-dimorphic expectancies and responses of other people. Such accommodation does, however, require time. It should be accomplished prior to the irreversible step of surgery. Sex-reassignment surgery should occupy a place in a person's life that corresponds rehabilitatively to hysterectomy in the life of a woman, or prostatectomy in the life of a man.

Differential Diagnosis

Effeminate homosexuality, masculinate or "butch" lesbianism, and episodic transvestism are conditions which should be considered in the differential diagnosis of transexualism. These variable manifestations of gender identity transposition may be regarded as constituting either a statistical typology, or as marking idealized points on a continuous distribution. One of the problems of differential diagnosis is that some diagnosticians postulate a typology, whereas the clinical phenomena are not polymodal, but statistically continuous in distribution. Confusion on this issue leads to unnecessary argument and dissent with regard to differential diagnosis.

The idealized type of erotically effeminate homosexual male derives his erotic pleasure from giving orgasmic satisfaction to another male. He simulates the receptive female and withdraws attention from his own penis. He may avoid orgasm with his male partner, and in the partner's presence may even be impotent. Stimulated by a replay of his sexual encounter in imagery, he may later masturbate alone to orgasm.

His affectations, mannerisms, carriage, interests, and attitudes may be effeminate. Although he may cross-dress as a drag queen routinely or only occasionally at parties, he is without a compulsion to do so. He often reports an aversion to vigorous competitive games and rough outdoor activities dating from childhood and recalls being labelled "sissy" by his playmates. In adulthood he has been able to make his peace with life as an effeminate homosexual; he does not have a compulsion to become a woman, and does not detest his genitals. In fact they are an integral part of his sexual identity.

The female counterpart of the effeminate male homosexual is the masculinate lesbian. In the idealized case her manners, movements, speech, and attitudes are typically masculine. She may dress as a man and seek to be a husband to her female lover. She often repudiates her breasts as a source of erotic pleasure and binds them as flat as possible.

The idealized type of male transvestite is heterosexual with respect to erotic partner. He is fetishistically dependent on dressing in feminine attire, or on the imagery of it for erotic arousal. He discovered his proclivity before or at puberty when he could masturbate to orgasm only while wearing or fondling women's clothing. In adulthood his cross-dressing may have come to involve a change in name and personality as well as wardrobe. Each cross-dressing episode is in response to an overpowering tension that builds up in the intervals between episodes, and which ideally is relieved by intercourse with a woman while wearing female garments. In the absence of partner consent, the male transvestite may have to rely on fantasy alone in order to have a coital orgasm. He cannot erotically divorce himself from either his penis or his transvestite wardrobe.

Bona fide transvestism either does not occur in females or is extremely rare, for it has not been reported in the sexological literature. Indeed it is a general rule that errors of psychosexual development leading to a paraphiliac image or object of sexual arousal are more frequent in the male. Most are unheard of in women.

The idealized transexual is someone who in early childhood differentiated an incongruous gender identity, and has always felt that nature made an anatomical mistake. The possibility of sex reassignment and the label "transexual" are discovered later. The idealized male-to-female transexual gets erotic pleasure from giving orgasmic satisfaction to the partner. In coitus and sex play he assumes the receptor role, receiving the partner's penis rectally, interfemorally, or orally. Preoperatively, the idealized male-to-female transexual's penis does not penetrate any orifice of the partner's anatomy, and penile stimulation is regarded as unpleasant and undesired.

The male-to-female transexual's fantasy may conform to the popular stereotype of the female as being sexually passive and accepting, slowly aroused, less prone to the initiation of sexual activity, and able to gain satisfaction from pleasing a partner. Adherence to this misconception is perhaps a function of the fact that many male-to-female transexuals have not experienced intercourse with a woman, and are, therefore, reliant on popular stereotypes. Many sex-reassigned male-to-female transexuals have had, and continue to have a sexual life with multiple male partners. A few establish themselves, in sex reassignment, as lesbians.

The idealized female-to-male, sex-reassigned transexual is erotically attracted to females. Like many ordinary women, he finds satisfaction in fidelity, and his sexual relationships are not too often casual or multiple. Also, like many women, he is dependent on intimate closeness for genitopelvic arousal. If he masturbates at all, it is infrequently. Presurgically, he regards penetration of his own vagina by a finger, a penis, or prosthetic device as intolerable, and is desirous of having male genitalia. Surgically, mastectomy has priority over genital plastic surgery. The breasts are a constant negative reminder of natal sex. Breast fondling either negates sexual arousal or is erotically unimportant. Coital imagery is of the self as male, without breasts, and usually complete with a penis, regardless of the sex of the partner.

In the idealized case, the conviction of transexualism dates from early childhood, although it also may evolve over the course of an individual's lifetime. For instance, in the fourth or fifth decade of life an apparent transvestite may find his episodes of femininity occurring with greater frequency and greater duration. The increasingly demanding female personality may come to insist on permanent repudiation of male clothing, and removal of the offensive male genitalia.

Effeminate homosexuality and butch lesbianism, as well as transvestism, may all be way stations en route to transexualism. If so, the differential diagnosis may be extremely difficult. Such people, above all others, owe it to themselves to live the real-life test for two years or more before surgery.

Social, Recreational, and Cosmetic Rehabilitation

A transexual beginning the real-life test may find it expedient in terms of earning power not to change the way he/she dresses at work, but only during off-work hours, until ready to embark on vocational rehabilitation.

Although the majority of patients are past masters at impersonating the other sex, a few exaggerate sexually dimorphic behavior patterns and require special counseling. For the female-to-male transexual this may mean toning down a macho swagger, and for the male-to-female transexual it may mean tutoring so that the daytime appearance is not that of a midnight whore.

The male-to-female transexual may begin electrolysis for the removal of facial and body hair. If carried out gradually and not completed until just prior to surgery, some hair follicles will remain should the real-life test be failed.

The female-to-male transexual may undergo mastectomy in order to flatten the chest. Should a return to the female role later be indicated, implantation mammoplasty will be possible.

Social rehabilitation may continue long after surgery, but prior to surgery the transexual must at the very least be comfortable and convincing in the sex of reassignment.

Establishing a New Public Identity

Early in the real-life test the transexual should establish a new public identity. Initially, this is a rather simple procedure since, by common law, any citizen of the United States has the right to change his/her name by personal decision, provided there is no intent of fraud or prejudice to others. Then the new name may be used on applications for library cards, credit cards, bank accounts, and various other items of identification.

When the transexual's public appearance as a member of the opposite sex becomes convincing, he/she will need a legal certification of name change prior to applying, in most jurisdictions, for an amended or reissued birth certificate. In some jurisdictions, bureaucratic regulations constitute no obstacle, whereas in others it still is not possible to get a change of sexual status on the birth certificate. In such a case, the help of an attorney is advisable in getting other documentary changes, as for example, passport or academic certificates.

Financial and Vocational Rehabilitation

Vocational and financial rehabilitation usually, though not always, begins before a new public identity has been established. Since work is gender-coded in our society, many transexuals begin their work career in an occupation suited to their transexual personality. Some of these people will arrange to declare their new public identity and remain in their place of employment. Others will decide to break with the past and change to a type of employment which they like better and find more in keeping with their sex of reassignment. Still others will change employment as part of a total program of breaking with the past so as to avoid stigmatization as a transexual.

It is enormously complicated for any person, transexual or otherwise, to live in total alienation from his/her prior personal history, constantly evading the chance of discovery. Most transexuals are well-advised not to make the attempt. If they are tutored in the public relations of transexualism, and how to explain their situation medically and psychologically, then they will probably be surprised at how well they are publicly accepted. Some transexuals experience a sense of triumph and achievement at "going public," and being not stigmatized but congratulated at work.

In those instances in which the patient does not expect to be financially autonomous, but to rely upon a parent or benefactor for support, it is necessary to familiarize this third party with sex-reassignment procedures and to secure assurance that support will indeed be forthcoming following surgery.

Familial Rehabilitation

At the time a transexual makes known his or her plans for sex reassignment, it is good policy to offer family counseling regarding the medical and rehabilitation aspects of transexualism. Younger siblings especially need to be included. So counseled, family members are better able to reintegrate the transexual into the kinship as a member of the opposite sex. The family can be an important source of psychological support during the progress of sex reassignment. If, even with professional counseling, no reconciliation proves possible, the transexual will have the opportunity to accommodate himself or herself to the lack of familial support or to rethink the reassignment decision.

In those cases in which the obsession for sex reassignment develops in later life, the transexual may be a spouse and parent. If so, reassignment is not indicated until the necessary personal, legal, and financial arrangements have been made. Counseling of the spouse and children is obligatory.

Hormonal Reassignment: Male-to-Female

Endocrine reassignment of the male-to-female transexual with estrogen and progestin results in hormonal castration which is reversible. The patient thus gains first-hand acquaintance with impotence and reduced libido, before the irreversible steps of surgical castration, penectomy, and vaginoplasty. Should the patient find the effect of hormonal treatment to be anything other than desirable, he should not be considered a candidate for reassignment surgery.

Hormonal feminization promotes a female appearance insofar as it brings about a feminine redistribution of subcutaneous fat. It also stimulates breast enlargement (gynecomastia), and may retard the growth of facial and body hair. If a return to the male role is indicated, the breasts may be flattened surgically, and the other effects may be reversed upon withdrawal of hormonal therapy.

Hormonal Reassignment: Female-to-Male

Hormonal masculinization of the female-to-male transexual with androgen induces suppression of the menses. Since breakthrough bleeding usually will eventually occur, permanent suppression requires castration or hysterectomy, preferably both.

The effects of hormonal masculinization include deepening of the voice and growth of facial and body hair. The effect on the breasts in minimal. The clitoris enlarges, but not sufficiently to permit masculinizing surgical reconstruction as even a very small micropenis. Its erotic sensitivity increases. The feeling of orgasm is reported as increased, with no loss of the female capacity for multiple orgasm.

Should a return to the female role be indicated after a trial of hormonal masculinization, the menses will return upon withdrawal of androgen therapy. Masculine hair growth may be reversed by electrolysis. An expensive and difficult procedure also makes possible the restoration of a feminine voice.

Associated Psychopathology

Psychopathic delinquency with lying and stealing may occur in association with transexualism. Less frequently, hallucinations, delusions, or suicidal depression may also occur. All such symptoms require therapy in their own right. It is preferable that they be brought under control prior to embarking on sex reassignment, as they are not relieved by reassignment per se.

Explanation of Surgical Procedures

Informed consent is a necessary prerequisite of surgery. This entails an explanation of the surgical procedures involved, and possible outcomes. Because sex-reassignment surgical technique is not yet standardized, the approach varies from surgeon to surgeon. Explanations must be individually tailored. However, a few generalizations are possible.

The male-to-female transexual can expect that the surgical admission will require approximately two weeks and, in the case of a two-stage procedure, an additional surgical admission for a week or longer. The body of the penis will be excised, the urethral tube shortened and implanted in the feminine position, and a vaginal cavity created in the musculature of the perineum and lined with penile skin augmented with skin grafted from the thigh. Postsurgically the patient must wear a form in the vagina for at least several months in order to ensure its patency.

The postoperative capacity for erotic sensation will depend on how the skin of the penis and scrotum are utilized in feminization, and on the particular hormonal regimen. The experience of orgasm may be a warm glow throughout the body or an orgasm of spasmodic intensity. The artificial vagina will supply a male partner with satisfying sexual feelings.

Surgical masculinization of the female-to-male transexual involves mastectomy (already discussed), and panhysterectomy, a relatively simple procedure in which the ovaries and uterus are removed. Should phalloplasty be decided upon there are two general approaches. Both are much more difficult than vaginoplasty for the male-to-female transexual, and produce a much less satisfactory end result. One involves the creation of a penis complete with urinary tube from abdominal skin grafts. As many as 15 surgical admissions over several years may be required in order to get a completely satisfactory urinary tube. In this procedure the clitoris is preserved intact, and retains its capacity to produce orgasm, but the numb roll of skin in which it is embedded is too flabby to effect sexual penetration, unless supported inside a hollow prosthetic penis.

The surgical alternative is to create a copulatory rather than a urinary organ. This procedure involves fashioning a hollow tube from an apron of skin peeled downward from below the naval. It also requires multiple hospital admissions. The clitoris is embedded in the base of the hollow tube as in the former procedure. For intercourse a prosthetic device must be fitted into the hollow tube.

Since sexual intercourse will be impossible without a prosthetic device regardless of the surgical procedure performed, the female-to-male transexual should be counseled as to the wisdom of making-do with a strap-on prosthetic penis, and forgoing the lengthy and complex procedures involved in phalloplasty.

A Promise to Cooperate in Follow-up Studies

Having embarked on the real-life test, some patients will decide that reassignment is not the solution they've been seeking to life's problem. Others will require a longer test period. For these, as for those who have passed the real-life test, and are still convinced in favor of sex-reassignment surgery, one final prerequisite remains. The patient must guarantee to cooperate in long-term follow-up studies. Transexuals eager to forget their preoperative past may balk at this requirement, but it is imperative if the procedure of sex reassignment is to remain acceptable as a proven form of therapy.

Outcome of Surgical Sex Reassignment

Though rare, it does happen that sex-reassigned individuals decide to revert to their original sex assignment. We have had personal interviews with three such individuals, and had correspondence from a fourth. In each instance, the patient planned his own timetable of sex reassignment so as to evade the two-year, real-life test.

Because the criteria of selection for sex reassignment have varied from institution to institution in the absence of proven standards, it is difficult to interpret much of the follow-up data in the literature. However, it is clear that when the two-year, real-life test is a prerequisite for sex-reassignment surgery, virtually 100 per cent of the patients benefit from surgery according to both subjective and objective criteria of evaluation. Thus, following surgery, job status stays the same or improves, sexual relationships tend to be more stable and longer lasting, and patients do not become psychotic. A history of arrests for solicitation may continue, but there is no increased incidence of law-breaking behavior. Patients report subjective satisfaction with sex reassignment, and indicate that if they had it to do over again they would make the same decision, even though the surgical outcome may have been a disappointment and, by the coital criterion, a failure.

Conclusion

By next century, research into the etiology of gender identity transposition may suggest new and better therapeutic approaches to transexualism. Insofar as sex reassignment provides the opportunity for the medical profession to maintain contacts with transexuals, and stimulates the systematic collection of data about transexuals, it will facilitate such research. In the interim, sex reassignment is the only demonstrably effective treatment—rehabilitative treatment, not curative. Truly preventive and/or curative treatment still awaits discovery.

Summary

Transexualism, once considered to be a sin and outside the realm of medicine, is now classified as an illness. Prenatal endocrine and postnatal social factors may be important determinants of gender identity transposition, as in transexualism, but in the final analysis the etiology is unknown. Whereas psychotherapeutic attempts to cure transexualism by altering gender identity so as to conform to the body have been unsuccessful, alteration of the body so as to conform to the gender identity through sex-reassignment surgery has proved to be an effective rehabilitative therapy. In the differential diagnosis of transexualism an important source of information is the tape-recorded, transcribed, and tabulated diagnostic interview. The differential diagnosis includes effeminate homosexuality, masculinate lesbianism, and episodic transvestism. The most important diagnostic test is the two-year, real-life test during which time the candidate for sex-reassignment undergoes social, recreational, vocational, economic, familial, and hormonal rehabilitation in the new gender role. The final prerequisite for the irrevocable step of surgical reconstruction is the patient's informed consent and agreement to cooperate in follow-up studies. When the real-life test is required prior to surgery, the outcome is positive according to both objective and subjective criteria.

Reference

Money, J., and Primrose, C.: Sexual dimorphism and dissociation in the psychology of male transexuals. *In* Money, J., and Green, R. (eds.): Transexualism and Sex Reassignment. Baltimore, Johns Hopkins University Press, 1966.

Comment

Most major American cities now have a gender identity clinic—a psychiatric-medical unit which offers guidance to persons concerned with their sexual identity, including the possibility of sex reassignment surgery. They appear to vary greatly in the range of diagnostic and treatment services offered and the sophistication and thoroughness with which they assess their clients before and following various treatment programs. Some are alleged to offer sex reassignment surgery virtually "on demand," and others consider surgery only after exhaustive assessment of the patient in his social and familial milieu. Psychiatric opinion on the condition termed transsexualism and its treatment also varies over a wide range. Some question the legitimacy of the condition itself, whether or not it is the proper concern of medicine, and whether surgical approaches have any rational or justifiable basis.

Drs. Money and Ambinder regard transsexualism as a medical (psychiatric) disorder. Leading authorities on the nature, diagnosis, and assessment of transsexualism and its treatment by sex reassignment, they have provided us with a clear and concise overview of the topic. Their central thesis is that properly screened and selected transsexuals may benefit substantially from reconstructive surgery when it is carried out in a comprehensive program which also pays attention to the patients' social, vocational, and recreational adjustment in their new sex role. An impressive aspect of Money and Ambinder's own program is the requirement that the patient assume his intended new sex role for a two-year, real-life probationary period before the irrevocable surgical changes in genital anatomy are carried out. This test, according to Money and Ambinder, greatly reduces the risk of including a patient who will later regret the anatomical changes and wish to revert to his/her original sex assignment.

Not all clinicians who have worked in the area of sex reassignment surgery are as sanguine as Money and Ambinder. Many programs do not conduct as thorough and sophisticated an assessment of the problem as Money and Ambinder describe, and many do not conduct essential long-term follow up procedures. Other investigators question the effects of the procedure on the patient's social and psychological adjustment—the only justification for doing the surgery in the first place.

In addition to more thorough assessment and follow up, there is a need for more comparative studies in which the effects of sex reassignment surgery are compared with those of alternative programs. Recently, there have been some preliminary but promising reports on the use of behavior modification programs for sex reassignment without the use of potentially destructive surgery. These and related approaches, which might include hormonal alterations, need to be developed, assessed, and eventually compared with programs which feature major surgical components.

JOHN PAUL BRADY, M.D.

Should Psychiatric Patients Be Given Genetic Counseling?

RAYMOND R. CROWE

University of Iowa College of Medicine

Is genetic counseling appropriate for psychiatric illnesses? Until recently most psychiatrists would probably have answered the question negatively. Considerable doubt existed over whether mental illness represented true "physical disease" in the same sense as other medical illnesses (Szasz, 1961). However, adoption studies and other genetic investigations have now firmly established a genetic basis for many of the major psychiatric syndromes (Crowe, 1975; Mendlewicz and Fleiss, 1974). In fact, in view of these recent advances, the first question might justifiably be rephrased to ask whether these illnesses differ in any important respects from a number of medical diseases for which a genetic basis has long been established and genetic counseling is customary.

Although the importance of genetics has been clearly demonstrated, the appropriateness of genetic counseling for psychiatric illness might be questioned on the basis of its ambiguous inheritance. It is far from clear how these diseases are inherited and to what extent environmental factors are involved. This situation contrasts sharply with the classic mendelian syndromes such as hemophilia, in which the transmission fits clear-cut genetic patterns. In reality, however, the genetic counselor cannot limit his practice to such clear-cut diseases but must counsel for a large number of disorders for which the underlying genetics are far from clear, and in some cases, an unequivocal genetic basis has not been firmly established. Diabetes mellitus provides a good example of this problem because it shares many features in common with psychiatric syndromes. In the first place, no biological test for the underlying predisposition is available and the disease cannot be diagnosed until glucose metabolism has been affected. The risk of developing the illness increases with age and there is no age beyond which it does not develop. The data support the importance of both genes and environment in causing the disease, but its inheritance does not follow any familiar mendelian pattern and the method by which the environment interacts with the genetic predisposition is not clearly understood (Neel, 1970). Finally, these problems are complicated by the fact that the disease is most likely heterogeneous, with the early-onset form representing a different disease with different genetics than the late-onset form. (See Science, *188*:347, 1975, for a review of the recent evidence.) Despite these problems, the disease is a common one and the need for genetic counseling frequently arises. Fortunately, data from large epidemiologic studies allow reasonably accurate risk estimates to be given and the pattern of inheritance provides a sufficiently close fit to certain mathematical models that for practical purposes (i.e., counseling) we can use these models as a working approximation. The analogy with diabetes is informative because it presents many of the same problems that will be encountered in counseling psychiatric patients and illustrates that these neither are unique to psychiatry nor preclude counseling.

A final question which must be considered is whether mental illness per se would contraindicate counseling. First, are psychiatric patients able to understand and use rationally the information they will receive in counseling; and secondly, will this information place an excessive emotional burden on them? Obviously, there are no easy answers to these questions, and mature clinical judgment is as important in genetic counseling as in any other branch of clinical medicine. Each patient must be assessed carefully with regard to both of these questions before proceeding. Here again, however, the problems are not unique to psychiatry and have a long precedent in genetic counseling. Dementia and emotional instability are prominent features of Huntington's chorea, but in spite of these problems, Huntington's patients are routinely counseled. It should also be borne in mind that psychiatric patients may be keenly aware of their family history and believe their risk of passing the disease on to their children to be much higher than it actually is. Mental illness, then, does not represent a contraindication to genetic counseling, and to the contrary, counseling may be beneficial in some situations by dispelling unjustified fears and prejudices about the disease. Although situations will arise which will demand considerable counseling skill and clinical judgment, these are not unique to psychiatry but have been dealt with in counseling for some time. Moreover, the psychiatrist should be ideally suited for dealing with these problems.

If psychiatric patients are appropriate for genetic counseling, then which patients should be counseled, and what should they be told? Before taking up these questions, it will be useful to review some basic principles of genetic counseling and the fundamental mechanisms of inheritance in man.

Some Principles of Genetic Counseling

Diagnosis. Genetic counseling begins with an accurate diagnosis. The importance of this cannot be stressed too much, for far greater harm will result from counseling for disorders of uncertain diagnosis than for disorders of uncertain heredity. This is especially relevant in psychiatry, where laboratory tests for verifying the diagnosis are unavailable and methods of diagnosing are likely to vary from clinic to clinic. If any doubt as to the diagnosis exists, every effort must be made to obtain all relevant information and establish a firm diagnosis before counseling. If still in doubt, don't counsel.

Family history. The genetic counselor must be skilled in taking an accurate and extensive family history from the patient and his relatives, and when necessary, by obtaining outside records. This information may aid in arriving at the correct diagnosis, as in Huntington's chorea, and it may be important in establishing the mode of transmission, as in a dominantly inherited form of presenile dementia. The information is recorded in standard pedigree form, which is elaborated in most standard texts on medical genetics and genetic counseling. Several of these are listed at the end of this article for the reader who would like to pursue this subject further.

Evaluation of the individual. This important aspect of counseling, which has been touched on in the introductory section, involves a careful evaluation of the individual seeking counseling in order to determine such matters as why counseling is being sought, how capable the individual is of comprehending and making rational decisions based on the information he is to receive, and the patient's level of understanding of genetics. This will determine which areas need to be stressed in counseling and whether counseling should be attempted in one session or several. Clearly, some individuals may come into the counseling session with considerable prior knowledge about genetics and the nature of the disease in question, whereas others may enter with little knowledge and fears based on frank misconceptions. Thus, the counselor must have a good "feel" for his patient before counseling is attempted or miscommunication may occur.

Risk versus burden. When the diagnosis and family history have been established, and the counselor feels that he understands the individual's prior knowledge and concerns, counseling can begin. As Murphy has pointed out, a realistic decision to have children or not must be based on two considerations: the risk and the burden of the illness (Murphy, 1973). Risk refers to the probability of any given child born to the couple being affected with the illness. Often couples will not be interested in absolute risk so much as how much their risk has been *increased* by having the illness in the family. Burden, on the other hand, refers to the severity of the illness and the hardship this is likely to impose on the individual, his family, and society. Thus, prospective parents may decide to take even a high risk if the burden is low, but only a low risk if the burden is high. It is important, then, that counseling include a discussion of the nature of the illness, its course and prognosis, and the effect of treatment, in addition to the assessment of risk.

The decision to have children or not. This decision properly belongs to the individuals counseled and should not be made by the counselor. Only they can assess the risk and burden as it pertains to their particular circumstances and arrive at a decision. The counselor's task should be limited to providing them with the factual information on which to base the decision and making certain that they correctly understand what they have been told. The decision requires time and thought and should not be rushed. Couples may need to return for further counseling sessions after having time to discuss the information between themselves, and this should be encouraged.

Assessing understanding. At the end of the counseling session, the counselor should satisfy himself that the individuals understand what they have been told. This is best accomplished by having them explain to the counselor the risk and burden of the illness as they understand it and their decision based on this information. It is also a good practice to write them a letter summarizing the counseling session for their records and future reference if questions rise.

Some Basic Principles of Genetics

The genetic counselor must be thoroughly familiar with the mechanisms of inheritance in man before attempting to counsel. A detailed discussion of these is beyond the scope of this chapter and the interested reader is referred to the references on human genetics and genetic counseling which are listed at the end of the article. This section is intended to present a brief overview of the basic mechanisms of inheritance to facilitate understanding of the sections to follow. Basically, inheritance can be subdivided into mendelian and multifactorial.

Mendelian inheritance. The human genotype consists of 46 chromosomes, 22 pairs of autosomes and one pair of sex chromosomes (male being XY and females XX). If a disease is caused by a dominant gene, the presence of this gene on either chromosome is sufficient to produce the illness. In recessive inheritance the defective gene must be present on both chromosomes in order to cause disease. This results in four types of mendelian inheritance. *Autosomal dominant* inheritance is characterized by (1) every affected individual having an affected parent, (2) each child of an affected parent having exactly one chance in two of being affected, and (3) males and females being affected in equal numbers on the average. Since every affected person must have an affected parent, persons born to unaffected members of the pedigree are not at increased risk for developing the disease. In *autosomal recessive* inheritance, affected subjects are born to two phenotypically normal parents who are both carriers of the recessive gene. The risk of being affected for each child born to such parents is one in four, and the risk of being a carrier is one in two. Finally, males and females are affected in equal numbers on the average. A phenotypically normal member of an affected sibship has two chances in three of being a carrier. The risk of being affected for each future child of such a carrier is equal to the probability that the carrier will marry another carrier (the carrier frequency in the population) times the probability of each child being affected given that this event occurs (one in four). For example, if the carrier frequency is 0.01, then the risk to each child born to a phenotypically normal member of an affected sibship is equal to the probability of that person being a carrier (2/3) times the probability of the spouse being a carrier (1/100) times the probability of each child being affected (1/4), which results in a risk of one in 600. By the same reasoning, the risk for a couple, both of whose families are free of the illness, works out to one in 4,000. Thus, in this case, the risk to each unborn child of a carrier is 7 times that of the general population but still very low. *Sex-linked recessive* diseases typically affect only males who receive the gene from their phenotypically normal carrier mothers, thus causing the disease to appear to "skip generations." The risk of being affected for any male born into such a sibship is one in two and for females the risk of being a carrier is likewise one in two. Males born to affected fathers are not affected, but all daughters are carriers. Finally, in rare *sex-linked dominant* inheritance females are affected twice as frequently as males, and father to son transmission is absent, although all daughters born to an affected father will be affected. When the affected parent is female, the transmission to her children behaves as an autosomal dominant.

In *multifactorial* inheritance an inherited diathesis to the disease is assumed to result from equal and additive effects of many genes rather than a single gene. This genetic diathesis is influenced by environmental factors, and the combined effects of both genetic and nongenetic influences determine the outcome. This form of inheritance may underlie continuous traits, such as blood pressure, or discontinuous traits such as cleft lip and palate. In the case of discontinuous diseases, an underlying continuously varying liability is assumed to exist but to be immeasurable given our present state of knowledge. When the liability exceeds a certain hypothetical threshold, illness will develop and below this threshold the individual will appear normal.

Clinically, multifactorial inheritance differs from mendelian inheritance in several important respects. First, the recurrence risks tend to be lower in multifactorial inheritance and the risks drop sharply as one becomes more distantly related to the affected subject. The risk to any child born into the family increases with the number of affected persons already in the family and with the severity of their illness. When one sex is less frequently affected, the recurrence risk is increased among the relatives of patients of that sex.

Unfortunately, in psychiatry few diseases fit neatly into either of the above categories of inheritance. Because of *genetic heterogeneity* the same disease may be produced by two or more genes or by different modes of inheritance. *Phenocopies*, or environmental reproductions of a genetic illness, may contribute to an unknown number of the total cases. *Incomplete penetrance* and *age-dependent penetrance* may render the underlying mechanism of inheritance impossible to determine. Finally, some diseases may run in families for purely environmental reasons. For these reasons, the counselor must rely on empiric risk figures whenever the actual mechanism of inheritance is not known with certainty. *Empiric risk estimates* are simply statements of the frequency with which the disease recurs among the relatives of persons known to have the disease. No assumption about the underlying mechanism of inheritance is implied, nor is it necessarily implied that the disease is genetic. Empiric risk figures are based on epidemiologic studies of affected families and represent average values for various degrees of relatives. For this reason, they differ from mendelian risk estimates in one important respect: mendelian risks are exact risks, whereas empiric risks are averages. The exact risk to an individual may be greater or less than the empiric risk, depending on the severity of the illness in his family, the number of persons affected, and possibly other unknown factors. Despite these problems empiric risks do provide a reasonable approximation to the risk an individual runs of developing an illness or having affected children. It is important, however, that the person being counseled understand the difference between empiric risk and exact risk.

One final problem which is particularly relevant to psychiatry is variable *expressivity*. This refers to the fact that the same genotype may be expressed differently in different persons. A person who has had multiple hospitalizations for affective disorder may have a sibling whose only manifestation of the illness has been an isolated mild episode. Likewise, one family member may have bipolar illness and others may experience depressions only. It is important that this phenomenon be appreciated by the person counseled so that the burden of the illness can be properly assessed.

Counseling for Specific Disorders

Now that some of the basic principles of genetic counseling have been considered, attention can be turned to the question of which of the psychiatric disorders may be considered appropriate for counseling. Although most of the major psychiatric illnesses are known to run in families, for the purposes of counseling, the discussion will be confined to those disorders for which large data sets exist. Most empiric risks to be quoted are based on averages from a number of studies. The individual studies vary due to differences in diagnostic criteria, sampling variance, and other factors. In some instances the morbidity risks vary between subgroups within the same study. These problems should not be troublesome, however, if it is remembered that most persons seeking counseling are interested in knowing roughly what their risks are rather than in precise risk estimates. Whether the true risk is 10 per cent or 15 per cent is not likely to be of critical importance. However, the discussion will be confined to first degree relatives, since the data are more reliable on parents, siblings, and children than on second and third degree relatives.

In counseling for specific diseases it is important that the individual acquire a basic understanding of how the disease is inherited if this is known. The prevalence of the disease in the population should be understood. This can be compared with the prevalence of the disease in families with an affected member. The discussion should include an explanation of how these risk estimates were arrived at and whether there are any modifying factors such as sex differences or number of affected persons in the family which need to be considered. Counseling should include a discussion of the disease in order to ascertain what the person's understanding of the illness is and to amplify on this or correct any misconceptions that may be uncovered.

Unipolar Depression

Unipolar depression will be defined as one or more episodes of depressive illness meeting the criteria of Feighner et al. (1972). Although diagnostic criteria used in various studies of depression have differed, this definition is sufficiently compatible with the majority of these studies to make the data in the literature applicable to patients who meet these criteria.

The genetics of unipolar depression present all of the problems encountered with psychiatric diseases. The mode of inheritance is not known, and furthermore, this category is almost certainly heterogeneous. One kindred in which the disease appears to follow an autosomal dominant pattern has been reported, but in other families the genetics have been unclear (Pardue, 1975). Helgason found the prevalence of depression (including bipolar) in the population to be 2.5 per cent among females and 1.8 per cent among males (Helgason, 1964). How does this compare with the frequency of this disorder seen in the first degree relatives of depressed patients? Gershon et al. have recently summarized the relevant family and family history studies of unipolar affective disorder (Gershon et al., 1976). These data, based on roughly 2000 subjects at risk of each sex, indicate a morbidity risk of 9.4 per cent among male and 13.5 per cent among female first degree relatives (i.e., parents, siblings, and children). This predominance of affected females has been found in most studies of depression.

Thus, the individual counseled should understand that depression is a common disease affecting roughly two per cent of the population and affecting females more frequently than males at a ratio of about three to two. Although the mode of inheritance is unknown, it is known to be familial with first degree relatives of affected patients running about five times the risk of the general population. The absolute risk is in the vicinity of 13.5 per cent for females and 9.4 per cent for males, which should be viewed as rough estimates and not exact risks in the sense of mendelian genetics. The wide variation in the frequency and severity of the illness as well as treatment results are well appreciated by psychiatrists and must be understood by the person counseled in order that the burden can be properly evaluated.

Bipolar Affective Disorder

This diagnosis refers to individuals who have had at least one episode of mania as defined by the criteria of Feighner et al., regardless of whether a depression has also occurred. Depressed patients with a positive family history of bipolar illness are likewise considered to be bipolar. As with unipolar depression, the genetics of bipolar illness are not understood. There is now considerable evidence that there are at least two genetically distinct forms of the illness, one being transmitted as a sex-linked dominant (Mendlewicz and Fleiss, 1975) and the genetics of the other being unclear (Goetzl et al., 1974). Unfortunately, this is not useful information for genetic counseling because it is impossible to determine clinically which cases are of the sex-linked variety. Over the past few years much has been written about sex linkage in bipolar illness, making it important that the problem of heterogeneity be fully appreciated. At the present time bipolar illness should not be counseled as a sex-linked disorder, because the counseling may be seriously in error if the family in question does not have the sex-linked variety of the illness.

Helgason's data indicate a population prevalence for bipolar illness of 0.8 per cent in the Icelandic population (Helgason, 1964). This is undoubtedly an underestimate, since we know from family studies that many bipolar patients manifest depression only and thus would have been counted as having unipolar illness (further evidence for the genetic heterogeneity of unipolar depression). Unfortunately, the family studies of bipolar illness show considerable variability in the morbidity risks reported. Five of these are reasonably consistent with morbidity risks for total affective disorder among first degree relatives ranging from 14.5 to 21 per cent (Angst and Perris, 1972; Perris, 1966; James and Chapman, 1975; Goetzl et al., 1974; Gershon et al., 1975). Others have found higher risks, however, with Winokur et al. reporting 35 per cent and Mendlewicz et al. 36 per cent for parents and siblings (children are excluded to make these two studies comparable with the others) (Winokur et al., 1969; Mendlewicz and Rainer, 1974). The studies which have reported morbidity risks in children have found surprisingly high ones (over 50 per cent), but since these figures are based on small samples and could be inflated by age corrections, the more conservative morbidity risks based on larger numbers of parents and siblings are felt to be preferable (Winokur et al., 1969; Mendlewicz and Rainer, 1974; Goetzl et al., 1974). A figure of 20 per cent is recommended as a reasonable reflection of the true lifetime morbidity risk for first degree relatives of bipolar patients, but it should be remembered that in some families the risk may be substantially higher. It will be noted that even these conservative morbidity risks are appreciably higher than those found among the first degree relatives of unipolar depressives, especially when compared with the base population risk for bipolar illness.

The preponderance of the data indicates that the morbidity risk is higher among females in affected families, and a recent review (Gershon et al., 1976) indicates a ratio of 3 to 2, although some (Winokur et al., 1969; Mendlewicz and Rainer, 1974) have noted considerably larger differences while others (Gershon et al., 1975; Perris, 1968) have failed to find this difference. In view of these discrepancies, it is probably best to use 20 per cent as the morbidity risk for both sexes.

Persons being counseled for bipolar illness should understand that the disease is strongly familial although the exact mechanism of inheritance is not understood. The fact that genetic heterogeneity exists should be appreciated as well as its implication: that morbidity risk may vary considerably from family to family. Since the genetic subtypes cannot be distinguished clinically at this time, we are forced to give a "ball park estimate" for the morbidity risk. The overall risk estimate recommended is 20 per cent, which is 20 times the population prevalence of around one per cent. The natural history of bipolar illness should be understood, in particular that it may be manifest as unipolar depression only. Finally, the success of current therapy and prophylaxis should be discussed.

SCHIZOPHRENIA

An accurate diagnosis for this disease is critical because other illnesses frequently present a schizophreniform picture and can be easily mistaken for schizophrenia, although their longitudinal course will not be that of schizophrenia and schizophrenia will not be found among their relatives (Stephens and Astrup, 1963; McCabe, 1976). The term schizophrenia here refers to "process" schizophrenia, which may be defined by the criteria of Feighner et al. as a chronic illness of at least six months' duration characterized by delusions, hallucinations, or disordered verbal production which cannot be explained by some other illness such as drug abuse or affective disorder (Feighner et al., 1972).

This syndrome is probably heterogeneous and there is evidence that the paranoid and hebephrenic subtypes differ in some important respects (Tsuang, 1975). In particular, hebephrenia appears to be a more severe illness with an earlier age of onset and carries a greater morbidity risk among relatives than paranoid schizophrenia. However, at the present time, the subtypes are not sufficiently established to be used in genetic counseling and it is preferable that schizophrenia be counseled as a single disease.

Although the genetics are not understood, the disease transmission fits a multifactorial threshold model well enough that this model may be used as a working approximation in genetic counseling (Gottesman and Shields, 1972). Because of this, a single morbidity risk for first degree relatives will not suffice, since the risk varies considerably depending upon the number of parents and siblings who are already affected. Smith has constructed a table of morbidity risks for multifactorial inheritance given various numbers of affected parents and siblings (Smith, 1971). Using a heritability estimate of 80 per cent, these morbidity risks provide a very close fit to those actually observed. The data reviewed by Slater and Cowie indicate that the risk to a child of a schizophrenic parent is 12 per cent, and that to a sibling of a schizophrenic is 8 per cent if neither parent is affected and 14 per cent if one parent is affected (Slater and Cowie, 1971). These risks are substantially higher than the population prevalence of the disease, which is usually found to be around 0.8 per cent (Slater and Cowie, 1971).

Thus, schizophrenia is a disease which fits closely to a predictive model. Nevertheless, the disease is probably heterogeneous and not all members of a family will be through the age of risk, thus leading to some inaccuracy in the data which is put into the model. Unlike treatment for affective disorders, treatment is palliative rather than curative, and complete remission is not to be expected. Nevertheless, the disease varies considerably in its severity, with some patients being only mildly affected.

The Dementias

Huntington's chorea is the most carefully studied of the dementias from a genetic standpoint. This is a rare disease with a prevalence rate in the range of four to seven per 100,000 population (Slater and Cowie, 1971). The disease is transmitted as an autosomal dominant with age-dependent penetrance. The mean age of onset is 44 years with a standard deviation of 11 years, and the risk of onset can be considered to be normally distributed (Murphy and Chase, 1975). This allows us to predict accurately the probability of being affected by a given age provided that a person has the gene. This adds an additional facet to counseling in that a person's initial risk of developing the illness is modified downward as he passes through the period of risk without developing it. All of the psychiatric disorders reviewed are characterized by age-dependent penetrance. The others differ from Huntington's disease in that their ages of onset are not as well worked out and furthermore suffer from all the problems of empiric risks. Attempting to use them in counseling would involve modifying empiric risks by more empiric risks, a practice which could lead to results falling wide of the mark. In Huntington's disease the counselor starts with an exact probability and modifies it with reasonably accurate onset data. The manner in which this information is used to modify risk estimates is dealt with in detail by Murphy and Chase, and the counselor should be thoroughly familiar with this technique before attempting to use it clinically (Murphy and Chase, 1975). The following example will serve as an illustration.

Let us suppose that the person at risk is a 44-year-old man whose father was affected with Huntington's chorea. The probability that the patient has received the gene is 1/2 and the probability that he has not received it is likewise 1/2. This is referred to as the prior probability. If he has the gene, the probability of living to age 44 without developing the illness is 1/2. If he does not have the gene, the probability is one. These are referred to as conditional probabilities. Now, the probability of receiving the gene *and* living to age 44 without being affected is 1/4 (1/2 times 1/2). Similarly, the probability of not receiving the gene and living to age 44 without being affected is 1/2 (1/2 times 1). These are referred to as conjunctional probabilities. Now, we are interested in the probability that our hypothetical subject has the gene (his posterior probability), which is equal to his conjunctional probability divided by the sum of the two conjunctional probabilities and is equal to 1/3 (1/4 divided by the sum of 1/2 and 1/4). If he continues to survive without being affected, this probability will progressively decrease, approaching 0 in senescence. The risk for each of his future children is simply 1/2 times his posterior probability, or 1/6 in this example.

Alzheimer's disease and Pick's disease are clinically indistinguishable, although the former is probably 20 times as frequent as the latter, making Alzheimer's the most likely diagnosis in any given case (Slater and Cowie, 1971). These diseases are genetically heterogeneous with autosomal dominant kindreds reported for both Alzheimer's and Pick's disease (Heston et al., 1966; Schenk, 1959), making a careful family history before counseling mandatory. The mean age of onset is in the fifth decade but unlike Huntington's chorea insufficient data are available to estimate an age of onset distribution. The best family data available come from the study by Sjögren et al., who report age-corrected morbidity risks of 15 per cent for parents and five per cent for siblings of affected cases (Sjögren et al., 1952). Moreover, the risk for siblings when a parent was also affected was 16 per cent, compared with 2.5 per cent when parents were unaffected. This speaks for polygenic inheritance in those kindreds which do not implicate a dominant gene.

In the case of the dominantly inherited illnesses precise risk estimates can be given, the risk being 1/2 for siblings and children and 1/4 for second degree relatives such as nieces, nephews, and grandchildren. In the remaining cases, those assumed to be polygenic, it is difficult to decide which risk estimate to use for first degree relatives. Sjögren et al. found a three-fold difference between parents and siblings of affected subjects, and the true risk probably lies somewhere between the two.

In *senile dementia* the baseline morbidity risk increases with age from 0.03 per cent at age 60 to 5.2 per cent at age 90. This age distribution is given in detail in a monograph by Larsson et al., who found that the morbidity risk among first degree relatives of affected subjects was 4.3 times that of the general population in each age group studied (Larsson et al., 1963). Although the genetics underlying the recurrence risk are unknown, this seems like a reasonable empiric risk for first degree relatives of affected subjects.

Conclusion

The foregoing sections have attempted to show that, with respect to genetic counseling, the psychiatric patient should be approached no differently from other medical patients. The argument has been illustrated by a number of diseases encountered by the psychiatrist for which counseling is likely to be sought, and on which sufficient data are available to make counseling feasible. If genetic counseling is to be extended to psychiatric patients, then what are our goals in counseling? In the case of the dominantly transmitted diseases of high morbidity (i.e., Huntington's chorea and dominantly inherited presenile dementias) we can hope to decrease the future burden to the family and society by preventing the occurrence of new cases in that family. In the case of the functional psychoses, which will constitute the majority of psychiatric patients counseled, the goals of counseling must necessarily be different. The risk and burden of these diseases are such that the parents would not necessarily choose not to have children. Furthermore, counseling may not be sought for family planning so much as to learn what to expect and be prepared for in their children. Finally, counseling may serve to dispel misconceptions about the inheritance of the disease which are based on family secrets rather than known facts. What we hope to accomplish in counseling psychiatric patients, then, is an increased understanding of their disease and its inheritance so that they may approach their responsibilities of planning and raising a family in a more enlightened fashion.

References

Angst, J., and Perris, C.: The nosology of endogenous depression, comparison of the results of two studies. Int. J. Ment. Health, *1*:145–158, 1972.

Crowe, R. R.: Adoption studies in psychiatry. Biol. Psychiatry, *10*:353–371, 1975.

Feighner, J. P., Robins, E., Guze, S. B., et al.: Diagnostic criteria for use in psychiatric research. Arch. Gen. Psychiatry, *26*:57–63, 1972.

Gershon, E. S., Bunney, W. E., Leckman, J. F., et al.: The inheritance of affective disorders: A review of data and hypotheses. Behav. Gent., *6*:227–261, 1976.

Gershon, E. S., Mark, A., Cohen, N., et al.: Transmitted factors in the morbid risk of affective disorders: A controlled study. J. Psychiatr. Res., *12*:283–299, 1975.

Goetzl, U., Green, R., Whybrow, P., et al.: X-Linkage revisited. Arch. Gen. Psychiatry, *31*:665–672, 1974.

Gottesman, I. I., and Shields, J.: Schizophrenia and Genetics: A Twin Study Vantage Point. New York, Academic Press, Inc., 1972

Helgason, T.: Epidemiology of mental disorders in Iceland. Acta Psychiatr. Scand. (Suppl. 173), 1964.

Heston, L. L., Lowther, D. L. W., and Leventhal, C. M.: Alzheimer's disease: A family study. Arch. Neurol., *15*:225–233, 1966.

James, N. M., and Chapman, C. J.: A genetic study of bipolar affective disorder. Br. J. Psychiatry, *126*:449–456, 1975.

Larsson, T., Sjögren, T., and Jacobson, G.: Senile dementia: A sociomedical and genetic study. Acta Psychiatr. Scand. (Suppl. 167), 1963.

McCabe, M. S.: Reactive psychoses and schizophrenia with good prognosis. Arch. Gen. Psychiatry, *33*:571–576, 1976.

Mendlewicz, J., and Fleiss, J. L.: Linkage studies with X-chromosome markers in bipolar (manic-depressive) and unipolar depressive illnesses. Biol. Psychiatry, *9*:261–294, 1974.

Mendlewicz, J., and Rainer, J. D.: Morbidity risk and genetic transmission in manic-depressive illness. Am. J. Hum. Genet., *26*:692–701, 1974.

Murphy, E. A.: Probabilities in genetic counseling. *In* Bergsma, D., Neel, J. V., and Paul, N. W. (eds.): Contemporary Genetic Counseling. Birth Defects: Original Article Series, V. IX, No. 4, April, 1973.

*Murphy, E. A., and Chase, G. A.: Principles of Genetic Counseling. Chicago, Year Book Medical Publishers, Inc., 1975.

Neel, J. V.: The genetics of diabetes mellitus. *In* Camerini-Davalos, R., and Cole, H. S. (eds.): Early Diabetes. New York, Academic Press, Inc., 1970.

Pardue, L. H.: Familial unipolar depressive illness: A pedigree study. Am. J. Psychiatry, *32*:970–972, 1975.

Perris, C.: A study of bipolar (manic-depressive) and unipolar recurrent depressive psychoses. Acta Psychiatr. Scand. (Suppl. 194), 1966.

Perris, C.: Genetic transmission of depressive psychoses. Acta Psychiatr. Scand. (Suppl. 203), 1968.

Schenk, V. W. D.: Re-examination of a family with Pick's disease. Ann. Hum. Genet., *23*:325–333, 1959.

Sjögren, T., Sjögren, H., and Lindgren, A. G. H.: Morbus Alzheimer and morbus Pick. A genetic clinical and patho-anatomical study. Acta Psychiatr. Scand. (Suppl. 82), 1952.

Slater, E., and Cowie, V.: The Genetics of Mental Disorders. London, Oxford University Press, 1971.

Smith, C.: Recurrence risks for multifactorial inheritance. Am. J. Hum. Genet., *23*:578–588, 1971.

Stephens, J. H., and Astrup, C.: Prognosis in "process" and "non-process" schizophrenia. Am. J. Psychiatry, *119*:945–951, 1963.

*Stern, C.: Principles of Human Genetics. San Francisco, W. H. Freeman and Company, Publishers, 1973.

*Stevenson, A. C., Davison, B. C. C., and Oakes, M. W.: Genetic Counselling. Philadelphia, J. B. Lippincott Company, 1970.

Szasz, T. S.: The Myth of Mental Illness. New York, Hoeber-Harper, 1961.

Tsuang, M. T.: Heterogeneity of schizophrenia. Biol. Psychiatry, *10*:65–74, 1975.

Winokur, G., Clayton, P. J., and Reich, T.: Manic Depressive Illness. St. Louis, The C. V. Mosby Co., 1969.

---

*General references on human genetics and genetic counseling.

Comment

Crowe clearly believes that genetic counseling is appropriate for psychiatric patients and their families. He notes that counseling begins with accurate diagnosis and that a realistic decision to have children or not must be based on two considerations: the risk and the burden of the psychiatric illness. The risk, he notes, refers to the probability that a child to be born will be affected by the illness; the burden, on the other hand, refers to the severity of the illness and hardship it will impose on the individual, the patient's family, and society. Clearly the decision to have or not to have children properly belongs to the individuals counseled and should not be made by the genetic counselor.

Crowe notes that the risk of developing unipolar depression is roughly 13.5 per cent for females and 9.4 per cent for males who have a first-degree relative with this disorder. He notes a risk of 20 per cent for an individual developing bipolar affective disorder if that individual has a first degree relative with this illness. Finally, he notes the risk to a schizophrenic parent of having a schizophrenic child to be approximately 12 per cent.

Few will argue with Crowe's brilliant review of a difficult topic. The need to collect additional data in this area with documented pedigrees of multigeneration families is high. Currently, there are sufficient data available to provide genetic counseling for the affectively ill and those afflicted with schizophrenia; however, with sufficient data, other conditions may lend themselves to genetic counseling. In the meantime, mental health professionals should make use of the data available which will enable clients to approach the responsibilities of planning and raising a family in a more enlightened fashion.

H. KEITH H. BRODIE, M.D.

Community Mental Health: Slogan or New Direction?

DANIEL X. FREEDMAN
University of Chicago

For discursive purposes, community mental health is an absolute metaphorical morass. It invites commentary about fundamental values, native virtue, the nature of man (up or down-trodden) and his sociocultural organizations, as well as what should be quite concrete issues of patient care—issues that will persist even in the current culture of "consumers" and competing professional and nonprofessional providers. Rarely encountered (Gardner, 1977; Musto, 1975) are probing analyses of issues of chronicity, the trade-off of urban ghettoes for back wards, the "problem" family and its multiple agency contacts, social welfare systems, fiscal accountability, or mental health as but one of several major service "industries." On the other hand, allusions abound to stigmatization as etiology, to the importance of professional non-identity, to the intrinsically high quality of services (simply and *only* because they are community based), and to training (or, more aptly, metamorphoses). On rare occasions the agenda contains inquiries into disease and dysfunction, the relative efficacy of treatment and treatment systems (in which utilization, accessibility, *and* outcome are honestly confronted), or professional competencies. Trivial assertions and self-serving haphazard countings are called evaluation (in which indirect dollar costs of novel therapies with undiagnosed clients are rarely estimated) and prevail over a handful of top-flight and serious investigations in the assessment area. If a content analysis of the topic were conducted we would also find discussion of the intricacies of congressional and presidential politics and the issues of groups competing for resources and maneuvering for sanction. And as a CMHC "advocate" has brilliantly analyzed it (Zusman, 1977a and 1977b), there is a set of untested old and new philosophical assumptions; these are contradictory and inexplicit and addressed to both technical and ontological beliefs, to "micro" and "macro" aspects of community mental health. This transitional characteristic further confuses the current scene.

As a slogan, this so-called topic was at its very outset, in 1963, a vehicle for announcing a noble caritas, a very American quasi-religious dream in which Lazarus (albeit, Emma) has re-arisen not only to receive but actively to retrieve the community's mentally tempest-tossed. With the Kennedy enabling legislation, NIMH's skillful leader (perhaps, in deserved triumph, a bit Dewey-eyed with the Jamesian human potential) proclaimed the aim of providing a climate for "... each citizen ... for sustained creative and responsible participation in the life of the community and for the development of his particular potentiality as a human being" (Musto, 1975). The spirit was infectious. APA's president concluded his oration in 1963, "Never was chaos so great; and never was paradise so near to reach of common folks like you and me" (Musto, 1975). Other founders were known to note that we had come to an era when institutions would no longer shape men but men would shape institutions.

There should be no doubt and no masking of the fact that 1963 marks not simply a legislative act creating federally sponsored community mental health centers and the advent of a bureaucracy to implement them, but the coming of a spasmodic moment in the developmental history of mankind. Having at the outset apparently dispatched mental illness (simply by being licensed to place the obviously effective instrument in the community), we were perceived as on the threshold of the harmonium of the optimal social arrangements for the optimal evolution of individual self-actualization. Of course, noble vessels are traditionally launched with champagne, and there is little harm in partaking of the bubbly so long as the crew and pilot can, in sobriety, chart the course and steer through the waiting storms. But it is disingenuous even to suggest that community mental health—whatever the topic connotes—was not a cause or movement. At its very origins it had both the ring and the considerable utility of a slogan.

There is, however, nothing incompatible in recognizing both a slogan and a new direction. On the contrary, they are inextricably and reciprocally linked social processes. The only problem is to define the direction and issues (a task whose time has probably not yet quite come). In a book devoted to controversies I must assume there is a fight in which I am expected to engage. But what to fight? Noble words or useful deeds? Aspirations to human decency? Or are doctrinal views of salvation to be in dispute? Theomachy is not, I hope, my fate. Nor is a fight always a positive human endeavor. Combat can have its casualties—and there are now over six hundred CMHC's funded. More than a billion dollars have been expended on them with enormous budgets annually at risk. Perhaps 25 per cent (1.1 million) of the people to receive mental health care within the year are seen in these federally funded entities. In terms of their location, of course, centers should have served the total mental health needs of almost 50 per cent of the population, if we were free to ask for a truly strict fulfillment of function. Nevertheless, there are funds, psychologists, social workers, paraprofessional personnel, and a few psychiatrists (an ever decreasing per cent—oscillating between 4 and 6 per cent of staff), as well as patients and clients who have much at stake. Both livelihoods and human welfare are involved.

These operations which bear the federal flag of CMHC have had an uneasy journey through the Nixon administrations (which determined CMHC to be a pilot project so successful that federal participation should be phased out). While the legislation of 1975 declared the CMHC a "national resource" which should be accessible to all, this enunciation (hailed by Stanley Yolles (1977) as the capstone of the entire USPHS-NIMH effort) may nevertheless have ominous indications as well. What is already a distinct two-class system of mental health care might, in the future competition for health care dollars and entitlement to NHI, be used to cleave the mentally ill from other health entitlements, leaving them with a partial care system, but one consolingly hailed as a national resource. In any event the federal program must look ahead to tight budgets, to reorganization of health funding, and of the federal relationship to both health service systems and welfare.

So if controversy has the outcome of hurting a thrust of what is still a fragile operation, there could well be victims. We should, then, perhaps downplay overall assessments of CMHCs as neglecting the aged, substance abusers, and increasingly serving less of the chronic major psychoses (Musto, 1975), as well as neglecting serious evaluation (Gardner, 1977). This catchment-based system meant to serve *all* has, in fact, preferentially met some of the undeserved (42 per cent of those served are from families with incomes under $2500). And if concern for the mentally ill is truly what is at stake, then whatever the definition of self-interest, careerist interest, and public interest, unfortunate outcomes—especially of rhetorical controversy—should be avoided. The ill all too long have been the pawn of those self-anointed who would save, serve, or deny them.

This, of course, puts us into a dilemma. For no matter how one estimates the risk of critique or probing analyses, concern about political consequences will confound candid discussion. To the extent that the latter is valuable, it may well have to be a casualty of this fear of risk; professionally accountable debate must perhaps find a closet! As I reviewed the recent literature on the topic, I would have to predict the reader may well expect not to confront in any convincing detail what the title of this book implies—at least for this particular topic. Rather, the guarded tone and explicit image is a plea to regard this adolescent, its mess, solipsism, and raucous rebellious ways, as a "phase" awaiting nature's rescue of maturation. Of course, all of us have known families that plead indulgence for their unruly preschooler, impatient latency child, unruly adolescent, and surly young adult in the hope that doubting friends who simply can't stand the racket will endure. Chronic "phase disease" might, of course, be the diagnosis of this common familial pattern of urging others to expect less of what they perpetually and wishfully overestimate as "more." Attending to and realistically expecting more of "less"—focusing on what is in fact possible—rather than hoping for more than can be forthcoming might be the cure.

So the problem with a slogan (originally a Scottish battle cry) is that it is shorthand to rally support around a pattern of practices and beliefs while it obscures inquiry and assessment. Its virtue is enlisting and reenforcing a high evaluation and assent of important constituencies. If mental illness were indeed the central concern of CMHC advocates, then public assent and support would be key. It is key not simply because of historical circumstance (the fact that the mentally ill have yet to take their place in commanding adequate resources among the range of competing human and health needs) but for another—and obvious—reason as well. Resources and participation of the community are inherently functionally necessary to the very recognition of mental dysfunction, to its consequences, and—sometimes—to its precipitation. This Darwinian fact—that man is a social animal and, sick or well, must be in transaction with the environment—should *not* convey any imputation that the milieu is therefore automatically the necessary and sufficient causal factor in mental illness. It is a precondition (just as blood vessels are to the function or dysfunction of the circulatory system). So apart from coma, we are behaving and in some linkage with our surroundings—and when we cease at the very end, our epilogue of burial (and relief or grief) are active psychosocial acts. I will refrain from further chorales dedicated to man and community and sung simply in order to rediscover the obvious linkage (that the head bone is connected to the neck bone, etc.). In brief, man indeed is embedded in his community, however he relates. But this hardly affords us a chart or mandate for differentiated treatment and cure.

It does remind us, however, that we must also view science as a social system for discovering and adjudicating knowledge and medicine as a social system—related to other tutoring and caring systems—which implements available scientific knowledge on behalf of the relief of suffering or painful deviation. This particular crucial consequence of our embeddedness in social systems is perhaps the least truly believed of all the current pieties on our community linkages. So simply to proclaim psychiatry's link with community processes as a new discovery from which all kinds of special knowledge about disease and disability and its skillful treatment *automatically* flow is hardly an intellectual triumph in the history of psychiatry and, in fact, functions as a distinct disservice. Nor in terms of high *moral* purpose do I see a distinctly "new direction" in community mental health (at least since Gheel, Pinel, and Tuke). Rather, as elaborated later, it is one of several reincarnations of moral treatment and a trend toward accessible offices, clinics, and wards over two centuries. This slogan and direction broadly refer to a primary and historic concern of the professions and community leaders to treat humanely a human disorder.

We should then both understand and not overestimate excesses. It is in the nature of politics that sanctioning beliefs be celebrated and only episodically examined. They require banners. But we surely should be canny enough to distinguish the essential rites of praise—a cultural act expressing communal aspiration and binding us, with our infirmities, to the uncertain future—from evaluation and design of efficacious practice. Anthropologists tell us much the same for the rain dances (which do not impede good agricultural practice).

My unease is that we have not been able clearly to speak of mental health *in* the community rather than community mental health centers as but one component or device to that end. We have been unable to get to the pragmatics of community health, since we must always connote new institutions with their credos and careers (if not credentials). We are prisoners of programmatic needs and rhetoric and may lose sight of the patient who is our charge. In tune with the times, our ahistorical momentum—required by revolutions that must construct their own patrons and mythologies—might lead the public to believe there was *no* mental health in the community prior to the federal act. More dangerous is the assumption that there is currently no community mental health that is not a nationally funded Community Mental Health Center.

Unfortunately, we did not originally promise what lay and psychiatric leaders had for over a century and a half espoused—the sound aim of bringing expertise and service into closer proximity to the consumer and hopefully to a supporting community.[2] It is worrisome—and in fact a major threat to whatever we think community mental health is—that we have not yet found the right colloquy and forum in which facts can be adjudicated, the issues of decision-making, goals, and implementation settled, and the questions debated of whether a new body of knowledge exists and whether a new profession or an evolution from our current knowledge base is desirable or useful. There are pressing real issues concerning quality of care, as well as the obvious demands (which are indeed having an impact) for accountability and fiscal control, if not quality control. I have seen no plan—if national health insurance were to be the fortunate heritage of the unfortunate mentally ill—that would indicate the treatment systems to which the purchaser of services would relate. To private practitioners? To psychiatric group practices with support systems? To free-standing mental health centers or to health-linked mental health centers? If this vague sense of unreality of our current status and mode of discourse is at all shared by others, then at some point we will have to bridge the chasm between specifically tested treatments and treatment "systems."

I believe, then, that we owe an enormous debt and we are equally paying an enormous price for the efforts of the distinctly public health minded leadership of NIMH to put into place a federal commitment to the mentally ill. One can view this attention to mental health in the community, and all the energy and excess that has gone with it, as but one more instance in the history of the effort to rescue moral treatment. Any historical perspective indicates the astonishing energy required simply to implement the arrangements in which moral treatment—whatever its content and form—would at least be possible. At the minimum, accomplishing this is what can be claimed for praise by those within and without government who advocated, lobbied for, and facilitated our present arrangements.

The mentally ill have always been a quasi-public responsibility; in the last analysis (sic) they are a community and public charge. The public health answer has been to view the governmental response on the model of tuberculosis. Thus, case finding was emphasized; community outreach was urged far in advance of any developed clinically and diagnostically relevant epidemiology. NIMH in fact underfunded this now burgeoning area for a number of years while the mandate to be as responsible for the hidden as for the self-referred case was strongly enunciated. All this was somehow equated with true prevention. The experience of both world wars has led to a confusion of accessibility and continuity of services with outcome and of all these with primary prevention of rates of the major psychoses. In fact for none of our wars have we sufficient investigations of the long-term outcome of what surely are humane and excellent short-term interventions and care. In both world wars, in which the emphasis on initial screening was extraordinarily high, the incidence of major psychiatric disorders was about the same for those armies which lacked this service. On clinical grounds, I believe in the importance of crisis intervention (especially with nonpsychotics), but on scientific grounds I deplore the lack of differentiated outcome data not only on hospitalization rates but later on diagnosable dysfunction. It would be gratifying to be able to answer public inquiry with sound knowledge. And it would be equally nice to be able to serve the public with humane services and to do so even where science is not yet able to equip us with the tools to prevent ultimately undesirable outcomes, let alone initial breakdowns.

The real thread, then, which carries an inexorable purpose far more compelling to program planners than a science base, was to commit the federal government to direct care for the mentally ill. This fight for a socialized psychiatric care system—far in advance of such arrangements for general health care—was evident in Dorothea Dix's drive for federal funds to state hospitals (Musto, 1975). That was vetoed by President Pierce in 1854. Through a series of landmark dates, this aim of federal commitment to patient care was "accomplished" in 1975 (Yolles, 1977). Thus, in 1930 the narcotics and psychiatric aspects of the UHPHS were coalesced into a Division of Mental Hygiene (and decoalesced, ironically, by Nixon's war on drugs in 1971); in 1946, the NIMH was authorized; in the mid-1950s the Joint Commission under Jack Ewalt began its work; and in 1963 the Kennedy act traded off a separate retardation effort for funds for the community mental health centers' construction. NIMH leaders staved off the attempts by NIH to allocate responsibility for services to the HEW bureaus authorized to administer them, and in 1965 mental health center staff became federally fundable. In 1967 the single-minded direction of NIMH succeeded in splitting it from the rest of health sciences at the insistence of the NIMH leadership; the organization became a bureau with more direct access to the Assistant Secretary of Health. State hospitals were viewed as the fundamental systems to be phased out over time in 50 states, and the gamble was that somehow the federal funds would be sufficient to provide the leverage. Psychiatrists were initially mandated by regulations to be in charge of the community mental health centers, but subsequent regulations shifted the rules and subsequent developments found few psychiatrists within CMHCs (and fewer within NIMH and its various components). Both the field and Congress were repeatedly told that the communities demanded these CMHC arrangements (a prophecy which, it was hoped, would be replaced by fact). The state hospitals and academia were both coaxed and fed—and hence distracted; the private practitioner was unthreatened. There grew, finally—with a minimum of professionalized direction—a disparate array of services alongside the expanding general hospital clinical operations that had been distinctly in place (as the Joint Commission had recognized in its report in 1961). There also grew constituencies of workers and local areas. By 1971 an APA reviewing body indicated that "therapeutic claims have often been unsubstantiated by experience and experiment. Our current knowledge . . . is still inadequate to validate comprehensive programs of prevention and treatment. . . . In the area of community mental health this policy (high priority for research) has not been implemented with the attention required by the newness of the programs and their scope" (Musto, 1975). In brief, the 120-year agenda that seeks above all a federal commitment to the mentally ill is surely to be respected, but the price in minimal technical and professional accountability in not linking the ill to health and welfare systems is surely yet to be assessed.

American psychiatry has thus always wrestled with the Sisyphean task simply of putting into place sound systems in which moral treatment could even occur—whatever specific treatments could be implemented. Thus, the Worcester State Hospital was founded in 1833, after careful demographic surveys, to implement the excellent combination of moral and medical treatments available in the leading private hospitals and to care for the state's ill as well as to reduce chronicity. As a system, the venture eventually met the question of sustained community funding and sanctioning. Almshouses or jails for the chronic population were no more desired by the perceptive leaders then than now, but the cure rates claimed by the movement Dorothea Dix led (the "cult of curability") evaporated, and the well-known cycle of public hope and neglect ensued. Less widely appreciated was the attempt in the mid-nineteenth century by the father of academic psychiatry—William Greisinger—to locate psychiatry (through bedside teaching) in the heart of the medical center in Germany and his design for outpatient clinics and specialized halfway houses in the community. He organized scholars and clergy and neurologists for seminars on the nature of man while emphasizing the available science base and advocating vigorous clinical scrutiny of mental illnesses. The grand plan of this designer (the Burgholzi, for example) involved a highly professionalized, medically linked psychiatry, but was fought by the rurally situated hospital superintendents whose agenda was the dreary complexity of administering and funding their institutions. The fact that different populations—conceptually important for psychiatry—are encountered in different settings at different phases of illness and recovery, and are inconstantly connected with the desirable expertise, remains one of the most perplexing and unsolved problems of contemporary mental health delivery.

At the turn of the century, American psychiatrists were largely alienists in rural citadels of insanity. American medicine had survived a 50-year attack by indigenous antiprofessional movements such as Thompsonism. Thompson, a New Hampshire farmer, sold a text (the original "family physician" was such) instructing on the use of herbals and practical measures and emphasizing the mother as the true physician. Self-help groups were to teach and practice (not unlike today's Alcoholics Anonymous); the movement stressed self-reliance, elevating conversation, and exercises. It succeeded in repealing the licensing laws for medical practice in most of the states. Allopathy and homeopathy struggled for belief of consumers, as did Christian Science. These efficient attacks on medicine did not subside until bacteriology and pathology and the germ theory were formally ensconced and the academic base for professional development designed at Johns Hopkins University. There Adolph Meyer, using his beliefs in the importance of the life pattern of the individual, and the developing dynamic therapies, clearly articulated by Chicago's Healy and the prevention-oriented child guidance movement (directed especially toward juvenile delinquency), spurred the development of a therapeutic rather than custodial emphasis. Psychiatric leadership joined with the Clifford Beers' movement, and the National Committee for Mental Hygiene became a major spur for the development of a therapeutically minded psychiatric presence in the community. APA's leadership, in concert with the Committee, enunciated a policy of comprehensive care in the community after World War I (where neurologists and endocrinologists as well as cultists and Christian Scientists competed). Healy, now in Boston, adapted the clinical pathological conference as a "case conference" in which different areas of expertise could be brought together to understand the child. Belief became prevalent that nipping an early maladjustment in the bud would prevent its linear development into major pathology.

Psychiatrists led in introducing nonmedical personnel during the 1920s, as John Burnham (1974) describes it. The Medical Director of the mental hygiene committee lectured psychiatrists entering the community on elitist attitudes; he must ". . . now take his place humbly with other workers . . . together they might extend the borders of knowledge and find solutions to problems that thus far in human history remain unsolved." Lloyd Stevenson in 1928 indicated there was no area of society which mental hygienists could not penetrate. All were welcome. A Buffalo psychiatrist noted that psychiatrists, psychologists, social workers, and clergy were so closely involved in their attempts to alter undesirable social traits that ". . . it is not easy for discussion to separate the function of each" (Burnham, 1974). This orgy of role transvestism was even caught in song, a parody of "Men of Harlech" in which each key member has a solo but ends in the chorus:

> Thus we pool each contribution,
> Synthesize a true solution,
> Engineer a revolution,
> Of personality.

Scholarships were granted for psychologists to train in community clinics, although it was noted that many left to engage in industry, schools, and private practice. Both the Depression and a general public disillusionment with claims to prevention which appeared to have no base initiated a backlash. By 1932, the presidents of APA—entirely unlike those of the earlier decade—explicitly attacked the incursions of paramedical personnel. The literature began to emphasize individual treatment by competent physicians. The team with the entire community as its playing field was in trouble, and

American psychiatry countered both the diffusion and competition with the device of accrediting psychiatrists through board examinations. The advent of malaria therapy and ECT emphasized medical skills. By 1940 the APA and National Committee for Mental Hygiene, which had shared offices, were separately situated, and while the team survived and indeed was utilized in World War II, roles were specified and medical direction clear. Burnham (1974) notes that just as medicine had been rescued, there was in psychiatry a ". . . notable movement to increase and upgrade psychiatric research . . . (as) a weapon in the hands of the M.D.s. They specifically attacked the scientific bases of other members of the mental hygiene team." Noting the enormous growth of both paraprofessionalism and cults in the 1930s and again in the 1970s, Burnham remarks that ". . . the momentum of the nonphysicians was so great that the question they raised was not merely one of economics but of the meaning of professionalism and, indeed, how secure any profession could be against invasion and eclipse in the last third of the twentieth century."

The fate of professions as guilds should truly be less our concern than whether we have something to offer for the mental health of the ill and the mental distress of the healthy. We have, I believe, far more in hand for delivering sound treatment and services than our programmatic debates, rhetoric, and political concerns of the moment permit us to see. The transgenerational clinical knowledge of the past 30 years based on intimate, intense experience with the persons who are patients and useful support systems (and well-developed in certain public, private, and academic center sectors) may eventually "model" (just as in 1833 the McClean Hospital and Institute of Living did for Worcester) treatment arrangements that are sound and work. Diagnosis of the condition, the person with it, his situation, his personality and social resources, and design of treatment with these dimensions in view may be increasingly available to persons in need; and new knowledge is there to be acquired, if it is wanted.

Obviously I believe that the programmatic and political mission of the NIMH has left us with some complicated problems for which the lacking ingredient of serious and responsible inquiry and assessments will someday be forthcoming. The agency became prisoner of its constituencies, and responsibility for professionally accountable treatments received, of necessity, less emphasis or priority than did advocacy. Linkage to a knowledge base that is not self-serving requires a primacy of scientific rather than political rules of adjudication. The reality of the resources that currently care for 75 per cent of patients cannot be treated as fiction simply because they do not fly the NIMH flag. The competing professions should—and no doubt ultimately will—have enough self-confidence and professional conscience to offer those services they can best provide, while opening their experience and knowledge base to public sanction.

Thus it appears to me that whatever community mental health is, both in slogan and in concrete practice, it is in transit. As any transit mechanism, it carries along with it a variety of baggage. If we knew—or could stipulate—its destination, we could better understand whether we dare risk the entire trip by focusing on the contraband in the luggage (or perhaps even the time bombs!).

This transit occurs at a time when the future design for all American health is under intense discussion. Fads (focus on "prevention," on discipline and exercise and abstinence from fun) are promulgated instead of development of "high technology" to treat efficiently and to prevent (Thomas, 1977). This arises because rationing of care and tempering of expectations of the medical system are as necessary economically for health care as for mental health care. Perhaps mental health experts might take some momentary comfort in the fact that the evolution of a sound policy for health care generally, and the particular forms of its delivery, are far from being saliently and dispassionately analyzed and discussed; I personally believe, though, that we are behind in the tortoise race to provide sound analyses of options. There is, indeed, what Aaron Wildavsky (1977) calls "the political pathology of health policy." In that general perspective, mental health is not outstandingly derelict in its confusions and perplexities, but it has not tapped the best of the minds that medical care issues engage. We have no reason for false comfort—such as the wistful belief that our long quasi-public health experience provides a clear basis for how general health problems can be sensibly arranged. There is no question that many psychiatrists and mental health workers have had practical experience in wrestling with community problems with which the rest of the health field is beginning to engage. But I do not believe that we have learned from our own experience as yet, nor that we have more than a few pragmatics to offer to the general debate on the future of American health delivery.

I believe, then, that if we can escape the environment of rhetoric (the opiate of the politician) and focus on our knowledge base, on our professional competencies, boundaries and limits, there is some chance that we will find the grounds from which some sensible solutions to the design of mental health in the community could emerge. We might well listen to Eli Ginzberg (1977), speaking of health generally, who reminds us that it is unlikely that a single standard of care would ever prevail,

> . . . as we have seen in the marked differentials between England and Scotland, and between urban and rural areas in the Soviet Union. A sensible objective of public policy in a democracy should be the improvement in the use of available resources within each area and subdivision, with some contributions from the pool of national resources to strengthen the position of areas with particular weaknesses. All services, including health services, are unevenly distributed . . . good theatres are more readily available along the Eastern seaboard. Competent lawyers . . . and most other professionals are most heavily concentrated in metropolitan areas. With the possible exceptions of postal and telephone services, no critical services are as readily available in rural as in urban areas.

And while he predicts health professionals may be headed for periods of acrimony with decreasing resources, he notes that we

> . . . must also consider whether we have or are capable of designing the social machinery needed to exercise tighter control over the uses to which health resources are put. The streets have not been made safe for the pedestrians; the schools have not learned to teach many pupils how to read and write; and corruption permeates much of our public and business life. In light of these failings in the provision of services, a call for moderation in the setting of health goals and for realism in the assessment of power

and decision do not represent a doctrine of despair and defeat so much as the plea for the role of reason in the search for a better society.

I believe that with an intention to do it we can assess our knowledge and that key strategies will emerge as we test them. This way of proceeding—this valuing of sobriety and professional and technical accountability—is really up to the community to require of us, if we cannot implement it. A joint sponsorship in which professional competencies and responsible community inquiry learn to collaborate is likely.

I am thus disinterested in controversy and far more intrigued with "resolution" in both the optical sense of the term (to render visible the competent parts) and that referring to the pathways by which puzzles are solved. For this I know of only one instrument—and that is rational discourse—and when we come to a time when funding for advocacy can subside to be replaced by investment in this fragile instrument, we may begin to utilize our history, our considerable experience, and our potential for problem-solving. We may then have less concern with slogans or whether a direction is new or old, but rather whether it is relevant and testable in the service of our mission. It will soon be time that we can hope with Emerson to "pierce this rotten diction and fasten words again to visible things."

References

Burnham, J. C.: The struggle between physicians and paramedical personnel in American psychiatry, 1917–41. J. History Med., *29*:93–106, 1974.

Freedman, D. X.: Can we put research to use? Keynote address, Highlights of the 17th Annual Conference, V. A. Cooperative Studies in Mental Health and Behavioral Sciences. St. Louis, Mo., March, 1972.

Gardner, E. A.: Community mental health center movement: Learning from failure. *In* Barton, W. E. and Sanborn, C. J. (eds.): An Assessment of the Community Mental Health Movement. Lexington, Mass., Lexington Books, 1977, pp. 103–115.

Ginzberg, E.: Health services, power centers, and decision-making mechanisms. J. Am. Acad. Arts Sci., *106*:203–213, 1977.

Musto, D. F.: Whatever happened to "community mental health"? Publ. Interest, *39*:53–79, 1975.

Thomas, L.: On the science and technology of medicine. J. Am. Acad. Arts Sci., *106*:35–46, 1977.

Wildavsky, A.: Doing better and feeling worse: The political pathology of health policy. J. Am. Acad. Arts Sci. *106*:105–123, 1977.

Yolles, F.: The future of community psychiatry. *In* Barton, W. E., and Sanborn, C. J. (eds.): An Assessment of the Community Mental Health Movement. Lexington, Mass., Lexington Books, 1977, pp. 169–185.

Zusman, J., and Lamb, H. B.: In defense of community mental health. Am. J. Psychiatry, *134*:887–890, 1977a.

Zusman, J.: The philosophic basis for a community and social psychiatry. *In* Barton, W. E., and Sanborn, C. J. (eds.): An Assessment of the Community Mental Health Movement. Lexington, Mass., Lexington Books, 1977b, pp. 21–34.

Comment

In this excellent chapter, **Freedman** notes that community psychiatry is really but one of several reincarnations of moral treatment consistent with the trend toward increased accessibility of mental health services over the past two centuries. He notes that to date community psychiatry seems to have promulgated fads instead of developing a "high technology" officially to treat and prevent disease, and that the field lacks a rigorous scrutiny or scientific reflection. He presents a notion that mental health workers have had a practical experience wrestling with community problems which the rest of the health field is beginning to engage and that we must view medicine as a social system—related to other tutoring and caring systems—which implements available scientific knowledge on behalf of the relief of suffering or painful deviation. His observation that an ever-decreasing percentage of the professional staff of community mental health centers [4 to 6 per cent] is composed of psychiatrists is clearly of concern to many.

Basically, this is a balanced presentation, devoid of any major bias. Since this chapter was written, the National Institute of Mental Health has embarked on a major effort to fund outcome research and evaluation studies of psychotherapy and drug therapy, several of which are being carried out in community mental health centers. This may provide the type of scientific reflection Freedman referred to as lacking in the past.

Given the recent introduction of the Mental Health Systems Act as developed from recommendations proposed by the President's Commission on Mental Health, it would appear, if this act is passed, that the delivery of mental health services will be expanded in the community setting, especially in rural areas, and emphasis will be placed on prevention and on delivery of services to children and to the elderly. I believe that Freedman would see this trend as consistent with his observation that the mental health field is continuing to develop new approaches for service delivery in the community which the rest of the health field may soon adopt.

H. KEITH H. BRODIE, M.D.

Should the Psychiatrist Have a Role in the Criminal Justice System?

DAVID L. BAZELON

Chief Judge, United States Court of Appeals for the District of Columbia Circuit

Psychiatry, institutional psychiatry in particular, stands today on the verge of a crisis of public confidence. Society's inflated expectations of psychiatry, fed in part by the profession itself, are being punctured on several fronts. Where once we believed in and institutionalized the psychiatrist's ability to predict and prevent the antisocial conduct of disordered offenders, we are now told that prediction (American Psychiatric Association, 1974) and, in most instances, effective treatment (Stone, 1976) are beyond present abilities and/or resources. Where once we were told that large numbers of marginally functioning persons, elderly persons in particular, were proper candidates for full psychiatric hospitalization, we are now told that many if not most are not helped by hospitalization and indeed would be better served in other, less liberty-restrictive settings (Dixon v. Weinberger, 1975). Where once we were told that psychiatrists could assist our determinations of criminal responsibility, we now hear distinguished psychiatrists calling for wholesale retreat from the fray (Stone, 1976).

Total retreat, to my mind, is neither a desirable nor a viable option. Psychiatry today, more than ever before, offers critical insights for our understanding of the mind and human behavior. Society has understandably, if somewhat naïvely, involved psychiatric expertise in an increasingly broad range of decisional processes. From criminal and correctional matters, from juvenile courts and involuntary hospitalization proceedings, psychiatric participation has spread to matters of employment in industry and government, to schools, and to preventive medicine in the community. Unquestionably, inclusion of the psychiatric perspective often enhances the sophistication with which such public and private decisions may be reached.

The danger, however, is that psychiatric participation in these decisional processes may ultimately slide by imperceptible degrees into psychiatric assumption of responsibility for the decisions themselves. Rather than confining themselves to those aspects of a problem for which they have expertise, psychiatrists may be seduced into taking responsibility for making judgments or assessing facts about which they have no special competence. As a result, not only does psychiatry become overextended, but society is deluded into believing that scientific, "medical" answers exist to a problem and that social, moral, and other determinants of the problem may therefore be ignored.

The critical point at which such dangers arise occurs when psychiatrists step beyond the traditional medical model of doctor and patient. When the doctor's employer is someone or some institution other than the individual whose mental functioning is at issue, the doctor must confront the effects his new masters have on the performance of his professional skills.

The issue, in essence, is one of candor and of the mechanisms we might devise to see that candor is assured. If public decision-making is in fact to be benefited by psychiatric input, then psychiatrists must be willing and able to state not only what they know but, more importantly, what they do not know. They must be attentive to biases arising from their professional theoretical orientation and from their personal values and beliefs. Finally, they must begin to recognize and divulge the conflicting interests they serve when they step beyond the traditional relationship of doctor and patient. Although these biases and conflicts of interests—these hidden agendas—must in the first instance be addressed by the profession itself, psychiatrists must also be willing to lay bare their contributions to the scrutiny of the ultimate decision-maker through such mechanisms as the adversary process.

Who's Calling the Tune?

The problem of hidden agendas can be seen most clearly in its extreme form. In 1967, I had occasion to visit the Soviet Union as a member of the First United States Mission on Mental Health. Although the seven-member team was concerned with a broad overview of Soviet mental health services, my own particular concern as the only legally oriented member was with forensic psychiatry. As an outgrowth of that mission, I later made a study of case reports furnished by the Soviets of the psychiatric commitment of political dissidents. Assuming that the case reports were authentic, they revealed obviously improper uses of psychiatry. The evidence supporting findings of psychopathology in the reports was tenuous at best, there were no behavioral manifestations of the alleged pathology to justify a conclusion of "social danger," and the facilities to which the dissidents were committed belied the asserted goal of treatment. In short, the medical label of "sick" had been used by Soviet psychiatrists to serve the political purposes of the state.

It occurred to me that the abuses I had encountered differed from American practice in motive and degree but perhaps not in kind. In case after case before my court I had seen the error of the Soviet psychiatrists benignly repeated: psychiatrists had, to one degree or another, abandoned their role as ally of the patient to serve institutional interests. The fact that these American psychiatrists lacked the more sinister motives of their Soviet counterparts offers me little consolation, for as Justice Louis Brandeis once wrote:

> Experience should teach us to be most on our guard to protect liberty when the Government's purposes are beneficient. Men born to freedom are naturally alert to repeal invasion of their liberty by evil-minded rulers. The greatest dangers to liberty lurk in insidious encroachment by men of zeal, well-meaning but without understanding (Olmstead v. U.S., 1928).

I do not suggest that American psychiatry is on the verge of participation in wholesale repression of political dissent. But my reasons for this conclusion have more to do with the political climate of the United States than with any confidence in our profession's recognition of the conflicting interests it serves. Isolated incidents in our history suggest the possibility of similar abuses in other, more politically heated times.

An example is the effort in 1958 of the Rev. Clennon King, then pastor of a church in Gulfport, Mississippi, to become the first black student at the University of Mississippi, only to be hustled off by state troopers, on orders from the Governor's office, to a commitment proceeding to the state hospital. After all, reasoned the man on the street, what sane black man would attempt to enter the University of Mississippi in 1958? To their credit, the state hospital staff were able to persuade the Governor's office that King was "without psychosis" and should be released. After twelve days' confinement and diagnosis, King was discharged to the custody of family members from Georgia who returned with him to their home.

A second example arose out of federal efforts to keep the peace when James Meredith became the first black to enroll at the University of Mississippi. Former General Edwin Walker was arrested October 1, 1962, on federal charges for contributing to the resistance to the federal marshals. Within 24 hours, General Walker had been transferred to the Medical Center for Federal Prisoners in Springfield, Missouri, and the Justice Department had obtained a court order to require him to submit to a psychiatric examination to determine his competence to stand trial. The order was based in part on the affidavit of a government psychiatrist who had never seen General Walker but suggested the need for an examination based on newspaper reports of his activities, a transcript of his testimony before a Senate subcommittee six months earlier, and some old Army medical records. The affidavit suggested the possible existence of paranoid mental disorder based in part on General Walker's strongly anticommunist statements. On November 22, 1962, the court declared General Walker competent to stand trial, and on January 21, 1963, the Grand Jury failed to indict him and the charges were dismissed. In the interim, General Walker had been portrayed in the press as insane (Szasz, 1965).

To a limited extent, service of the political and social status quo is endemic to the concept of mental illness itself. Mental disease is a "cross-dimensional concept," reflecting in addition to medical judgments "moral, legal, actuarial, or political" judgments as well (Fingarette, 1972). One who drinks alcohol to excess over a long period of time may be judged sick or not sick depending on who is judging and the purpose for which he is making the diagnosis. The fact that psychiatrists may have special skills in diagnosing and treating such conditions does not by itself render the decision as to illness a purely medical one. Similarly, in the well-known Blocker case, a weekend meeting of staff psychiatrists at St. Elizabeth Hospital resulting in a decision to call psychopathy a mental illness for purposes of Blocker's insanity defense related only marginally to the medical issue presented by the patient (Blocker v. U.S.). The degree to which Blocker and many others are considered mentally ill is dependent upon the diagnostician's social, political, and cultural reference points and the degree to which the patient's behavior and ideation depart from those norms.

Although the "cross-dimensional" nature of the mental illness concept creates some potential for abuse even in the traditional doctor-patient relationship, those dangers are minimized and made tolerable by the nature of that relationship. For there the patient has come to the doctor to engage the doctor as an ally or agent to help the patient deal with what the patient has at least tentatively identified as a medical problem. By the same token, if the patient ceases to believe the problem is medical or becomes dissatisfied with the doctor's approach in some way, the patient may terminate the relationship. To be sure, the patient may be so impressed with the mystique of the doctor's expertise that he may be swayed to a great degree by the doctor's assessment of mental illness, an assessment governed in part by the doctor's personal beliefs and professional orientation. Although such dangers are not to be taken lightly, they are held in check somewhat by the doctor's training in the traditions of the doctor-patient relationship and by the patient's ultimate power, if not actual ability, to control the relationship.

When the patient no longer controls the relationship and is no longer free to disregard the doctor's assessment of mental illness, however, the dangers of hidden agendas are greatly increased. Furthermore, there is an additional factor threatening distortion of diagnoses: the interests of the institutions seeking the doctor's services. Thus, for example, a psychiatrist employed by a state hospital for the "criminally insane" who conducts court-ordered examinations of persons raising the insanity defense in a criminal trial must deal with many masters. His professional theoretical orientation may dictate a broad or narrow view of mental illness. Soviet forensic psychiatrists, for example, at least in non-political cases, appear to take a narrow, largely organic view of mental illness (Bazelon, 1970). His personal values, especially his views on the causes of crime, are clearly implicated, whether he be of the law and order mentality or of the view that all crime is sick. Additionally, he must deal with the interests of his various constituencies—the hospital which employs him, the court which seeks to render a legal-moral decision on criminal responsibility, and society at large. The hospital is concerned with such matters as bed space, whether the defendant, if returned as a patient upon a finding of non-responsibility, will be the sort of patient the hospital can handle effectively, and the extent to which it can afford to expend its resources on the court-ordered examination, to name only a few (Pugh, 1973; Chambers, 1972). The court, although theoretically obligated to make its own determination of the moral issue, may be eager to have this thorny question resolved for it under the guise of a "medical" expert opinion (Pugh, 1973). Society may wish to keep the offender off the streets for as long as possible and may informally hold psychiatry partially accountable for any failures to achieve that goal.

In such a setting, the nonmedical determinants of a diagnosis of mental illness increase in importance. Values of the political and social status quo as defined by the new institutional clients, as well as the physician's own internal values, contribute significantly to the definition of norms against which the patient's behavior is measured. Such values may not all be irrelevant to the ultimate decision which is to be made—in this example, the decision of criminal responsibility. But they are values and factors beyond the medical expertise of the psychiatrist. The psychiatrist who conceals such factors in his expert opinion not only taints the decisional process by usurping the function of the appropriate decision-maker—in this example, the jury—but also undermines the credibility of his profession in the public arena. He allows his profession to be prostituted, just as Soviet psychiatrists have done, to achieve decisions for which other institutions in society should bear responsibility. And he allows society to deceive itself as to the true nature of the issues involved and to avoid facing the real and difficult questions of the state's power over the individual.

It is tempting for the psychiatrist in perfect good faith to insist that his professional attitude and his humanitarian concern for the welfare of the patient allow him to overcome bias and conflict of interest. But psychiatrists are also human, and the pressures of conflicting interests are often subtle and intense. Where we might be willing to trust the psychiatrist's professionalism in the context of a relationship which the patient is free to terminate, we (and the profession itself) cannot afford to extend that trust where the patient has no control and where, in fact, competing interests hold the real power.

If we are to facilitate the real contributions psychiatry can make to public decision-making, we must develop techniques for confronting and sorting out the institutional interests which intrude upon the psychiatrist's proper function. Some of those techniques can and should be instituted by the profession itself. As a first step, let me presume to offer the following suggestions.

First, the profession can begin by frankly confronting the existence of competing interests at work when psychiatric practice steps beyond the traditional doctor-patient relationship. Various types of conflict of interest settings—one example would be the handling of court-ordered examinations for the insanity defense—can be identified and analyzed for the ethical dilemmas which they pose. Guidelines for professional conduct might be debated and instituted. In short, the first step must be recognition and acceptance of the problem so that solutions might ensue.

Second, psychiatrists working in conflict of interest settings should keep careful and detailed records of their conduct of a particular patient's case. Keeping records serves both to remind the psychiatrist continually of his obligations and to provide a basis upon which others might review his conduct.

Third, peer review mechanisms should be established by which professionals situated outside the conflict of interest setting can evaluate the performance of the psychiatrist.

Fourth, the patient must be forthrightly advised at the outset of particular conflicts of interest besetting the psychiatrist. For the psychiatrist to encourage a free flow of communication from the patient as though the traditional doctor-patient relationship existed is nothing short of fraud. If such disclosure inhibits the ability of the psychiatrist to obtain information for the institutional decision-maker, then it is for the decision-maker, not the psychiatrist, to bear the consequences.

Beyond these techniques which the profession itself can employ to refine its input into public decision-making, the decision-making bodies themselves must have mechanisms to assure that they are addressing the appropriate issues in their use of psychiatric expertise. It is here that the legal model of the adversary process provides some guidance for coping with these new uses of psychiatric skills.

Morality and the Decisional Process

Persuading the psychiatrist to learn to love the adversary process of the courts is like persuading the old Tories to appreciate self-determination. Yet I firmly believe psychiatry's aversion to the legal process to be in large part the result of misunderstanding of the nature and goals of that process. Courts are continually handling a wide range of complex and esoteric subjects, from the problems of nuclear power to environmental questions to the intricacies of economics. In so doing the courts are not attempting to substitute their own spurious expertise for that of the scientists and professionals. To do so would be to commit the same error I see many psychiatrists making in seeking to shoulder the moral responsibility in criminal trials. Rather, courts seek assurance that the contributions of the professionals on a particular issue are within the bounds of their expertise and are based on a rational consideration of all the information and alternatives available.

In my view, the law is not a static order built on certitude, but a dynamic order built on process. Rather than providing wisdom, it offers a structure for seeking wisdom. Courts work through cases, actual conflicts which must be resolved whether or not all the information which we might wish to have is available. Policies may change as new cases and the passage of time bring more information to bear on a particular question. In this way the law grows, shedding old conceptions for new ones as new facts and values emerge.

Applying my model of law as process, I became deeply concerned in my first few years on the bench with our mechanistic application of the criminal laws. Time after time appeals by defendants from the lowest socioeconomic-cultural strata of society were brought before my court without our ever seeking to understand the causes of their behavior or whether our punishment schemes were at all relevant to the problem. It seemed to me amoral, if not immoral, to be imposing moral blame in case after case when we neither knew nor were even attempting to know the roots of the behavior we condemned.

The criminal trial seemed to me an ideal forum for raising such issues.

Each case presented the opportunity to conduct a kind of post-mortem of a particular crime. The community, as represented by the jury, was involved as decision-maker to assess against its concept of moral blame the career and conduct of the defendant. With each new presentation of facts and values, the community through the jury could gain further insights into the problem of assessing blame. As a byproduct, the community could learn more about the causes of crime and how those causes might be addressed, either through the application of criminal laws or through other social programs.

The most available avenue for conducting such an inquiry was the insanity defense. In substituting the Durham rule (the accused is not responsible for his act if it "was the product of a mental disease or defect") (Durham v. U.S., 1954) for the M'Naghten (the accused is not responsible for his act if he lacked understanding of the "nature and quality" of his act, or did not know that his act was wrong) (M'Naghten Rule, 1843), we sought to broaden the inquiry beyond cognitive functioning to encompass modern dynamic theories of personality. Our goal was simply to allow the jury a more complete picture of why the accused acted as he did, in order to render the moral judgment of blame as informed as current knowledge of human behavior would permit.

Although the Durham case broadened our trial inquiries somewhat, it soon accumulated in practice all the problems of its predecessor. Psychiatrists, often encouraged by trial judges, testified in conclusory terms which concealed many of the hidden agendas discussed above. Jurors knew little more about those they judged than they had before, and indeed were often deluded into thinking that the psychiatric conclusion foreclosed any further investigation on their part into the moral issue of criminal responsibility.

Nor has our experience with psychiatric testimony in other areas such as juvenile proceedings and civil commitment been any better. Different jargon and different labels are used with the same effect: concealment of the difficult issues of the state's power to deprive individuals of liberty.

I joined my court in discarding the Durham formula in 1972 (U.S. v. Brawner, 1972), but dissented from its adoption of the American Law Institute test for insanity. In its place, I suggested that we instruct the jury that the defendant be held not responsible "if at the time of his unlawful conduct his mental or emotional processes or behavior controls were impaired to such an extent that he cannot justly be held responsible." The value of such a test would be to focus the jury on the ultimate issue of moral responsibility while directing the psychiatric expert to provide information to the jury on the defendant's behavioral impairments. Whether the accused can be considered "mentally ill," from whatever frame of reference, is irrelevant to me. What the jury needs is raw information about the defendant's behavioral controls, be it psychiatric, social, or cultural information, upon which it might base its assessment of moral blame.

From the example of criminal responsibility, one can derive broader principles of the use of psychiatric testimony in the courtroom. First, it is imperative that psychiatric and other information from the behavioral sciences continue to flow into the decisional process when society attempts to decide what to do with persons whose ability to cope within social norms is impaired. A decisional process which ignores relevant, available information is not morally defensible. Although we have to decide how to resolve particular cases without waiting for all relevant information to be discovered, we are at least bound to investigate all avenues currently available.

Second, it is essential that the decision-maker not have the issues of state power and individual liberty obscured by testimony which overreaches the bounds of the witness's legitimate expertise.

Third, it is essential not only that the decision-maker confront what relevant information is known, but also that it be aware of what is unknown. Only then will the process attain the humility which is critical to a just determination of the balance between individual and state. We cannot cope with uncertainty and we cannot move forward toward certainty if we are deluded into thinking we have ultimate answers at hand.

Lastly, in evaluating the psychiatric and other information provided, the decision-maker must be able to see clearly the extent to which such information may be colored by individual and institutional bias. To preserve the legitimacy of its own process, the court must insist on the opportunity to probe witnesses' testimony for bias to determine the appropriate weighting of that information in the final decision.

To these ends, the process of cross-examination by adverse parties is the law's principal mechanism for sifting through the competing facts and values presented in court. Parties adversely affected by a particular witness's testimony carry the burden of testing that information for its completeness, its factual basis, and its coloration by personal, theoretical, and institutional values and beliefs. Psychiatric use of conclusory labels thwarts this process and leaves the decision-maker unable to weigh accurately the facts and values presented and to confront honestly the issues at hand.

If psychiatrists follow my advice to "let it all hang out," they will make our job in the courts immeasurably more difficult. We will be forced to face a number of difficult issues for which we have no ready solutions. What, for example, is society to do with a dangerous offender who cannot be held responsible for his past criminal conduct, yet is not now "sick" and for whom no particular course of treatment or rehabilitation is available? I do not know. But I do know that courts and other public decision-making bodies cannot begin to resolve such questions, for which they are ultimately responsible, until they are provided with relevant and accurate data upon which to base the first tentative steps toward a wise and just solution. So long as psychiatrists presume to decide such questions for us by incorporating into their medical judgments factors beyond their medical expertise, they will be subject to the kinds of charges we currently levy against Soviet psychiatry. Their integrity as scientists and their public image will suffer, and their usefulness in helping those whom they are dedicated to helping will be diminished.

References

American Psychiatric Association: Clinical Aspects of the Violent Individual, Task Force Report 8. July, 1974.

Bazelon, D.: Introduction. *In* Davidson, H.A.: Forensic Psychiatry. New York, Ronald Press, 1970, pp. vii–xxvii.
Blocker v. U.S., 274 F.2d 572 (D.C. Cir., 1959).
Chambers, D.: Brief Amicus Curiae. U.S. v. Brawner, 471 F.2d 969 (D.C. Cir., 1972).
Dixon v. Weinberger, 405 F. Supp. 974 (D.D.C., 1975).
Durham v. U.S., 214 F.2d 862 (D.C. Cir., 1954).
Fingarette, H.: The Meaning of Criminal Insanity. Berkeley, University of California Press, 1972.
M'Naghten Rule, 8 Eng. Rep. 718 (1843).
Olmstead v. U.S., 277 U.S. 438, 479 (1928) (Brandeis, J., dissenting).
Pugh, D.: The Insanity Defense in Operation: A Practicing Psychiatrist Views Durham and Brawner. Washington University Law Quarterly, vol. 87, 1973.
Stone, A.: Mental Health and Law: A System in Transition, New York, Aronson, Jason, Inc., 1976.
Szasz, T.: Psychiatric Justice. New York, Macmillan, Inc., 1965.
U.S. v. Brawner, 471 F.2d 969 (D.C. Cir., 1972).

Comment

Judge Bazelon, in his excellent article, notes that psychiatric participation in the court may slide by imperceptible degrees from participation in the decisional processes to the assumption of responsibility for decisions. He notes that psychiatrists, rather than confining themselves to a specific body of knowledge about which they have expertise, may be seduced into taking responsibility for making judgments or assessing facts about which they have no special competence. This has resulted in psychiatry's overextending itself, with a secondary casualty that society is deluded into believing that scientific and medical answers exist to forensic problems and that social, moral, and other determinants of these problems may be ignored.

Judge Bazelon reminds us that the forensic psychiatrist is influenced by the institutions which he serves and the social, political, and cultural reference points of his time. Thus, he notes that psychiatrists have many times abandoned their role as ally of the patient to serve institutional interests, thus depriving the psychiatrist of credibility. Bazelon notes that if we are to facilitate psychiatry's contribution to the court, we must develop techniques for sorting out and confronting the institutional interests intruding upon the psychiatrist's proper function. He advocates a peer-review mechanism in which professionals outside the conflict-of-interests setting evaluate the performance of the psychiatrist, who should keep careful and detailed records and should advise the patient concerning the particular conflicts of interests to which he may be subjected in examining the patient.

Most would agree with Judge Bazelon's observations. It should be emphasized that the psychiatrist can make a number of contributions in the spectrum of services delivered through the criminal justice system. Those few who have dared venture into this system have received few rewards, possibly owing to a controversy surrounding their role. More emphasis has been given lately to the role of the psychiatrist as a consultant to the judge once a verdict has been established. This would allow mental health input to sentencing and rehabilitation which could be beneficial to the defendant.

H. KEITH H. BRODIE, M.D.

Should Psychiatrists Be Medically Trained? Let's Consider the Alternatives in Light of What the Psychiatrist Does*

MARTIN T. ORNE

The Institute of Pennsylvania Hospital and University of Pennsylvania

The generally accepted definition of psychiatry is exemplified by that offered in the abridged Oxford dictionary: that branch of medicine dealing with mental, emotional, or behavioral disorders. On the face of it, it seems strange indeed for anyone to question the necessity of medical training for the practice of medicine. Certainly no such question was raised until the early 1950s. In this discussion we will try to understand how this question arose, the implications it raises for various views of psychiatric practice, the consequences it has had for the status of psychiatry in American medicine and among the public at large—consequences which are only now becoming obvious—and, finally, what we might learn from such a discussion about the future of our field.

The development of psychiatry as a discipline

The role of the psychiatrist as a physician who dealt with psychoses, severe neuroses, and functional somatic symptoms evolved during the early part of the century until, by the end of World War II, these three functions were accepted as an integral part of psychiatric practice. By that time psychiatry had established itself as a separate discipline distinct from neurology. While there were several different patterns of psychiatric practice, the main division was between two groups:

---

*The substantive research upon which the theoretical outlook presented in this paper is based was supported in part by grant #MH 19156 from the National Institute of Mental Health and by a grant from the Institute for Experimental Psychiatry.

I am indebted to A. Gordon Hammer for his many conceptual contributions, and to William M. Waid for his substantive comments in the preparation of this paper.

1. Those psychiatrists committed to the view that the major psychoses would ultimately be identified as organic and/or genetic in origin, who, while using a variety of psychotherapeutic approaches, nonetheless saw biologically oriented procedures as the real treatment. This group, which included many neuropsychiatrists, eclectic psychiatrists, and traditional mental-hospital-based psychiatrists, identified themselves with biological psychiatry and, until the mid 1940s, represented psychiatric orthodoxy.

2. Other psychiatrists who viewed the psychodynamic approach as central to psychiatry. The etiological factors that mattered were seen as developmental and psychodynamic in nature. Explanatory mechanisms for psychiatric symptoms were sought in the life experiences of the individual. Though differences between neuroses and psychoses were clearly recognized, the latter were generally interpreted as involving psychological traumas, particularly loss and other interactive deficits, at a very early period, while the neuroses involved similar psychological stresses at a later time in an individual's development. Even psychosomatic illnesses were seen as yet another type of consequence which followed from specific psychodynamic etiologies. Obviously, if the etiology of all psychiatric conditions involves psychological trauma, it is hardly surprising that the only appropriate treatment becomes psychodynamically oriented psychotherapy.

Though one might expect that the basic division within psychiatry might lead to different attitudes toward medical training, orthodox psychoanalysis as well as most of the derivative psychodynamic schools shared the commitment to medical training with their colleagues in biological psychiatry.

The therapeutic process (psychoanalysis or dynamic psychotherapy) was seen as a delicate medical treatment requiring extensive special training, acquired like other medical skills by both formal training and extensive apprenticeship, for its proper execution.

The Acceptance of Dynamic Psychiatry by the Medical Establishment

As long as psychiatry was seen as a narrow specialty dealing with the diagnosis and treatment of deranged individuals, the field had little impact on medicine in general. Medical students had only a few hours of training in this specialty. However, in its development psychoanalysis had captured the interest of artists and writers, and a good many novels, plays, and movies were greatly influenced by its theories. The concept of psychological causation was all but taken for granted by modern writers, and psychiatry successfully redefined its role, not merely as treating deranged individuals but, even more important, as helping the relatively mildly neurotic individual to lead a more effective, more satisfying, more successful life.

One of the crucial decisions that was made by the American Psychoanalytic Association was to limit its membership to psychiatrists. Thus, psychoanalysis by definition became a medical treatment and a medical science, a point of view that was eminently congruent with the conceptual model upon which it was built. This decision helped provide the basis for its later wholehearted acceptance by academic medicine.

Probably the single most important factor in this acceptance was the success with which psychodynamic psychiatry asserted its claim that it represented a rational scientific approach based on well-established theories in contrast to the crude eclecticism which characterized much of the contemporary psychiatry of the day. Psychoanalysis seemed to provide a rational diagnosis of psychiatric disorders, somewhat analogous to medical diagnoses based on a sound knowledge of physiology, and seemed to provide a treatment based on that diagnosis.*

During the decade following World War II, psychodynamic treatment became equated with psychiatry. Although there were some active biological psychiatrists, they were all but eclipsed within much of academic medicine. Textbooks of general medicine included discussions of psychoanalytic views, and even the Merck manual—the intern's bible—carried extensive sections on psychodiagnosis and treatment. During this period psychiatry became a very popular medical specialty and psychosomatic medicine came to be accepted as an integral part of the modern medical center. Psychiatric consultation became accepted by other medical specialties as a necessary medical service, and the number of individuals in psychiatric training rapidly increased to meet the growing demands for psychiatric services—demands generated by the growing awareness of functional disorders and neuroses by physicians in other specialties.

This recognition was coupled with a new-found respect for the specialty of psychiatry and the realization that a considerable group of patients could be helped by psychiatrists. Equally important, however, was the increased visibility of psychiatry among large segments of the public who sought psychiatric help directly because of a self-perceived need for help of this type. During this period the demand for psychiatric services continued to exceed the availability of trained individuals. Further, psychiatrists themselves saw their training as relevant to an increasing number of problems which went far beyond those of treating individual patients.

The Medical Model in Psychiatry

Though psychodynamically oriented psychiatrists in the early 1950s tended to reject the significance of hereditary factors for the etiology of psychoses, were reluctant to utilize psychotropic agents or other biological treatments, and carefully avoided becoming involved in the patient's physi-

---

*It should be kept in mind that medicine has appropriately been concerned not only that its treatments be effective but that they also be rational and based on valid scientific principles. There have been many instances in the history of medicine where individuals providing irrational therapies based on unacceptable premises seemed for a time to be more successful, e.g., homeopathy. In the long run, however, acceptance by established medicine depended upon an acceptable theory as well as evidence of success. For example, Christian Science, while often effective in providing relief of functional symptoms, has obviously not become acceptable medical treatment.

cal difficulties, they nonetheless shared basic assumptions with those psychiatrists who were more clearly biologically oriented.

All psychiatrists emphasized the rational scientific basis upon which their procedures rested. Though there was considerable disagreement within the field about etiology, diagnosis, and appropriate treatment, there was a clear consensus that it was necessary to have an understanding of etiology; it was essential to diagnose the patient's disorder and to base a rational treatment upon this diagnosis.

To summarize the basic points relevant to the medical view of psychological illness:

1. Psychiatrists, regardless of their persuasion, perceived themselves as physicians treating patients suffering from some form of disorder. The diagnostic manual was seen as providing useful categories which would allow classification of any difficulty afflicting an individual who might be seen by a psychiatrist. In developing the manual, care was taken to provide for the various orientations that characterized contemporary psychiatry.

2. In all matters of health, the medical profession had, by common consent, defined what constituted illness and health. The extent of the physician's definitional role is seen if one considers that under most circumstances an individual is not considered dead until pronounced so by a physician. Similarly, psychiatrists were seen as those members of the medical profession who defined whether an individual was mentally healthy or sick, a matter which determined whether the individual was capable of making a will, managing his own affairs, or even being allowed to come and go as he pleased. The courts generally sought and accepted psychiatric opinion on such matters, and in a real sense the psychiatrist determined who was psychotic, who was neurotic, and who was within the normal limits of mental health. In an analogous way, the psychiatrist was the one who determined when a patient needed treatment and what treatment was required. He then usually became the therapist and ultimately the judge of when the patient was well. Though the nature of the diagnosis and treatment might vary with psychiatrists of different orientations, the exercise of these functions was considered by essentially all psychiatrists not so much as their prerogative but rather as the necessary and appropriate exercise of their professional responsibilities.

3. As in all medical treatment where the physician takes on specific moral and legal responsibilities when he agrees to minister to a patient, in the same way psychiatrists took medical responsibility for the treatment of their mentally ill patients. Clearly, if a patient became overtly suicidal, the psychiatrist viewed it as his obligation to prevent the patient from committing suicide. Not to do so in the face of a high likelihood of such an event was seen as a clear dereliction of duty. Just as the physically ill patient who becomes delirious may need to be restrained temporarily to prevent him from doing damage to himself, so would the depressed patient require analogous help lest he do something in his morbid state of mind which would certainly have been against his wishes once he had recovered from this depression. The issue of medical responsibility is at the very core of

the physician's role in society. While such responsibility was accepted by both dynamically and biologically oriented psychiatrists, there were important contradictions between some tenets of psychoanalytically oriented treatment and the view that the psychiatrist was ultimately responsible for the patient's welfare. This troubling paradox was dealt with in different ways by a number of authors, but in general it was deemed appropriate that psychiatrists should avoid becoming responsible for the neurotic patient but could not avoid an obligation to protect both the individual and society in the case of psychotic patients. Szasz (1961) was the first to articulate clearly the inherent contradictions in such a position and used it as the basis for a concerted challenge to current psychiatric practice.*

4. The medical model conceives of signs and symptoms as superficial manifestations of underlying pathological processes. An excruciatingly painful big toe which brings the patient to his physician is recognized as reflecting the systemic disorder of gout, which in turn is treated biochemically, effectively bringing relief. This conceptual model was carried over into psychiatry. Consequently, both subjective symptoms and behavioral signs were taken as evidence of an underlying pathology which needed to be treated. Specific symptomatic relief was generally considered an inappropriate goal, much as the application of a local anesthetic to relieve the gouty toe would hardly be considered an appropriate treatment. Though the concept of symptoms reflecting underlying disorders was almost totally accepted by psychiatrists until very recently, there was of course considerable disagreement about the nature of the underlying processes, with some psychiatrists focusing upon genetic and biochemical etiologies, others emphasizing psychobiological consequences of specific stressors, and psychodynamically oriented psychiatrists tending to look to developmental and interpersonal etiologies. While the psychodynamic psychiatrists accepted the model of illness, the basic sciences which would contribute to their elucidation were seen to be more closely related to psychology, sociology, cultural anthropology—all disciplines which concerned themselves with the study of mechanisms which were postulated to be basic to the patient's clinical problems.†

5. One corollary to the medical point of view seems particularly important in terms of more recent developments. Illness has always been viewed

---

*While Szasz's position is in many regards logically consistent and points to areas where there have been instances of serious abuse, he merely pushes upon the courts the responsibility for deciding the difficult questions of the degree to which an individual has the right to harm himself, the extent to which the psychiatrist has an obligation to protect his patient from harming not only himself but others, and a variety of related questions for which the courts had sought advice from psychiatry.

†It was this realization that led to one of the early challenges to the appropriateness of medical training for psychiatrists. Dr. Lawrence Kubie (1950) proposed that a new kind of degree in the healing arts, a doctorate in medical psychology, be established, which, like dentistry, would teach the basic sciences and allow the graduate to obtain a license to use those drugs appropriate to his discipline, but in addition to general medicine the training would include much psychology, sociology, and anthropology and thus be specifically tailored to provide the background which was relevant from the point of view of psychodynamic psychiatry.

as the enemy by the medical profession. Thus, it is hardly surprising that psychiatrists saw themselves as opposed to mental illness in all of its manifestations.

While a number of psychiatrists had recognized that the creative urge was uncomfortably closely related to some aspects of psychopathology (see Hartmann, 1964; Kretschmer, 1948; Kris, 1952), the experience of a psychotic episode was never seen as desirable or productive.

The physician's role in society and the medical model in psychiatry. One can hardly leave a discussion of the medical model in psychiatry without recognizing the tremendous social importance which medicine has in modern society. Physical illness is the one event which can excuse just about every kind of behavior in modern society. There is little or no blame attached to the soldier who falters in battle because he is physically ill; there is no social obligation from which one is not excused because of physical illness. Some courts accept illness as an appropriate reason to delay any form of trial, and medical excuses are even accepted by the IRS!

Modern society is justly proud of its enlightened humanitarianism. While anthropologists point out that other societies such as the Hopi lack the concept of physical illness, ascribing all illness to either witchcraft or bad thoughts, we are quick to dismiss such a naïve view with a smile and some self-satisfied thoughts about the irrationality of such a position. It might be well to consider, however, that modern society's enlightened view of illness is by no means necessarily totally rational. Ample research has shown that motivated individuals with very high fevers can carry out a wide range of performance tasks with little or no perceptible decrement (Alluisi et al., 1971). In practice, what excuses an individual rarely involves proof that he is incapacitated by an actual test, but rather it is sufficient to be seriously ill and have a physician attest to the fact that undertaking a certain activity might have untoward consequences for the individual's health. Whether or not the illness is sufficiently incapacitating to justify being excused from whatever would otherwise be required is a decision made by physicians according to appropriately conservative criteria—in the sense of protecting the patient more than worrying about his obligations. In most instances, the word of even a single reputable practitioner is rarely challenged.

As one considers the medical model in psychiatry, one cannot ignore the social significance illness has in our society and the high degree of acceptance of medical statements by a broad range of institutions. Thus, the psychiatrist gains considerable credibility within our society by the simple fact that he is a physician. Though physicians as a group do not now enjoy the unambivalent admiration of most Americans that was common some 30 years ago, their statements continue to have a high degree of credibility. (Ironically, the high incidence of malpractice suits is partly at least related to the high degree of belief in the physician's inherent ability to be correct and assure good therapeutic outcomes.)

The Changing Role of the Psychiatrist

During the period following World War II, psychiatry had come of age as a specialty. It was suddenly accepted not only by academic medicine but also by other academic disciplines. Psychiatrists were eagerly sought after and listened to in departments of psychology, anthropology, sociology, literature, industrial management, and political science. It is hardly surprising that they saw their training as relevant to an increasing number of problems which went far beyond those of treating individual patients and began to encompass most of the social ills man was heir to—war, prejudice, aggression, crime, as well as other forms of social deviance.

While a significant segment of psychiatrists were re-evaluating their role and saw themselves as more closely allied with humanism and the social sciences, a number of other factors also combined to encourage a split of psychiatry from the rest of medicine. It will not be possible here to trace each of these developments and the complex interrelationships; rather, we will only touch upon some of the trends. There were three main thrusts involved: (1) the intellectual challenge to the medical model stemming from psychology and the development of psychological therapies; (2) the development of social psychiatry, ultimately leading to the community mental health center where psychiatric services were provided by mental health aides or counselors with little formal training or education; (3) the challenge to the concept of mental illness from within some segments of psychiatry, which in the service of a new humanism sought to redefine the subject matter of psychiatry as helping people deal with problems of living.

The intellectual challenge. From the very beginning psychoanalysis sought to develop a psychological science. Though Freud appropriately felt that nineteenth century psychology had little to offer the psychotherapist, he also recognized the importance of developing a psychology which could form the scientific basis for psychotherapy. While much of psychoanalysis developed outside the academic context, it rapidly began to have an impact on the developing science of psychology. Thus, Freud's lectures in 1911 at Clark University were given under the auspices of the department of psychology, and there was some continuing interest in psychodynamic aspects by the psychologists of that period. Other outstanding medical therapists at the turn of the century emphasized that they were practicing medical psychology. Pierre Janet in France and Morton Prince in the United States are particularly clear examples. Thus, Morton Prince, a medical therapist, founded the *Journal of Abnormal Psychology,* which ultimately was given to the American Psychological Association. In those early years, Freud, Jung, Adler, and other medical psychotherapists thought it appropriate to train nonmedical therapists, and a small number of psychologists chose psychoanalysis or psychotherapy as a career. These individuals were trained in traditional psychopathology and tended to think in terms of the medical model. They were few in number and were not perceived as a threat to those relatively few psychiatrists who were interested in the psychotherapeutic treatment of troubled individuals.

The first real challenge came from a different tradition of psychological therapy. Carl Rogers, a psychologist trained in the child guidance movement—an interdisciplinary treatment approach which originated in the 1920s—eventually accepted an academic appointment in clinical psychology with responsibility for a counseling center. It was within the tradition of counseling psychology that Carl Rogers (1942) wrote his remarkably successful book on nondirective therapy.

Rogers put forth a number of ideas which dramatically challenged the medical model in treatment. He argued that it was not necessary to diagnose the patient's difficulties. Instead, it was sufficient to provide an atmosphere of unqualified positive regard for the client (emphatically not the patient) and in such a context the individual would resolve his own difficulties. He provided an upbeat view of man where the individual was seen as basically healthy and his difficulties relatively easily resolved—provided he had the opportunity to reflect upon them in an appropriate setting. In particular, he felt that the client would need to understand his feelings, and to facilitate this process the therapist should sedulously strive to reflect the patient's feelings without making any interpretations or comments. Not only did Rogers propose that such a process would be therapeutic, but he also insisted that as long as the therapist provided the appropriate positive emotional setting the mere act of reflecting feelings would allow the patient somehow to get to understand his problems and work through a constructive solution for them. In contrast to the medical model, Rogers argued that the therapist does not know best, nor should he attempt to second guess what the patient ought to do. He genuinely felt that the patient could and would learn the unique solution to his problems by having his creative capacities liberated by working with someone who truly respected him as an individual and sought truly to understand his feelings.

Not only did Rogers provide the first important novel psychotherapeutic approach not based on a medical model, but he also initiated the first major research effort to explore the factors affecting success in psychotherapy. In a series of pioneering studies he and his colleagues (1954) demonstrated that the appropriate emotional tone was crucial to therapeutic progress, that therapists who talked less were more effective than those who talked more, and so on (see Truax and Mitchell, 1971). Thus, Rogers not only provided a technique of psychotherapy developed by a psychologist, but also offered systematic evidence concerning the factors affecting therapeutic effectiveness. It is hardly surprising that his work attracted wide attention within the psychological academic community, and, though it was virtually ignored by psychiatrists, rogerian therapists established themselves in counseling services of a large number of institutions and some became private practitioners. Rogerian therapists did not generally agree to see psychotic individuals, nor did they view themselves as trying to help severely incapacitated individuals. In restricting their activities to individuals not defined as sick, they distinguished what they were doing from medical treatment and obviated the need for what they viewed as pigeonholing individuals in some diagnostic category.

In time rogerian therapists inevitably sought to treat an increasingly wide range of troubled individuals. They did not, however, ever come to feel the need to concern themselves with diagnostic categories. Probably because rogerians addressed themselves mostly to their academic colleagues and published largely in the context of counseling psychology, the profoundness of their challenge to the medical model in psychotherapy did not come to the attention of psychiatrists until recently, when rogerian thinking, as one of the important roots of humanistic psychology and, in particular, as the basis of T-groups, helped usher in some of the more recent popular developments of quasitherapies. It seems all the more relevant in view of this recent development to consider Rogers' historical position about psychotherapy, a position which has undergone remarkably little change through the years, though it is perhaps difficult for the observer to identify the eminently proper, establishment-oriented counseling psychologists (who often held important administrative roles in universities) and the hip, counterculture-oriented T-group leader as sharing the same intellectual heritage.

In structuring the therapeutic relationships Rogers carefully eschewed taking any responsibility for the patient's well-being, insisting that it was his role merely to help the patient comprehend his feelings and to provide the setting where he would be able to carry out his difficult work of reappraisal. Rogers never claimed expertise in the sense of knowing what was wrong with his clients. On the contrary, he exuded a sublime belief in the patient's ability to heal himself and was firmly convinced that in the context of the therapist's unswerving respect for his feelings, the client would come up with the solutions best adapted to his needs. In direct contrast to the medical model, there was no diagnosis and no concept of medical responsibility. Even when a client threatened to commit suicide, Rogers would not deviate from this position. In no case did he feel entitled to take responsibility for the patient; rather, he would steadfastly act in accordance with his conviction that the patient would resolve his own problems and the expectation that he would see him at the next appointment.*

---

*Considerable controversy followed his playing a tape of a course of therapy with a client who indeed sounded extremely suicidal, where many colleagues felt it was not justified to allow him to leave the office. Rogers argued that he did not have the right to do otherwise, that the patient would have to solve his own problems, and that to take responsibility for him would be an unpardonable infringement which might cause serious harm. It does appear, in that case at least, that Rogers' faith in his relationship with his client and in his client's basically healthy core was justified.

It should be noted, however, that Rogers maintained that even if the patient had committed suicide he would still not have had the obligation nor even the right to prevent him from leaving his office. By the same token, he would have argued that it would have been counterproductive to advise the patient that he should not commit suicide.

It is not intended here to argue the merits of client-centered therapy. Certainly in proper hands it can be a more formidable therapeutic procedure than is generally recognized within psychiatry, nor, as a practical matter, is the difference between selective reflection of feeling and properly timed explicit interpretation as great as might be supposed at first glance. The important matter is the radical difference in the manner in which the role relationship between therapist and patient is conceptualized. By external criteria the rogerian therapist is still defined as an expert, and he certainly maintains the accouterments of an appropriate office, clients seen by appointment, professional status, and the like. Nonetheless, in explicitly refusing to provide any advice whatsoever, refusing to take any responsibility for the patient's behavior, and insisting that decisions at all times are the patient's responsibility, the approach is truly nonmedical.

Rogers' pivotal role developed certain attitudes within psychology and had profound effects on a number of the newer psychotherapies which emphasized the primary importance of feelings in the therapeutic process and the refusal to accept responsibility for the patient's welfare (various forms of Gestalt therapy, rational emotive therapy, aspects of psychodrama, and so on). Nonetheless, neither the therapies nor the quasitherapies whose origins can be traced back to the influence of Rogers' ideas nor the psychotherapy research which owes its beginnings to Rogers' influence have had much impact on psychiatric thought. Until relatively recently, the fact that these therapies were generally applied to individuals who had not defined themselves as patients and that psychotherapy research usually involved psychologists as therapists unfortunately prevented the studies from being recognized as salient by most psychiatrists. It is only recently that T-groups, Gestalt therapy, sensitivity training, EST, and a myriad of other popularizations of these various procedures have achieved phenomenal popularity within our culture and have therefore come to the notice of the psychiatric community. In some areas these various approaches have begun to provide serious competition as alternatives to psychiatric help that troubled individuals might choose to take.

An entirely different challenge to dynamic psychiatry developed from Eysenck's (1952) classic criticism which emphasized the lack of evidence documenting the effect of psychotherapy and suggested that, regardless of the therapist or his technique, one third of the patients get better, one third get worse, and one third remain unchanged. Though this critique attracted much attention, it did not basically challenge the medical model of treatment; it merely took the practitioners to task for failing to be effective physicians. Only when this critique was combined with the renewed interest in behavior therapy, which served to provide an alternative for troubled individuals, did it begin to pose a serious challenge to psychodynamic psychiatry.

It seems unnecessary to review the history of behavior therapy in this context. (See Birk et al., 1973; Herson et al., 1975; Yates, 1975 for appropriate reviews.) There is a growing understanding and awareness of behavioral approaches in psychiatry. From the point of view of this discussion, there are two aspects of behavior therapy which make it relevant:

1. It challenges the medical model as it rejects the notion that symptoms inevitably reflect an underlying process. In the case of phobias, for example, the symptom may well be the illness. Removal of that symptom does not usually appear to result in other symptoms as would be predicted by the psychodynamic model; rather, that improvement may produce unexpected and unanticipated improvements in other areas. While behavior therapy itself is in the process of maturing as a field, there is some awareness that certain symptoms do indeed reflect underlying problems but that the specific and direct treatment of some psychiatric symptoms is clearly effective and appropriate. Further, even in instances where one is dealing with a major psychosis, significant salutary changes can be brought about by behavior therapy. Thus, the success of behavior therapy in some areas of psychiatry in bringing about enduring relief of symptoms serves to challenge the basic validity of the dynamic model as explaining all psychopathology.

2. Behavior therapy has provided an alternative model for psychopathology derived from theories of learning. It proposes that just as we have learned motor skills and coping mechanisms, we also learn maladaptive processes which descriptively fall into the category of psychopathology. To the degree that one can successfully conceptualize significant aspects of psychopathology as problems of learning, one inevitably puts the treatment of these disorders into the domain of learning and out of the domain of medical therapy as usually defined. The basic science relevant to behavior therapy is presumed to be academic psychology, and its treatments take their roots in psychological experiments.

Not only is behavior therapy a treatment developed by psychologists, but it appears to be based on sound theory derived from a solid body of scientific knowledge. It matters less whether these claims are fully justified than the fact that they have been successfully asserted. Most importantly, this view has gained credence not merely among the general public but within large segments of the scientific community itself.

Though behavior therapy challenges some aspects of the medical model, it emphatically does not challenge other significant aspects. Thus, the role relationship between the behavior therapist and his patient is closely analogous to the relationship of the nonpsychiatric physician and his patient. He is the expert, administering a treatment with the patient's consent. He defines what constitutes improvement and how it shall be evaluated. He is carrying out a treatment that is presumed to be rational and specific. He has taken a careful history and keeps careful notes on the patient's progress. Thus, while behavior therapy challenges the psychodynamic view of the medical model, in many regards it is eminently compatible with the medical approach. One important similarity that is easily overlooked is the extent to which there is consensus about the kinds of difficulties that are symptoms and should appropriately be modified. Just as there is no doubt in a physician's mind that a fever or an increased blood pressure represents something to be remedied, so is there little question in the behavior therapist's mind that a phobia, a psychotic symptom, or anorexia constitute symptoms that one should strive to eliminate.

The challenge of social psychiatry and the community mental health movement. During the 1950s the demand for psychiatric services increased as the medical profession came to accept the psychiatric services and the public at large increasingly sought out such help. As soon as a new psychiatric clinic was opened, it developed a backlog of patients who had to wait months or even years before they could be accepted for treatment. Epidemiological studies, such as *Mental Health in the Metropolis* (Srole et al., 1962), revealed a profound and shocking incidence of severe disturbance among the population of a large city, and the Joint Commission on Mental Health proposed concerted action to help relieve the problem of widespread incidence of psychiatric difficulties.

The Community Mental Health Act represented a mammoth effort to provide psychiatric services on an unprecedented scale. Reflecting the widespread dissatisfaction with the large mental hospital as a warehouse of human misery, far away from the patient's former associations, a new impetus was given to provide early treatment in the patient's community, preventing if possible the initial hospitalization and keeping the individual within the community. The community mental health center was intended to obviate the need for prolonged custodial care and to allow the gradual phasing out of the large hospitals, to be replaced by treatment-oriented institutions of manageable size. When one considers the magnitude of the problems of building and staffing new institutions, recognizing that the staffing needs of these institutions far exceeded the available number of psychiatrists, clinical psychologists, and social workers, it is surprising that they were not less effective than was actually the case.

It is not possible here to review the aims, achievements, and failures of community psychiatry—only to focus on three aspects which profoundly affected psychiatrists' self-perception.

1. It quickly became apparent that there simply were not enough psychiatrists to be primary providers of services. Whereas psychiatric clinics had been staffed by residents, there were not nearly enough residents to staff the mental health centers, nor were there enough clinical psychologists or social workers. Leaning heavily on promising results with highly selected, unusually mature older women reported by Margaret Rioch (Rioch et al., 1963), the concept of the mental health worker rapidly evolved. Part of the justification derived from the remarkable lack of success which middle-class psychiatrists encountered in attempting to treat lower-class patients. They simply were unable to identify with the incredibly deprived and often emotionally barren backgrounds of these persons, and were frightened and often dismayed by the widespread physical violence within their lives. The notion that individuals could be found who might lack formal academic training but had the maturity and appreciation of the subculture necessary to empathize with and help the troubled minority member from a deprived environment made a virtue of necessity. Unfortunately, in most instances the selection of the mental health worker in no way parallelled the care which Margaret Rioch had taken, nor were these individuals given the prolonged supervision and extensive training that provided the initial promising results.

There is no doubt that there are many devoted, committed, and hard-working professionals on the staffs of community mental health centers seeking to provide the best possible service to their patients. Unfortunately, the yardstick by which the amount of work carried out is measured involves the number of patient hours provided, and it is hardly ever considered whether the training or the skill of the individual who actually has contact with the patient is adequate. In most instances, such an arrangement will rapidly create the situation where virtually all services are provided by those individuals with the least training, since they apparently are the most cost-effective workers. The highly trained individuals on the staff are reserved for supervision, training in the treatment of special problems, and representational functions vis-à-vis other agencies.

2. The psychiatrist's role in the context of a mental health center tended to involve a broad range of nonmedical functions, including consulting with a wide range of agencies and the nominal supervision of a large number of paraprofessional workers. At the same time the psychiatrist's medical functions tended to become quite routine, often seeming to involve an exploitation of the psychiatrist's license to practice medicine in order to prescribe psychoactive drugs that the nonmedical staff thought were needed. Under these circumstances it is hardly surprising that the psychiatrist would perceive his psychiatric functions as largely unrelated to medicine, while his medical role was at best technical, requiring relatively little of his training and skill. In a community mental health center there was no question who would do therapy, and it was very clear that medical training was not the crucial skill in making the therapy successful. By the same token, the psychiatrist was made forceably aware of his limitations and the importance of social and cultural factors. Many psychiatrists working in community mental health centers found it difficult to remain comfortable about their professional identity. Unavoidably, the fact that the bulk of treatment was carried out by essentially untrained individuals would tend to denigrate the psychiatrist's function as a psychotherapist and diminish his pride in the hard-won skills that he had achieved in the practice of psychotherapy. It becomes increasingly difficult to insist that psychotherapy is a medical discipline while simultaneously assigning patients to paraprofessionals for treatment.

3. The impact of the community mental health center has thus been to deprofessionalize the enterprise of psychotherapy as such. In many ways the psychiatrist virtually became superfluous. Psychotherapeutic functions were being filled by paraprofessionals, the administrative functions were gradually taken over by administrators, and the educational, supervisory, and representational functions were increasingly filled by social workers and psychologists. While a physician was needed to prescribe drugs, this function could be—and at times has been—filled by general practitioners. The medical aspects of the psychiatrist's skills had relatively little value in the setting, and in terms of identification, those psychiatrists who stayed with community mental health centers tended to move further and further away from an identification with medicine. A small group of psychiatrists

have indeed established new role models in social psychiatry and have become effective by seeking to work through a number of institutions such as the schools, the welfare system, industry, the courts, and so on. The sphere of action of these colleagues is far removed from the usual medical model, and one might appropriately ask to what extent medical training itself specifically facilitates the work of these social psychiatrists. Probably, for these colleagues, the most benefit that medical training provides is to legitimize their status while their substantive skills are more closely related to those of the anthropologist, the sociologist, and the psychologist, combined with the skills of modern management.

There is no mental illness—only troubled individuals with problems of living

Perhaps in reaction to the large mental hospitals and to the often disastrous effects of labeling an individual as mentally ill (Rosenhan, 1973), an increasingly powerful tendency to reject psychiatric classification and to deny the concept of mental illness became apparent. Szasz's (1961) position represents a relatively scholarly attack of this kind. Taking the model of hysteria and extending it to schizophrenia, he argues that all manifestations of major psychoses are largely iatrogenic. Those which cannot be laid at the physician's door can at least be blamed on the culture.

Others have emphasized the pathogenic aspects of modern society and argued that one cannot be well if the society as a whole is sick. Perhaps the most popular argument of this sort has been put forth by Laing (1957), who treats schizophrenic patients by helping create a milieu which tolerates their psychopathology and allows them to experience their psychoses as an aid to their ultimate development. Psychopathology in such an environment is not to be feared but rather to be understood, empathized with, and integrated in a creative way. The appeal of such a point of view to the idealist as well as to the social reformer was great indeed. In interesting ways some very gifted individuals have sought to make these views work. It is hardly surprising that some antiestablishment themes are easily discerned in this position, and it is worth noting that one of the most constructive aspects of the counterculture movement has been its tolerance for deviance of all sorts, including mental illness. It is understandable why the philosophical and political implications as well as the demand for tolerance of individual differences would appeal to the creative instinct and attract members of the counterculture, providing one of the most socially constructive rallying points.

It is too early to judge the true merits of Laing's position and its variants. Undoubtedly there is some justification for rejecting premature labeling and considering alternative approaches to mental illness. Above all, it seems desirable for society to develop greater tolerance for deviants, even those who are not wealthy enough to be called eccentric. Nonetheless, the rejection of systematic efforts to classify, predict, and understand mental disorders seems a large step backward. As much as we might like to believe that love and tolerance will conquer all, the evidence that they are a sufficient treatment for schizophrenia remains wanting.* Similarly, the assumption that it is ever good to encourage a full-blown schizophrenic episode is undocumented. If the assumption were correct, to encourage the psychosis to develop in the course of treatment would be a draconian measure, and if the assumption is incorrect, it would be the worst kind of mishap.

It is not intended, however, to go into the merits or demerits of this view, only to point to its effect in contributing to the identity crisis of psychiatry. Those of us who think about what we do and why we do it have always been troubled by the greater number of questions than answers that characterize our field. To now find our most basic notions under attack is troubling indeed.

The challenge to the established order and the distrust of rationality. As long as the cultural values were essentially stable, the psychiatrist's basic role within the culture was reasonably clear. Certain kinds of deviancies were defined as medical problems and dealt with as such. While such a solution was not necessarily satisfactory and might lead to new problems (as, for example, the use of indeterminate court sentences for the treatment of sex offenders), on the whole the psychiatric approach appeared to be an enlightened substitute for the punitive control of deviancy which preceded it. Psychiatrists were characteristically both products and carriers of middle-class values. It was usually assumed that health and a reasonable adjustment to the cultural norm were inevitable concomitants. While psychiatrists tended to hold liberal views, they tended to take the basic values for granted. There were always isolated radical individuals who challenged the psychiatrist's liberal assumptions and argued that psychiatry is basically a tool of the establishment and a modern means of supporting the status quo.

As the unpopular Vietnam war increasingly polarized society, this type of criticism became increasingly strident, with extreme groups accusing various groups of psychiatrists, psychopharmacologists, dynamic psychiatrists, and behavior therapists of being apologists for the establishment, seeking to eliminate dissent hand-in-glove with other repressive elements of society. The scandals about the political use of psychiatric commitment in the Soviet Union have not served to make any of us more comfortable and seem to lend credence to the possibility that psychiatric methods can indeed be used in the service of totalitarian regimes. Similarly, the documented effectiveness of coercive persuasion as a political tool in China, and some of the similarities which can be drawn between that process and some psychotherapeutic efforts in a hospital setting, cannot help but make us uncomfortable.

It is not that many of us have had any serious questions about what we ourselves do in actual practice; rather, these issues have made us aware that it is virtually impossible to practice psychiatry without making innu-

---

*It is interesting that depression, being a disease of older people, is rarely treated in the same way as schizophrenia, which occurs in young individuals.

merable implicit value judgments. When criticized for supporting non-American researchers with government research grants, our Secretary of Health, Education and Welfare was able to assert that it mattered little whether it was an American or a Russian that found a cure for cancer. We would all benefit. The issue is considerably more complex when we contemplate psychiatric treatment. What constitutes mental health for a member of a commune may be quite different from what constitutes mental health for the junior executive.

With the development of so-called alternative life styles, the determination of whether certain types of adjustments are healthy has become increasingly difficult. This is often referred back to the question of how a healthy individual can successfully adjust to a sick society.

It would, I believe, be inappropriate to view some of the current influences on psychiatry in isolation from the profound anti-intellectual bias that has developed throughout the western world. It is not surprising that psychiatry would be profoundly affected. Thus, while the subject matter of psychoanalysis has always been the unconscious, and psychodynamically oriented psychiatry is inevitably focused on unconscious motivation, its goal was well enunciated by Freud when he said, "Where id was, ego shall be." The mainstream of dynamic psychiatry did not encourage the expression of emotion for its own sake. Similarly, the supportive therapy practiced by biological psychiatrists and the work of modern behavior therapists emphasized rational approaches to treatment. Recently, however, a number of movements which have impinged upon psychiatry to varying degrees have emphasized the virtue of affect for its own sake and the importance of dealing with irrationality on its own terms. We have already commented on the work of Laing in this regard. However, this view is equally pronounced in the various Gestalt therapies, in the increasing popularity of some reichian approaches, and in the encounter or T-groups as well as the far more extreme variants of this genre. The importance both of scientific proof that a method works and of professional expertise is minimized.

In this context the rapid spread of the use of drugs solely for the purpose of altered subjective experience among the youth and counterculture is also relevant. Whatever else the drug experience may do, it inevitably allows the individual to escape the constraints of accurately perceiving the real world. Often the same individual takes "uppers" and "downers" as well as hallucinogenic drugs. It seems unlikely that he is seeking a specific type of high as much as some kind of new sensation. While the reasons for drug use in our society are complex and some intoxicants have been in use since before recorded history, the deliberate and widespread use of hallucinogens is a new development. Though the specific long-term effects of these agents remain controversial, they inevitably involve an individual's purposive decision to distort his perception, experience, and feelings. It does not seem accidental that the use of agents designed to temporarily induce irrationality is closely linked with other evidence of the wish to reject social norms. The cultural values that are espoused by these segments of the counterculture emphasize the rejection of the work ethic, a lack of obligation to be one's brother's keeper, the assertion of an individual's right to do his own thing almost to the exclusion of a concern for its effect on others, and the view that feeling is in the final analysis more important than reason.

The psychiatric community was initially intrigued with reports of the effects of hallucinogens, and there were some efforts to use them therapeutically. However, vis-à-vis the drug culture and its various manifestations, most psychiatrists felt peculiarly helpless. The success of psychiatric treatment of runaways, dropouts, and active participants in the drug culture is limited at best. The bulk of the psychiatric community was torn between an intellectual commitment to encourage growth development, creativity, and experimentation and a frightening awareness that this new social phenomenon defies ready explanation in psychiatric terms.

The ambivalence of the psychiatric community toward the drug culture is not surprising. In a true sense this group showed the close link between the rejection of rationality as a necessary good along with the rejection of many other values of traditional society. Psychiatrists as a group tend to share some of the concerns expressed by the counterculture but, despite the important differences between dynamic psychiatrists, biological psychiatrists, and behavior therapists, there is a shared commitment to seek rational solutions to man's problems. The sharp controversy about what constitutes the most appropriate scientific approach is matched by an equally profound consensus that a scientific approach is needed. It appears to me that a significant trend which crosscuts the various orientations of psychiatry is the rejection of the scientific method and the emphasis on experiential learning. The greater acceptance of Laing's views, on the one hand, and the T-group, the marathon therapies, the reichian approach, on the other hand, among groups who identify more closely with the counterculture makes sense in that these trends within psychiatry appear to be reflections of the larger anti-intellectual, antiestablishment trends within society.

Though there is little doubt that some very important positive insights have emerged from our colleagues in humanistic psychology and the renewed awareness of the importance of affect, it also seems evident that we cannot afford to give up the search for satisfactory criteria by which progress can be evaluated and the means of phrasing our knowledge in terms that can be understood by others. However, psychiatry today finds itself not only confronted with rapidly changing values within society but also with having to deal with challenges to the most basic notions upon which any scientific discipline must rest. Thus, while most of us have been concerned about the relatively inadequate way in which psychiatry lives up to its scientific ideals, we now find that some of us point with pride at these very inadequacies and reject the notion that we should ever base our work on scientific knowledge.

What Shall Be the Appropriate Training for the Psychiatrist?

An effort has been made to sketch some of the diverse trends within modern American psychiatry. Not only is there disagreement about how scientific psychiatry should proceed, whether our basic sciences are physiology, molecular biology, neurochemistry, and electrophysiology, or whether they should more appropriately be sought in the social sciences, but even our definitions of what constitutes illness vary, and the relevance of diagnosing illness has been challenged in some quarters. Finally, there are very wide differences in how the role of the psychiatrist in society is conceived.

One of the reasons for the review of these issues is to make clear that the differences in the role that the psychiatrist plays in different contexts cannot be dealt with simply by analogy to different medical specialties. Thus, the training of a community psychiatrist demands a range of skills which are almost totally divorced from those required of the psychopharmacologist which, in turn, are radically different from those needed by the behavior therapist. It is in such a context that we must weigh the relative merits of different kinds of training for the psychiatrist.

Traditionally psychiatry has been a medical specialty, and as such medical training was a prerequisite to the beginning of specialty training. Not only is medical training difficult to obtain and requires a great deal of effort and commitment from the student but, in contrast to other medical specialties, its relevance to the day-to-day practice of many psychiatrists is far from clear. Further, it has been argued that by focusing the psychiatrist's attention on diseases of the body, medical training may actually be counterproductive. Thus, the search for physical causation may prevent a full, appropriate appreciation of psychological causation. The search for physical factors causing derangement within the individual may prevent the recognition of effects caused by a maladaptive social system, and so on. Finally, given the shortage of physicians in general and the difficulties of expanding the number of places in medical schools, questions have been raised about the advisability of allocating a large number of training opportunities to individuals who will make limited use of their training. One might well wonder why a community psychiatrist, working as a consultant with a school system, needs to have attended medical school; similarly, why should a behavior therapist be required to know how to deliver a baby or hold a retractor during a gallbladder operation? The psychotherapist's skills demand the kind of experience in interpersonal relationships and an appreciation of the nuances of psychological causality which some have argued is deterred by the kinds of attitudes that characterize the doctor-patient relationship usual in medical practice.

Part of the difficulty of assessing the appropriateness of different kinds of training for the psychiatrist is the large number of subspecialties within the field. The differences between the day-to-day activities of psychiatrists in different subspecialties are often greater than the similarities. It seems necessary therefore to consider what the core area of psychiatry is and what basic skills should be common to all psychiatrists. For the purposes of this discussion we will consider the evaluation and treatment of individuals who are sufficiently disturbed to seek help—or who sufficiently disturb others to be sent for help—as the core skills which all psychiatrists should have mastered.

As soon as such a heuristic position is spelled out, each professional is quick to point out the obvious importance of his particular discipline. "Is it not absurd," the psychologist will ask, "to have psychiatrists without any training in the systematic study of behavior?" He may go on to say, "Does it seem sensible to have those individuals who expect to treat abnormal behavior lack any understanding of the normal individual? Can you imagine a pathologist who had failed to study normal histology or a surgeon without a knowledge of anatomy?"

The sociologist will ask, "How can you begin to evaluate an individual without a full appreciation of demographic variables?" He will emphasize the significance of the individual's unique background, the structure of his family, the impact of role expectations, job opportunities, social pressures, and changes within the family, perhaps in response to broader social trends. He may well ask how psychiatrists can hope to understand the significance of a patient's actions without a broader appreciation of deviancy within our society, recognizing that the same problem treated by the psychiatrist might, under slightly different circumstances, be "treated" by the police, the courts, or the penal system, and under still other circumstances be tacitly tolerated in some communities (e.g., incest). The anthropologist will argue that without an understanding of other cultures it is inevitable that we confuse the social arrangements of our own society with what is normal, instinctive, right, or desirable. Similarly, he will point out that many attributes highly valued in one culture are seen as pathology in another: that one tends to assume the role which is normal for a man, a woman, a child, or an adult is somehow preordained, whereas, in fact, these roles show a remarkable degree of plasticity across cultures, and so on.

If, after consideration of such viewpoints, one decides that psychological training, augmented by familiarity with some of the other social sciences, ought to be the basic training for psychiatrists, the physician will ask how one can possibly hope to treat mental disorders without a thorough understanding of the myriad of physical causes of psychological difficulties. Certainly he would say that one would need to make the differential diagnosis between hyperthyroidism and an anxiety state, between a hysteric seizure and epilepsy, and between depression and postinfectious debilitation, as well as to recognize other instances where organic problems present as psychological symptoms.

The fact of the matter is that knowledge of each of the disciplines is relevant to the psychiatrist's function. It is true that the psychiatrist needs to understand what constitutes normal behavior, ideation, cognitive processes, and the like; that he should have a true appreciation for the systematic study of psychological processes, both normal and disturbed; that he should be able to quantify his findings and test their validity in a systematic fashion. Certainly he needs an understanding of the social system within which he works, nor should he believe either that his personal values are of necessity the best guides for his patients to follow or that everything he finds personally offensive is of necessity serious pathology. By the same token, he must also have an appreciation of how organic factors can cause psychological symptoms and have the ability to properly utilize psychotropic agents in his work, not to mention a broad understanding of basic medical science. Ideally, then, he should have training in each of the formal disciplines we have touched upon and, of course, if he is to do psychotherapy, he should have acquired that skill by dint of extensive training and supervision.

Psychiatry as it is currently conceived has its roots in a large number of disciplines, each of which is important for the psychiatrist's development. We need to recognize, however, that it simply is not possible to demand an in-depth knowledge of each of these areas. To do so would further extend the length of training required of the psychiatrist. From an economic and social point of view, such a solution would hardly be acceptable.

Because of these difficulties, the suggestion was originally put forth by Lawrence Kubie (1950) that a special curriculum be developed for psychiatrists analogous to the way special training has been developed for dentists. By eliminating those aspects of medical training least likely to be relevant to the psychiatrist's work and substituting more relevant training in psychology and the social sciences, he argued, a better use of the students' training period would be made. Certainly this general notion requires careful consideration.

In the succeeding section we shall seek to compare some of the advantages and disadvantages of the three most likely alternatives which have been proposed as appropriate training for psychiatry: medical training, training in psychology and related social sciences, and some new curriculum, leading to a new kind of degree and involving a hybrid training of medicine, psychology, and the social sciences.

The Current Training of Psychiatrists

At the present time, those individuals who ultimately become psychiatrists will have taken premedical courses in college, usually with a strong emphasis on biology and biochemistry because most college premedical counselors feel that this gives the student the best opportunity to gain entrance to medical school. Relatively few students take advantage of the opportunities to obtain a thorough grounding in psychology and the social sciences or a broad liberal arts education during their college years. The psychiatrist-to-be then enters medical school, which emphasizes the basic and clinical sciences necessary to graduate a student capable of dealing effectively with a broad range of medical problems.

While in recent years in many medical schools psychiatry has been able to obtain a somewhat larger number of hours than was the case some years ago, and more medical schools now include a few hours of behavioral science during their preclinical years, the major task facing the student is to master the skills necessary to be a general physician. In theory at least, the student on graduation should be capable of handling the duties of general medical practice. Since in such a context psychiatry must of necessity play a limited role, it is not surprising therefore that the focus of medical school is on the acquisition of knowledge which is not directly relevant to psychiatric practice. Further, despite the efforts to introduce the concept of psychological causation as an integral part of the medical curriculum, the overall program must maintain as its focus the identification of organic causes to explain the signs and symptoms with which patients present. Usually there is little more than lip service paid to the recognition of psychological factors and their effects on patients, except perhaps to explain those cases where no organic etiology can readily be identified.

All too often the presumptive diagnosis of psychological factors is presented in a pejorative manner in a medical setting and related to patients who are unattractive or unpopular, the "crocks" of the medical clinic. (Regretably, it is precisely this type of patient who is often not properly worked up and in whom organic factors are overlooked.) It is not surprising that few medical students are able to integrate psychiatric principles into their medical thinking. Though the number of hours devoted to psychiatry in the curriculum may have increased, the perceived significance of psychiatric principles remains quite limited compared to other aspects of medical training.

Though some medical schools do provide a considerable amount of elective time, making it possible for an interested student to obtain additional exposure to psychiatry, such exposure is almost always at a purely clinical level and does not include any systematic training in psychology or the social sciences. Rather, it is the beginning of the apprenticeship by which the psychiatrist ultimately obtains his training and professional identity.

After the completion of medical school and some medical internship,* the true training of the psychiatrist begins. From the onset of his residency the student is asked to treat troubled individuals, usually on an inpatient service. By this time, the psychiatrist-to-be will at least have acquired some feeling of identity as a physician; he will be capable of conducting a reasonable physical examination and obtaining a medical history but will have had very little training or experience in the treatment of psychopathology. It is typically in the context of working on an inpatient service in psychiatry that he becomes familiar with psychopathology, begins to appreciate the effects psychotherapeutic interventions can have even on individuals who are severely disturbed, and comes to recognize the effects of a therapeutic milieu. The training of a psychiatrist is in a true sense an

*This requirement, which had been dropped in order to shorten the length of training, is for a variety of reasons being partially reinstated.

apprenticeship. While good residency programs offer some formal courses and attempt to encourage the resident to familiarize himself with the literature of his field, the most significant aspect of training remains the day-to-day care the resident gives to his patients, accompanied by both formal and informal supervision by preceptors, service chiefs, senior residents, his colleagues, and other staff within the therapeutic setting. The training obtained prior to the beginning of residency has only limited relevance to the training which occurs during residency. Whereas it would be hard to conceive of someone without medical training taking a residency in internal medicine or surgery, it is possible for someone without any medical background to participate in virtually all the activities of a psychiatric residency.*

The resident, when he completes his training, will have acquired an identity as a psychiatrist. He will have learned to conduct a psychiatric examination designed to assess the psychological functioning of a patient and to classify him according to the current diagnostic scheme. He will have become familiar with a variety of therapeutic approaches and developed an appreciation for the effects of psychotherapeutic intervention. He will have seen a large number of troubled individuals, some troubled children, and have been responsible for the care of many of these individuals with varying degrees of supervision by senior psychiatrists.

Though the psychiatrist will have acquired these skills, it is entirely possible that he will never have had a single course in psychology, sociology, or anthropology. His appreciation for what constitutes normal behavior will be based almost entirely on his personal life experience with people whom he considers normal and whom he has, of course, not studied the same way and under analogous circumstances to those under which he studies his patients. From this idiosyncratic data base he will extrapolate how the patients he sees ought to be if they were "normal." In most training programs the resident will have become familiar with one or another theory for the understanding of psychopathology. However, if he has been trained in a psychoanalytically oriented program, he will have had almost no exposure to behavioral approaches. Further, he may be totally unfamiliar with concepts of learning which are basic to behavioral approaches. Similarly, if he has been trained in a family therapy tradition, he may have little experience with individual therapy and less concern about making a precise diagnosis of the patient's difficulties. A residency oriented to biological psychiatry will provide experience in careful observational diagnosis and drug and other organic therapies but may virtually ignore dynamic factors both within the patient and in his interaction with his family.

Current psychiatric training, in other words, begins after the trainee has obtained his medical training and involves an apprenticeship. While there are, of course, some basic principles which are communicated in virtually

*One residency with which I am familiar trains a small number of psychologists along with psychiatric residents and, except for the administration of drugs, there is no material difference in how these individuals are trained or the duties to which they are assigned.

all residencies, the nature of the training is highly specific to the kind of patients who are treated and all too often lacks a comprehensive framework within which it is taught. There are approaches which are taught to the resident in a reasonably systematic fashion, such as psychoanalysis, group therapy, behavior therapy, psychopharmacology, and so on, but to the extent that the psychiatrist develops a broad systematic overview of his field, he is required to do so largely on his own. While medical training helps to provide the skills to assess biochemical and physiological theories, he lacks many of the intellectual tools which have been developed by psychology and the social sciences to deal with the kinds of issues that concern the psychiatrist.

An Alternative to the Medical Model

If it is true that the core of psychiatric training begins with the residency and medical training is not particularly relevant as preparation for such a residency, why should medical training be required? Would it not make more sense for psychiatrists to be thoroughly grounded in an understanding of psychological mechanisms as they occur in normal individuals, to develop the kind of intellectual tools which allow one to assess a psychological theory, much in the way medical school helps the physician to assess an organic theory of disease? Instead of learning about physical illness, his time would be well spent in developing an understanding of the laws governing learning, cognition, and motivation, theories which are rigorously stated and can thus be systematically evaluated. Similarly, if the psychiatrist is to understand the effects of interpersonal interactions, would he not benefit more from a systematic understanding of social psychological principles? Would he not need an understanding of sociological factors and their effect on health and illness, or the effects different cultures have on the development of personality structures?

For reasons such as these, the virtues of psychological training as the appropriate preparation for the conduct of psychological therapies have been vigorously put forth. While in the abstract such a view can hardly be faulted, the issues become somewhat more complex as one seeks to design an appropriate curriculum. Just as it was necessary to consider current training for the psychiatrist, it is necessary to consider the kinds of training available in psychology. Since World War II the discipline of clinical psychology has gradually evolved from its original interest in the understanding of psychopathology and its diagnosis to encompass and focus upon the modification of psychopathology either by way of the dynamic psychotherapies, client-centered therapy, behavior modification, or some of the more recent approaches focusing almost exclusively on feelings.

The claim for legitimacy. Just as the psychiatrist established his legitimacy by way of his medical training and leaned heavily on the prestige of his colleagues in other specialties, the clinical psychologist established his legitimacy on the basis of the intellectual achievements of his experimentally oriented colleagues. Until relatively recently the training programs for clinical psychologists demanded that the student develop a broad understanding of the discipline of psychology, that he pass qualifying examinations in a number of established areas, and that he become intimately familiar with the research techniques by which psychology has sought to put its theories to the test. The clinical psychologist, like any of his colleagues in other parts of the field, was required to carry out an original, meaningful, and methodologically sound piece of research as his dissertation in order to obtain his Ph.D. As a consequence, a major portion of psychological training involved becoming a psychologist, and a relatively small portion of time was devoted to the task of becoming a clinical psychologist.

It is probably fair to say that the most prestigious programs were those which made the greatest demands in terms of general psychological knowledge, and it was felt that the in-depth, applied aspect of clinical psychology could easily be acquired on a postgraduate basis. One important aspect of clinical psychology training involved an internship in which the training followed the apprenticeship model far more closely than is usual in graduate school. For a number of reasons, however, the psychological intern was rarely in a position fully analogous to that of the psychiatric resident. An important distinction is that the resident has already earned his doctorate and is a licensed practitioner, whereas the psychological intern is generally in his third year of graduate training, obviously lacks the title of doctor, and has no prior experience in dealing with patients. The beginning resident, while lacking in psychiatric skills, would have had some experience in taking care of sick individuals.

The usual time devoted to obtaining a doctorate in clinical psychology was four years; the internship year was fully taken up by the task of acquiring basic clinical skills, learning something about applied diagnostic procedures, and becoming familiar with some basic procedures of psychological therapies. The major portion of the final year would have to be devoted to the dissertation, and if the student hoped to make a truly meaningful contribution, a greater expenditure of time would be needed. Whatever systematic training was to be part of the program would have to fit primarily into the first two years, with, as we have already noted, a major portion devoted to the task of becoming a psychologist.

Once clinical psychology had successfully established itself as a profession, the conflict between psychologists oriented primarily to clinical practice and those interested in clinical problems but with more strongly academic orientations was soon joined. It was cogently argued that a broad knowledge of general psychology, an understanding of statistics, a knowledge of research methodology, or the experience of having carried out a meaningful dissertation had very little to do with the effectiveness of the student as a clinician. In the short run, at least, the most important experience for the student was an understanding of technique and supervised practice. Further, clinical students found it both tedious and difficult to study the large body of knowledge in such traditional areas as perception, psychophysics, physiological psychology, and especially statistics. The dissertation requirement was in many instances seen as a necessary evil. In many departments of psychology, clinical students were notorious for submitting dissertations which would not be acceptable in any other area.

The conflict between psychologists in areas other than clinical seeking to maintain standards of their field and the pressure to turn out clinical practitioners led to a variety of partial resolutions. To preserve the integrity of the Ph.D. while at the same time to do away with the requirements for dissertation, languages, and statistics, a degree of doctor of psychology was introduced in some institutions. More recently, schools of professional psychology have been developed to accommodate a more applied training program which would focus even less on the traditional areas of psychology. While it is not possible in this context to review in depth the changes within clinical psychology training programs, and indeed opinions remain strongly divided within the field of psychology in general and clinical psychology in particular about which approach is most desirable, the changes seem to illustrate a conflict between two basic points of view.

The first recognizes that clinical psychology's legitimacy owes a great deal to the acceptance of psychology as a science. It insists that the clinical psychologist-to-be must first and foremost learn how to think like a psychologist, because this provides the essential intellectual tools to allow him to gain perspective on his day-to-day activities. While this view acknowledges the importance of technical skills, it also recognizes that the field of clinical psychology has changed a great deal over the past 30 years and only those individuals with a broad background were able to adapt effectively with the changing field. Finally, it is recognized that clinical psychology's strength depends upon its continual renewal by progress in the larger science of psychology. Therefore, if clinical psychology became truly autonomous, it would lose not only its legitimacy but also its future.

The opposing position emphasizes that training in academic psychology has no discernible relevance to the effectiveness of a clinical psychologist either as a therapist or as a diagnostician. The proponents of this view argue that the need for services is sufficiently great and the time of training already so unduly extended that we cannot afford to load the curriculum of future clinicians with material of largely historic interest and thereby deprive them of time devoted to the truly relevant aspects of training. The fact that some of the requirements, such as statistics, have been a stumbling block to some individuals who eventually became effective clinicians is used as an argument that the requirement is counterproductive. The fact that the median number of publications by clinical psychologists is zero is used as an argument that it is wasteful to train future clinicians in those skills which are needed to contribute meaningfully to the literature of the field, and since most clinical dissertations do not lead to publication and often are seen as merely an onerous stumbling block to be overcome, they feel the requirement should be eliminated and the student's time would be better spent in honing his clinical skills, which would allow him to best serve his future clients.

It would appear that just as psychiatry derived much of its credibility from the fact that it was practiced by physicians, clinical psychology derived its credibility in large part by being practiced by individuals who had achieved a doctorate in the basic scientific discipline of psychology. Yet, in each instance the relevance of many aspects of the training is not immediately apparent to some practitioners, and pressures are exerted seeking to eliminate some of the "unnecessary" hurdles in the way of someone's wishing to practice psychiatry or clinical psychology. Later the significance of a therapist's right to call himself "doctor" and the consequences of easing the task of obtaining such a title will be discussed in more detail. Suffice it to say that in this matter, as in most others, there is no free lunch.

In considering whether psychological training is a viable substitute for medical training for the psychiatrist-to-be, one needs to ask whether we are discussing a more or less traditional program in clinical psychology, which provides a broad background, or the highly applied emphasis of the schools of professional psychology. It seems likely that the latter type of training would, like present day psychiatric training, not provide the broad understanding of psychological issues and theories which would help the student gain perspective on his field. Of greatest concern, however, is the fact that the very same issues that are raised against the appropriateness of medical training for the psychiatrist are now being raised by some clinical psychologists against training in general psychology as not being relevant to the practice of clinical psychology. Though I personally would strongly disagree with either view, it seems important to recognize how difficult it is to document the relevance of any basic training program for an individual who is concerned with providing psychiatric care, broadly defined.

A Hybrid Training for Psychiatrists

Many of the difficulties characterizing both medical training and the graduate program in psychology could be obviated if the suggestion put forth by Kubie (1950) some years ago could be adopted and a special degree of Doctor of Medical Psychology could be offered within a medical school setting. It is hard to quarrel with the view that the psychiatrist is required to learn more physical medicine than he will actually use, and that some of this time could be well spent in acquiring relevant training in psychology and the social sciences. In principle, the idea can hardly be faulted. The development of such a program would have to take place somewhat analogously to that of dentistry. At one time the rudiments of dentistry were taught in some medical schools, and only with the development of the field did dental schools and dental curricula evolve. Certainly today there would be little support for the view that dentists ought to complete medical training to be fully qualified. While there is some overlap in the basic sciences between medical and dental training, there is a high degree of consensus about the large body of specific relevant training and skills that the future dentist must acquire.

It is on this very issue of consensus that the hybrid curriculum breaks down. Thus, if one asked a number of outstanding psychiatrists to plan a curriculum leading to a degree in psychiatric medicine, it is highly unlikely that one could obtain consensus from among psychiatrists of different theoretical orientations. The biological psychiatrist would probably demand medical training, supplemented by additional emphasis on biochemistry, pharmacology, and genetics. The psychodynamically oriented psychiatrist would lean toward a program along the lines of that proposed by Kubie, which emphasizes psychoanalytic training, psychology, and the social sciences as well as some core medical training. The social psychiatrist would focus more on epidemiology and the social sciences, whereas the behavior therapist would insist on a solid background in learning theory and classical conditioning. There simply is not the consensus necessary to design a program which would provide the basis for a new discipline that is not a specialty of a larger discipline such as medicine or psychology but a true discipline in its own right.

This problem is by no means unique to psychiatry but can best be understood in a broader perspective in the history of science. New disciplines arise whenever there is a sufficiently large body of knowledge upon which there is basic consensus within the field to justify the new area of science. For example, biochemistry and nuclear physics are two fields that emerged in recent times and are clearly delineated as disciplines. In contrast, there were several efforts to create the discipline of social relations. Harvard, for example, combined sociology, social anthropology, social psychology, and clinical psychology as a new field and began to offer degrees in social relations. Though the department had outstanding faculty and attracted excellent students, the field did not come together as a coherent whole, and after some 10 years the department was disbanded and its components reconstituted along more traditional disciplinary lines. While similar attempts in other universities persisted for longer periods of time, no real field evolved because there was a lack of consensus about what constituted this new discipline, and members of such departments tended to identify themselves more closely with colleagues in the academic disciplines whence they came than colleagues within their own interdisciplinary department. It appears that present-day psychiatry lacks the kind of consensus necessary for the evolution of a new discipline truly independent of medicine. Unless this condition existed, however, any effort to put together such a training program would be doomed to failure. Unless the program caught on, graduates of the program would find themselves without acceptance either by medicine, by psychology, or by the social sciences, and they would then lack the kind of backing essential for effective professional practice.

How justified is medical training for the psychiatrist?

The preceding discussion has tried to demonstrate that none of the proposed training programs begin to provide a good grounding in all of those areas which may reasonably be considered basic to psychiatric practice. While most psychiatrists are likely to agree with the need to add certain specific educational experiences to the training of the psychiatrist, the precise nature of this additional knowledge will vary with the theoretical predilection of the psychiatrist being asked. Despite the fact that the training of psychiatrists requires at least seven years (four years of medical school and three years of residency), it would hardly be possible to design a program to train psychiatrists in all of the areas which may ultimately be deemed relevant. Nonetheless, the fact that even a seven-year training period fails to provide a graduate with the knowledge which would seem desirable makes it all the more reasonable to ask why the training should take so long when the clinical psychologist's basic training is completed in four years. What benefits does medical training provide the practitioner to justify an additional three years of training as well as the extremely arduous demands that have typically been required of those admitted to medical school and have characterized medical training in years gone by.

There are a number of self-evident arguments which have been put forth to justify the requirement that psychiatrists complete medical school before being admitted to residency training in their chosen field. These include an emphasis on the role organic factors may play in bringing about specific psychological experiences, how what appears to be an anxiety may actually be due to hyperthyroidism, how a temporal epilepsy may mimic episodic thought disorders, and so on. Again, it is obvious that medical training is useful for the appropriate use of psychotropic agents whose role in psychiatric treatment is likely to increase as more powerful drugs with even more specific effects on psychological symptoms are developed.

It is not intended to minimize the advantages of medical training regarding these issues. However, it is by no means clear that these benefits are sufficiently great to justify the expenditure of effort needed to acquire a medical degree for those individuals who do not go into biological psychiatry. One might well argue that the amount of knowledge required in modern medicine is sufficiently great that collaborative treatment efforts are becoming the rule rather than the exception. Consequently it might be far more efficient for practitioners of psychotherapy, for example, to work collaboratively with medical colleagues without themselves having had to acquire such training. One biological psychiatrist might deal with the medical diagnostic problems and the administration of organic therapies in collaboration with a number of nonmedically trained psychiatric practitioners, leading to a more effective utilization of manpower.

While there is no doubt that medical training facilitates an appreciation of organic issues and provides some definite, specific information occasionally useful even for the practitioner of outpatient psychotherapy, the actual use that is made of medical knowledge in outpatient psychotherapy is limited. Except for those colleagues who specialize in drug therapy, many psychiatrists have a very limited knowledge of psychopharmacology at a level that might easily be acquired by nonmedically trained individuals. Finally, even in those instances where medical training would seem important for the psychotherapist—the occasional patient with hyperthyroidism,

Addison's disease, brain tumor, and the like—there is no assurance that such a condition will be recognized by the medically trained psychotherapist who may have a low index of suspicion, particularly if the patient has been referred by an internist. An argument could even be made that an individual without medical training who has been taught to look out for certain conditions, lacking the false sense of security provided by largely forgotten medical training, might be more likely to investigate the possibility of relevant physical factors affecting his patient.

It seems to me that the real benefits of medical training for all psychiatrists involve a number of issues that are rarely explicitly discussed. These additional aspects of medical training which, in the final analysis, seem to justify the expenditure of time and effort can be summarized as follows: (1) The medically trained psychiatrist has the option of combining psychological and organic treatments without being restricted by a limited licensure. (2) Medical training makes the psychiatrist a member of a larger discipline, facilitating communication with medical colleagues in other specialties and allowing for integration into an overall health care system. In addition to specific knowledge, professional training serves the function of (3) legitimizing the professional knowledge and skills vis-à-vis his patients and society at large, and (4) providing him with the attitudes and beliefs of his profession which serve as guides to behavior that is acceptable to his profession and society at large. It is these four upon which we will seek to expand.

Medical training as a means of providing the psychiatrist with a choice of treatment. While at one time the split between psychodynamic and biologically oriented psychiatry was very sharp, I know of no contemporary psychiatrist, regardless of his orientation, who has either never employed psychotropic drugs as an adjunct to treatment or who has sedulously avoided using all forms of psychotherapy. Thus, today the merits of combining therapies, at least in some cases, are almost universally accepted in the field. As has been pointed out earlier, it is, of course, possible for a nonmedical psychotherapist to collaborate with a medical colleague in order to provide the benefits of both psychological and organic treatments. However, it would be difficult to avoid being influenced by the fact that one is trained to provide psychological therapy but must work collaboratively to provide drug treatment. One of the reasons I personally chose to obtain medical training was because it seemed important to me to avoid placing myself in a situation where I might be biased against a given therapeutic approach because of being legally prohibited from utilizing it.

It is, of course, true that bias is unavoidable, since each of us will interpret available data slightly differently. Nonetheless, it seems likely that decreasing the reality obstacles to employing a variety of treatment modalities will decrease the likelihood of systematic bias. Consider as an example the change that has taken place over the past 20 years among medically trained psychotherapists. In the late 1940s psychoanalysts were almost unanimously opposed to the use of medication as an adjunct to treatment, a view they shared with clinical psychologists. With the increasing effectiveness of drug therapy, it is the consensus among psychoanalysts, as we have noted earlier, that medication is an appropriate adjunct in suitable cases, while there is considerably less agreement in this regard among our colleagues in clinical psychology. It seems difficult to avoid the conclusion that the legal right to employ psychotropic agents when indicated makes it easier for the medically trained psychotherapist to change his attitude toward their use.

Now, more than ever, psychiatric therapy is in a state of flux, and new therapeutic approaches are constantly being evolved. It seems likely that a dispassionate appraisal of the merits and demerits of a given approach will be more likely achieved by professionals who have the widest possible degree of freedom in employing any procedure that may prove to be safe and effective.

The merits of medical training to facilitate communication with other specialties. The differences between the day-to-day activities of different medical specialists are often greater than the similarities. The more specialized the branch of medicine, the more difficult it is for the physician to keep up with progress in other fields. This is as true for the roentgenologist, the dermatologist, and the allergist as it is for the psychiatrist. While colleagues in these and in many other fields would encounter much difficulty in again passing their national board exams, they nonetheless share an exposure to a core curriculum of medical training. Though much of the detail will have been forgotten, and few colleagues in the above specialties would contemplate carrying out even the simplest surgical procedure, communication is greatly facilitated by their shared training. With relatively few questions, it is possible to follow a case history outlined by a colleague in another specialty. Thus, even a cursory analysis will show that a good deal of medical training is not relevant to the practice of most specialties. No one has yet suggested that the concept of medical school be abandoned simply because a shared training is essential in order to meaningfully communicate with physicians in different fields.

For these reasons, even if one were to argue that medical knowledge were totally irrelevant for the psychiatrist (a view with which I would certainly not agree), it would still be of great importance in facilitating communication with medical colleagues. The integration of the psychiatrist into the modern medical center would simply not have occurred without this shared background. Thus, while some clinical psychologists may work in medical settings, they tend to relate through a department of psychiatry which forms a bridge. Similarly, some psychologists may work in a department of neurology, providing special expertise in the diagnosis of organic disorders, but here again their input is through the neurologist who finds the psychologist's contribution worthwhile and makes it a part of his own workup. While a similar relationship exists with other nonmedical professionals who are part of a modern medical center, such as clinical biochemists, bacteriologists, biomedical engineers, and so on, each of these relates either to a specific medical specialty or to a small subset of medical specialists and simply does not have the same kind of broad interaction which characterizes most medical specialists' roles vis-à-vis their colleagues.

Thus, medical training serves the psychiatrist in making possible his acceptance by his colleagues and his integration into medical practice as a whole. It provides a ready access to needed information from any of the specialties. To the extent that psychiatric therapy is to be an integral part of other forms of medical treatment, such integration is essential; to the extent that it is seen as a totally different kind of service which must be identified and sought out by the patient independently, it becomes less important.

The need for the therapist's ability to be legitimized. A number of authors, most notably Frank (1961), have emphasized that in all societies healers must go through a process of legitimizing their abilities. Usually this involves arduous training for some form of priesthood, and in addition it may be necessary to demonstrate one's gift by evidence of supernatural favor. Though from the physician's point of view he practices rational and scientifically based medicine, it is worth keeping in mind that the patient rarely is able to judge the scientific merits of the procedure. For example, the reasons underlying some of the simple aspects of a physical examination such as percussion are not understood by most patients but are accepted by them on the same basis as the Navajo Indian accepts the treatment by his native singer—faith.

The average patient believes in "science" in much the same way as the native patient believes in witchcraft. In other words, these are special professional skills, explicable to those individuals who have by dint of hard work and training achieved competence to evaluate what goes on. Nor is the modern man's faith in science nearly as secure as we might like to believe. The difficulty in eliminating the cancer quacks, not to mention the psychoquacks, is ample evidence of modern society's ambivalence.* Nor ought we to fault the layman for being taken in by the chiropractor who uses some machine with flashing lights to detect "cancer," since it is by no means easy for the layman to differentiate between the scientific and the pseudoscientific procedure, and the chiropractor who has the right to call himself "doctor" is careful not to emphasize the distinction between himself, an osteopathic physician, and a medical doctor.

As has been emphasized earlier, the physician's role in modern society is a uniquely powerful one, and despite a lack of full understanding and some ambivalence, the public tends to trust the physician's judgments on medical matters. The psychiatrist has in the past used the medical degree successfully to augment his prestige and lend credibility to his observations concerning troubled individuals, taking advantage of the physician's acceptance as the culturally defined authority on matters of health.

In a number of areas, the shortage of physicians and the inevitably relatively high cost of services by highly trained individuals has led to the

---

*Note, for example, that six states have legalized Laetrile despite repeated, carefully documented negative results.

development of health professionals other than physicians who compete with some medical specialists as providers of some specialized services.

It seems clear, however, that the medically trained physician is acknowledged by contemporary American society as the most desirable health care provider—all other things being equal. The medical degree inspires the greatest confidence and has the highest degree of social acceptance. This is not surprising insofar as the medical degree is known to be the most difficult to obtain. Medical schools are widely recognized as being the most highly selective professional schools, making them the most difficult to gain entrance to. Medical training is generally recognized as being the most arduous, making the greatest demands, both intellectually and in terms of actual work expended. Finally, medical training, combined with specialty training, takes the longest time to acquire of any professional training in our society.

Those professions which are known to be the most difficult to enter, make the highest demands upon the trainee, and require the longest period of training tend to be the most highly valued. Similarly, those priesthoods which are most selective, require the most of the neophyte, and whose training period takes the longest and involves the greatest amount of sacrifice are typically able to command the greatest respect.

Thus, even if medical training were totally irrelevant to the task of the psychiatrist, it would still be of considerable advantage to the practitioner to have established his legitimacy by his medical credentials. While we as psychiatrists are understandably concerned with emphasizing the specific skills of our profession, the public's attitude toward the physician is a major asset. A wise old uncle can and often does play an important supportive role within the family. His status within the family—inevitably affected by his status in society as a whole—will often be important in making it possible to be of help to those who consult him. Though such an individual may have acquired through his experience and learning a degree of understanding and empathy for the problems of others—he may even have learned to listen and seek to understand rather than seek to give gratuitous advice—nonetheless he will tend to be significantly less effective than a psychiatrist with no greater interpersonal skills, simply because the latter's role has been legitimized by society. The wise uncle may categorize behavior as foolish and may empathize with someone whom he considers troubled or perhaps even a peculiar person; his statements do not, however, define someone as sick or healthy.

The question remains whether medical training can be replaced by an easier, less time-consuming, and more relevant alternative. Thus far we have discussed the not inconsiderable sociological benefits of medical training for the psychiatrist. Does that mean, since medical training merely serves to legitimize the psychiatrist's work, that another form of training, less time-consuming and more efficiency acquired, involving more specific skills germane to the psychiatrist's duties, would serve equally well?

In considering such an argument, it should be clear from the outset that there is a contradiction in the view that equal status can somehow artificially be conferred by virtue of a training procedure which is inherently less demanding, intended for a profession which is inherently less selective. As has been emphasized earlier, members of a community tend to be keenly aware of the amount of investment which a particular type of training involves. One has but to look at the evolution of professions in the United States over the last 30 years to see how quickly it is decided to make the selection criteria more rigorous, the training more difficult and arduous, and to increase the length of time required. This has been true of every emerging profession, whether it be nursing, social work, occupational therapy, speech therapy, or for that matter, osteopathy. In each instance, as the training demands increase—without necessarily a commensurate increase in relevant performance of the graduates—the status of the profession increases. This increase is typically expressed not only in intangible status but also directly in terms of income. The real beneficiaries of this process are, of course, not the new professionals who are compelled to undergo the increasingly longer periods of training (of questionable relevance to the professional's ultimate activities), but rather the existing professionals who are prescribing the increased period of training, since they obtain the benefits of the new-found status without having had to pay the price.

The Medical Approach as Providing a Stable Value Orientation in a Changing Culture

Though the knowledge involved in having delivered a certain number of babies has little specific relevance to psychiatry, having participated in this activity has much relevance to being a physician. Again, while the sad, frightening, and harrowing experience of having a patient die while ministering to his needs hardly involves the acquisition of knowledge, it is precisely the kind of experiential learning which ultimately helps an individual to better understand the role of the physician.

In the context of being overloaded with facts, having to face the inevitability of not knowing enough, and the need to nonetheless make decisions, facing the anxiety associated with failing to prevent the eventuality of death, and participating in the act of birth, seeing our fellow man reduced to his biological core in the face of pain and suffering and finally restored to a civilized, self-possessed human being with dignity as he recovers, we inevitably face experiences which are shared by other physicians but rarely by other members of society. To make it easier to deal with such issues, medicine has over the centuries evolved a set of values which have continued to stand it in good stead despite tremendous changes in the structure of society at large. Swearing the Hippocratic oath may strike us as quaint and anachronistic, yet it serves to remind us how remarkably similar are some of the issues faced by the physicians of ancient Greece and those today and how we continue to use an essentially stable code of ethics as a guide for action.

It is worth noting that the physician's values were different from those of other members of society. He typically had the role of the noncombatant on the battlefield, and was often allowed to treat, and heal if he could, enemies whom others would have been required to slay. He was permitted to breach taboos which were placed upon other members of society, and his relationship with his patient was typically defined as going beyond a simple contract.

That the ethos of medicine and the values it embodied transcended physical illness was already clear in the writings of Hippocrates. Though the distinction between physical and mental disorders was not clearly articulated until relatively recently, the ancients had a considerable degree of understanding for what we would call today psychological factors in illness. Perhaps the most important single aspect of the medical ethos for the development of modern psychiatry has been the physician's role as a secular healer who was not expected to pass moral judgments on his patients' behavior, but rather to address himself exclusively to the restoration and maintenance of his patients' health. In this regard, an alternative basis for judging behavior was created, not in terms of right or wrong but rather in terms of health and sickness. Although the physician is inevitably a product of his time and culture, his role allows—demands even—that he have tolerance and understanding for behaviors and customs that are different from his own. Physicians often traveled a good deal and rose to positions of influence from relatively humble origins. In many ways, the physician saw himself not only as a member of a particular class or nation but as one of those whom society designated as healers, willing and eager to add to his skill from the knowledge of others. In this regard at least, his perspectives transcended the xenophobia of his particular culture.

In many regards the manner in which medicine solved some of the highly complex moral and ethical problems with which each practitioner dealt in his day-to-day activities provided an extremely useful framework within which to deal with deviancy. The fact that the physician's role makes him somewhat of an outsider and requires him, to some degree at least, to be a cultural relativist provided a remarkably stable guide to behavior. The medical ethos, evolving as it did over a long period of time under a wide variety of different political systems and in the face of changing social mores, has adapted to both dramatic changes in the effectiveness with which medical treatment could heal and drastic changes in the life styles where it is practiced.

The physician was able to maintain his role by remaining essentially apolitical, separating his medical activities from what would otherwise be his obligations as a citizen. Further, it was often necessary to divorce, as far as possible, religious obligations from the requirements of medical practice. With rare exceptions it was possible for the physician to behave in accordance with medical ethics, being excused from conflicting obligations either to the state or to God which would be expected from other members of the society. For example, a prisoner might be treated harshly, but if he became sufficiently sick for the authorities to call in a physician to treat him, it was generally expected that the physician would do what he could to help the patient who, while under his care, could and did receive better food and gentle treatment. Once the prisoner was no longer sick, however, the physician was not expected to have any say about his subsequent treatment. It was possible for the physician to minister to the sick, disregarding the patient's status and the extent to which he might or might not be in favor with the prevailing political authorities—provided he limited his activities to healing. While he might have sympathy or compassion for his patients' lot in life, he was expected not to abuse the freedom which society accorded him.

It was a relatively easy matter to separate one's political convictions and religious beliefs from the practice of medicine as long as one was treating physically sick individuals. Physicians also concerned themselves with epidemiological issues and, once the effectiveness of the public health procedures became clear, they tended to become accepted regardless of the particular political system which prevailed. Since disease tended to spread to all segments of society, it is easy to understand why medical measures tended to gain acceptance.

Through the centuries physicians have practiced supportive therapy. It seems likely that the bedside manner of the nineteenth-century physician was in some ways better than that of his modern counterpart simply because he had less to offer by way of specific therapy and could ill afford to deprive his patients of the therapeutic effects associated with faith and expectation of cure. The development of modern psychiatry took place under the general umbrella of medical practice. It is difficult to imagine how any other umbrella would have permitted anyone to publish descriptions of sexual perversions in nineteenth-century Germany, or the details of sexual fantasies in nineteenth-century Austria, the epitome of the Victorian society ruled by "his most Catholic majesty, the Holy Roman Emperor." It was possible within the context of the medical umbrella for Freud to ignore the taboos of his day, to avoid concern with right and wrong and substitute instead the concepts of health and illness. The medical role allowed the psychoanalysts to take insights from other scientific disciplines as well as the humanities without losing the advantages and status that academic medicine conferred upon them. The entire practice of psychoanalysis and psychodynamic psychiatry took place wholly within the context of established medical traditions. These traditions were adopted even by the nonmedical analysts and certainly guided the work of the psychodynamic psychiatrists in the United States.

On the surface the medical ethos appears to avoid the pejorative value judgments which pervaded Victorian society and seemed to allow the physician to transcend those restraints. Certainly to some degree this was true; more careful analysis, however, shows that the definition of health and sickness inevitably reflected the value system of the psychiatrist which, while often different from that of society at large, involved no less a value judgment—though at times a less obvious one. Thus, the psychiatrist would carefully avoid calling a patient bad or evil; instead he might diagnose "moral insanity," or the patient's behavior might be termed "acting out," or he might be described as having a "character disorder." It is easy in retrospect to show how complex value judgments invariably crept into psychiatric therapies, or to use a current cliché, that psychoanalysis was basically sexist, or that psychodynamic psychiatry continued to be a product of and was consumed by middle-class society. Nonetheless, it is all too easy to overlook the fact that the medical umbrella provided the opportunity to develop viewpoints at sharp variance with those that were currently acceptable for the society of the day, and despite some contradictions, it provided a framework within which clinicians were able to work effectively, interacting successfully not only with their patients but also with their medical colleagues outside of psychiatry and with society at large.

The Psychiatrist as a Social Reformer

As has been pointed out earlier, the epidemiological approach applied to dynamic psychiatry must suggest that social problems are at the root of most psychological difficulties. Further there is a tendency for colleagues with liberal persuasions to be attracted to the social sciences in general and, as physicians, to psychiatry in particular. In working with individual patients, the therapist's biases may reflect themselves in the patient's response; nonetheless, what the patient says and does will tend to place some reality constraints on the therapist's beliefs about causative factors of his patient's difficulties. Unfortunately, the further we become removed from the treatment of actual patients, the easier it becomes to project our convictions onto the social system, particularly if we have no easy way of testing their validity. The distinction between the psychiatrist as a concerned citizen and the psychiatrist speaking as a trained specialist—analyzing the cause of various individual problems—is all too easy to overlook. The willingness, for example, of a significant segment of American psychiatry to diagnose Goldwater as disturbed prior to the 1964 election without access to the kind of material which would normally be considered essential for such a diagnosis is an unfortunate case in point. Similarly, we have been urged by colleagues to take positions as *psychiatrists* on a broad range of social issues which have great political significance but are far removed from both clinical practice and the area of our expertise. These tendencies have at times had particularly catastrophic effects on the functioning of some community mental health centers.

It would be well to remember that the unique role of the physician was made possible only by the physician's careful delineation of his professional responsibility. As long as he stayed within his area of special knowledge he could do much to make life more worthwhile. Psychiatry, of necessity, must deal with some issues which have political implications. If this is true, we must exercise more rather than less care that what we say is thoroughly documented and entirely within our special expertise. We can and should speak out as citizens for what we believe, but we must be careful not to confuse our role as psychiatrist with that of citizen. This confusion is likely to have much to do with the decrease in credibility that we have experienced in the profession. The medical ethos demands that we act responsibly, and if we fail to do so we will forfeit in time the benefits society accords the physician's role.

At some level colleagues who feel they do not wish to forfeit the opportunity to push their personal views by using their professional status recognize this paradox. It is likely that the wish to separate from medicine is related to the wish for greater rather than less license to comment as social philosophers on social and political issues. As one examines the changes within American psychiatry over the past 20 years, it is difficult not to become convinced that we have all lost a great deal as some of us have moved farther away from medicine; further, that the confusion of political conviction and professional judgment has become increasingly costly for the future of psychiatry.

At the present time I know of no alternative to the medical ethos which provides as meaningful a guide to action in a complex and changing society. It is by no means a perfect solution, but it has stood the test of time. The combination of the humanism inherent in the concept of the art of medicine and the devotion to the search for solid knowledge inherent in the concept of the science of medicine continues to be the compromise most widely accepted by the public. While some particular social or political view might have greater appeal to relatively small segments of our discipline, none of these seems to provide a sufficiently broad umbrella to encompass the field as a whole.

Conclusions

Having reviewed where we have been, the problems facing psychiatry today, and the role of medical training in the development of psychiatry, I have become increasingly convinced that we do not have a viable alternative to medical training. I fully recognize that much of medical training has little relevance to the psychiatrist's day-to-day functions. However, the same can be said for all proposed alternatives. At this time no evidence exists which would allow us to choose among the various kinds of training that have been proposed as alternatives.

The hope to develop quick and easy training for specific skills that are particularly relevant to psychiatry and that will result in a broadly trained clinician who can successfully attain high status within our society is by its nature doomed to failure. The arduousness of the training itself has much to do with the status it confers. The breadth and lack of specificity has much to do with preparing the psychiatrist for a future practice which is bound to be vastly different from what he does today, and finally and probably most important, medical training provides an effective, well-developed guide for the physician's actions which has stood the test of time and remains appropriate for clinical practice to the present day.

An analysis of the challenges facing psychiatry suggests that the solution is not to move farther away from medicine, though we can and should learn from other disciplines whenever appropriate. Rather than moving away from medicine, we need to work to rejoin it. This means accepting the strictures that have always applied to the physician—that he not confuse his personal sympathies with his professional duties. Similarly, at a time when anti-intellectualism is increasingly widespread throughout the world, we need to be doubly cautious not to confuse appealing ideas and good intentions with proven competence. Fortunately, medicine as a whole will continue to strive to increase the scientific basis of its activities. By moving closer to medicine, we can make certain that we in psychiatry do likewise. This does not mean that we should neglect the significance of feelings, ignore unconscious motivation, or diminish our continuing efforts to be sensitive to the needs of our patients. It does mean, however, striving to put our beliefs to empirical test and becoming increasingly disciplined in the evaluation of what we do.

The changes that have taken place within American psychiatry and within the life style of the culture at large have contributed to the identity crisis we face as a profession. In our efforts to solve this crisis, we will need to partake of much relevant knowledge that has been generated in psychology, sociology, anthropology, and related areas—fields which are not generally considered medical disciplines. However, this in no way should lessen the importance of medical training which is shared with other physicians who also owe increasingly large debts to basic scientists in other fields. The unique contribution of psychiatry is likely to be not the creation of a science but rather bringing to bear a variety of disciplines on the clinical problems of psychiatry. As we recognize the area where we can contribute uniquely and begin to accept the limitations of our discipline, it is likely that we will become increasingly effective in its practice. Here too we can benefit from the model of other fields of medicine. One might hope that the psychiatrist of tomorrow will not seek to solve all problems of society but will instead successfully and efficiently be able to treat what we today call the major psychoses and the psychoneuroses. Whether these maladaptive syndromes are ultimately defined as medical illness, a form of social deviancy, or problems in living should not affect the psychiatrist's ability to seek out effective procedures derived from any or all basic sciences. While medical training is by no means sufficient to this task, it does form the basis for communication with other members of the healing arts and still remains the most effective preliminary training program to provide the kind of basic knowledge, social legitimacy, and eclectic tradition that allows the broadest range of therapeutic modalities to be integrated into the psychiatrist's therapeutic armamentarium.

References

Alluisi, E. A., Thurmond, J. B., and Coates, G. D.: Behavioral effects of infectious diseases: Respiratory Pasteurella tularensis in man. Percept. Mot. Skills [Suppl. 2], *32*:647–668, 1971.

Birk, L., Stolz, S. B., Brady, J. P., et al.: Behavior Therapy in Psychiatry. Task Force Report No. 5, American Psychiatric Association. Washington, D.C.: American Psychiatric Association, 1973.

Eysenck, H. J.: The effects of psychotherapy: An evaluation. J. Consult. Clin. Psychol., *16*:319–323, 1952.

Frank, J. D.: Persuasion and Healing: A Comparative Study of Psychotherapy. Baltimore, The Johns Hopkins University Press, 1961.

Hartmann, H.: Essays on Ego Psychology. New York, International Universities Press, 1964.

Hersen, M., Eisler, R. M., and Miller, P. M.: Historical perspectives in behavior modification. *In* Hersen, M., Eisler, R. M., and Miller, P. M. (eds.): Progress in Behavior Modification, Vol. 1. New York, Academic Press, Inc., 1975, pp. 1–17.

Kretschmer, E.: Geniale Menschen, 7th ed. Berlin, Springer Verlag, 1948.

Kris, E.: Psychoanalytic Explorations in the Arts. New York, International Universities Press, 1952.

Kubie, L. S.: Practical and Theoretical Aspects of Psychoanalysis. New York, International Universities Press, 1950.

Laing, R. D.: The Politics of Experience. New York, Ballantine Books, Inc., 1957.

Rioch, M. J., Elkes, C., Flint, A. A., et al.: National Institute of Mental Health pilot study in training mental health counselors. Am. J. Orthopsychiatry, *33*:678–689, 1963.

Rogers, C. R.: Counseling and Psychotherapy. Boston, Houghton Mifflin Company, 1942.

Rogers, C. R.: Client-Centered Therapy. Boston, Houghton Mifflin Company, 1951.

Rosenhan, D. L.: On being sane in insane places. Science, *179*:250–258, 1973.

Srole, L., Langner, T. S., Michael, S. T., et al.: Mental Health in the Metropolis. New York, McGraw-Hill Book Company, 1962.

Szasz, T. S.: The Myth of Mental Illness. New York, Hoeber, 1961.

Truax, C. B., and Mitchell, K. M.: Research on certain therapist interpersonal skills in relation to process and outcome. *In* Bergin, A. E., and Garfield, S. L. (eds.): Handbook of Psychotherapy and Behavior Change: An Empirical Analysis. New York, John Wiley & Sons, Inc., 1971.

Yates, A. J.: Theory and Practice in Behavior Therapy. New York, John Wiley & Sons, Inc., 1975.

Comment

Before offering an answer to the question, "Should psychiatrists be medically trained?" **Dr. Orne** places this question in sociohistorical perspective by tracing the development of psychiatry as a medical discipline. It was only after World War II that American psychiatry, with its new dynamic orientation, was accepted by establishment medicine. Psychiatry came to be seen as operating within the "medical model" and as having its own rational, scientific basis. It was seen as having an important and legitimate role in general medicine, i.e., in consultation psychiatry and in the management of psychosomatic disorders, in addition to its traditional concern with "mental illnesses." Psychiatry was surely a medical specialty. Then came a series of challenges to the centrality and even the relevance of medicine to the mental health field. These included the nondirective psychotherapies of Carl Rogers and others, behavior modification therapy with its emphasis on the learned basis of psychiatric disorders, and the social and community mental health movements. The most recent challenges come couched in antiestablishment terms and often include a distrust of rationality—mental illness is a myth, an appropriate adjustment to a sick society, or a concept invented to justify repressive political or social acts. Although these challenges have different origins, varying degrees of legitimacy, and disparate adherents in the culture, they have produced an identity crisis within psychiatry and some confusion in the public mind as to the nature and role of this branch of medicine.

All this has led to a questioning of the relevance of medical training to psychiatric practice. Are mental and emotional disorders medical illnesses or problems of living? In any case, how much knowledge of general medicine and medical skills does the psychiatrist retain after a few years of practice limited largely to psychotherapy?

Orne briefly mentions some of the traditional arguments for the medical training of psychiatrists: the value of being knowledgeable about the role that biological factors play in emotional experience, being able to combine psychological and organic treatments, ease of communication with medical colleagues in other specialties, etc. Orne also argues the case for the medical training of psychiatrists from some unexpected points of view. He points out that the efficacy of healers in all cultures depends in part on their having a culturally legitimized and sanctioned role, which usually includes priestlike features. Western culture confers this role on the physician. The public trusts the physician's opinion in medical matters, since he is the culturally defined authority. If psychological disorders are viewed as medical concerns, then the medically trained psychiatrist is generally regarded as the most appropriate and potent healer available. Thus, aside from the obvious advantages of medical training in practicing a profession which may require differential diagnoses of medical disorders and the prescribing of medicines, Orne argues that the very demanding nature of the education and training of the physician and his role in the culture adds to his efficacy as a healer.

Orne stresses another reason for the medically trained psychiatrist. This is his function in maintaining a stable value orientation in a changing culture. Here Orne analogized with the value of a liberal arts college education even though the specific content of courses is soon lost in areas outside one's continuing fields of interest. What is important is the appreciation and understanding we gain of how scholars approach and view their subject matter. We retain also the ability to acquire specific content rapidly, since we know how to go about it. It is the attitudes toward knowledge and learning that are important. Similarly, medical education and medical experience instill in the physician-psychiatrist an appreciation for the complexity of the human machinery and the human life in its psychological, social, and cultural dimensions. This is acquired largely as a function of the physician's role—direct experience with the human condition in sickness, deprivation, loss, and death. An ethos evolves from the training and experience that medicine provides which constitutes the best guide to action in a complex and changing society. Orne believes that the humanism inherent in the concept of the art of medicine and the commitment to the rational search for new knowledge inherent in the concept of the science of medicine provide the best guide available for the future of psychiatry.

Most professionals would agree on the necessity for the psychiatrist in the mental health care system, i.e., a physician with additional training in the diagnosis and treatment of mental and behavioral disorders. They differ sharply, however, on the desirability of medical training in the education of psychotherapists generally. While Orne would place the physician-psychiatrist at the head of the mental health care team, his broad and extensive training making him or her the appropriate leader of the mental health effort, other health care professionals argue that it is precisely the physician-psychiatrist's superordinate position which makes him ill-suited to this role. The elitist psychiatrist makes effective team work impossible and in addition unwittingly discourages the patient-client from accepting appropriate responsibility for his own mental health care. Further, persons taking this point of view point out that the competent practice of psychotherapy does not require medical training and it is wasteful of our medical education resources to do so.

There are two additional views of the appropriate role of the psychiatrist. One view is that the psychiatrist should have no role, i.e., the psychiatrist should be allowed to become an extinct species. The essence of this view, forcefully argued by Dr. E. Fuller Torrey in this book, is that those persons with behavioral abnormalities who suffer from actual medical (physiological) disorders should be treated by neurologists and those whose problems have no significant biological basis should be treated by psychologists, social workers, and other nonmedical persons, since the treatment task is in fact one of re-education.

The remaining view makes some of the assumptions inherent in Torrey's position. Many of the persons treated by psychiatrists have problems of living and problems related to their life styles for which the proper "treatment" is re-education not requiring medical knowledge and experience. However, the decision that a patient is in this category is not always easy to make. Indeed, there are a large number of patients who have symptoms suggestive of organic disease but who in fact suffer from purely nonorganic (functional) disorders or persons who in fact have a disorder that has a basis in part in disturbed physiology but in whom the predominant symptoms are in the behavioral or psychological realm. The training of psychologists and other nonmedical professionals is not adequate for this task. Similarly, neurologists and internists, at least as currently trained, also are not competent to make informed diagnostic and treatment decisions in many of those cases. It is only the psychiatrist with his unique training in biology, general medicine, and some aspects of applied social science who has the potential to carry out with competence the highly complex problems of differential diagnosis and the formulation of an effective treatment plan. In this model, however, the psychiatrist would not presume to do everything as well as or better than everyone else in the mental health profession. Rather, his training would focus on the demanding task of differential diagnosis and selection of a treatment program, working in a consultant and liaison capacity with other physicians in cases where the major problem is a medical illness and in the area of perhaps the greatest need and promise—systematic research into the biological, behavioral, and social origins of emotional and mental disorders and the development of more effective methods of treatment. However, most day-to-day therapy would be carried out by other well-trained professionals, such as the social worker with special competencies in supportive psychotherapy and in facilitating the patient's transition from hospital to community. Others could include the master's level psychologist with special competencies in behavioral procedures, new professionals with special training in family therapy and group techniques, etc. The number of psychiatrists in this model need not be great, but they would have to be differently trained than is general practice today. Acquiring and maintaining medical diagnostic skills, especially in neurology and internal medicine, would be essential. Essential also would be a working knowledge of *all* treatment methods that have demonstrated efficacy in some clinical situations: pharmacotherapy, supportive psychotherapy, behavior modification procedures, family therapy techniques, etc. Of course he would not devote substantial time to employing most of these but would know well their indications, contraindications, and compatibilities. Finally, his training would include sufficient knowledge and experience in research to permit him, at times collaborating with other scientists, to advance knowledge in the field. Such a psychiatrist would head the mental health team, not, however, by virtue of his greater prestige or his priestly mantle or because he is competent to do everything everyone else can do in the team. Rather, it would be because his special skills and competencies, not present elsewhere in the system, are essential to make the critical diagnostic and treatment decisions in the best interest of the individual patient.

JOHN PAUL BRADY, M.D.